MEDIEVAL PERCEPTIONS OF MAGIC, SCIENCE, AND THE NATURAL WORLD

BORDERLINES

Further Information and Publications

www.arc-humanities.org/our-series/arc/bl/

MEDIEVAL PERCEPTIONS OF MAGIC, SCIENCE, AND THE NATURAL WORLD

Edited by
CAROLINA ESCOBAR-VARGAS
and ANNE LAWRENCE-MATHERS

ARC HUMANITIES PRESS

British Library Cataloguing in Publication Data
A catalogue record for this book is available from the British Library.

ISBN (hardback): 9781802700411
e-ISBN (PDF): 9781802702019

www.arc-humanities.org
Printed and bound in the UK (by CPI Group [UK] Ltd), USA (by Bookmasters),
and elsewhere using print-on-demand technology.

CONTENTS

LIST OF ILLUSTRATIONS

ACKNOWLEDGEMENTS

THIS BOOK SPRANG from a set of conference sessions organized by the Reading Graduate Centre for Medieval Studies at the International Medieval Congress, University of Leeds, 2021. Those discussions led to contacts and exchanges with an expanding group of experts on related subjects, and ultimately to the present volume. The editors would like to thank firstly all the contributors, whose illuminating research has made this such a wide-ranging and—we hope—ground-breaking volume.

Secondly, we should like to thank the team at Arc Humanities Press who have been with us from the start, and especially Danna Messer, who made invaluable contributions at a crucial moment.

Special thanks go to Caroline Bourne, who not only contributed an inspiring chapter, which brought navigation and sea travel into the scope of the volume, but also undertook invaluable editorial tasks at a difficult stage in the process. Caroline's patience, sharp eye for detail, and capacity for hard work are outstanding and we thank her sincerely.

Anne Lawrence-Mathers and Carolina Escobar-Vargas

INTRODUCTION

CAROLINA ESCOBAR-VARGAS

WITHIN THE PAGES of this volume, we embark on an intellectual journey through the expansive terrain of Medieval Magic, Science, and the Boundaries of the Natural. At its core, this exploration navigates the intricate themes of boundaries, liminal spaces, and the ever-shifting categories that defined the intellectual landscape of the Middle Ages. Throughout this time, conceptions of nature and its perceived opposites—the miraculous, the supernatural, the wondrous, and the magical—constantly underwent a dynamic interplay of expansion, contraction, and redefinition. As we delve into the nuanced tapestry of medieval thought, we seek to unravel the profound implications of these conceptual shifts, which resonate not only as markers of evolving attitudes and ideas but also as echoes of the continual interaction between humanity, nature, and the divine.

As we trace the contours of the Middle Ages, a narrative unfolds where boundaries blur, where liminal spaces become crucibles of transformative understanding, and categories prove to be not static but fluid, subject to the currents of intellectual evolution. In the late-1970s, the French medievalist Jacques Le Goff presented a thought-provoking work that delved into the intricate categorization of supernatural phenomena in the twelfth and thirteenth centuries in the Latin West. Le Goff proposed a framework wherein supernatural phenomena were divided into three distinct categories defined by the Latin adjectives *mirabilis*, *magicus*, and *miraculosus*.[1] This conceptualization reflected a medieval worldview where God had intricately set up His creation according to discernible patterns and principles of His own design. These patterns and principles constituted the rules of nature, a regularity that defined the known order of the world—a world that could be comprehended through diligent study and keen observation. Thus, for some, the pursuit of knowledge during the Middle Ages was, in essence, the pursuit of God.

However, within this structured framework, the possibility existed for occurrences that transcended the natural order, phenomena that could be identified as being *praeter naturam*, meaning beyond nature or supernatural. Miracles, wonders, and magic found their place within this supernatural category, each differentiated by their presumed origin. Miracles were exclusively attributed to God, magic was intrinsically associated with demonic activity, and wonders were believed to emanate from hidden causes within nature itself, although there were instances in which they were seen to defy nature or go *contra naturam*. While Le Goff's categorization provides a compelling starting point

1 Le Goff, *Imagination*, 30.

Carolina Escobar-Vargas is an Associate Professor of Medieval History at the Universidad Nacional de Colombia, Sede Medellín.

for discussion, a closer examination of the evidence reveals that alternative perspectives on the supernatural existed within the medieval milieu. This acknowledgment prompts us to explore the rich tapestry of medieval thought, recognising the diversity of beliefs and interpretations that contributed to the complex intellectual landscape of the time. It invites us to delve into the nuanced expressions of the supernatural, acknowledging the varied lenses through which individuals in the Middle Ages perceived and engaged with God's creation.

In particular, as suggested by Robert Bartlett, scholasticism offered a distinctive framework characterized by an all-encompassing category of nature that included everything except miracles. According to the thirteenth-century theologian Thomas Aquinas, miracles were phenomena that, if left to follow their true nature, would produce a different result, and thus could only be attributed to the power of God. Nature, in this view, was conceived as a system devised by God, beyond himself, serving as His creation. This systematic approach positioned the miraculous in opposition to the natural, as it depended on the natural but surpassed it—existing above (*supra*), beyond (*praeter*) or against (*contra*) nature.[2]

Within the confines of this scholastic system, primarily dedicated to exploring the causes and effects of phenomena, the natural was systematically juxtaposed with the divine. The divine encompassed the miraculous, relegating other causes of wonder to the hidden recesses within nature. Phenomena with concealed natural causes could emanate from occult properties within nature, a concept articulated by another thirteenth-century theologian, William of Auvergne, who referred to it as natural magic. Alternatively, these phenomena could find attribution to demonic activity. Demons, being entities within the framework of creation but distinct from humans, possessed the capability to manipulate nature in ways that appeared wondrous and inexplicable. They did so in order to tempt and deceive humanity. In such instances, the boundary between

2 Aquinas, *Scriptum super Sententiis*, lib. 2 dist. 18 q. 1 art. 3 c.: "Haec autem quandoque sunt supra naturam, quandoque praeter naturam, quandoque contra naturam. Supra naturam dicitur esse miraculum, quando natura non potest in ipsam substantiam facti, sicut divisio maris rubri, suscitatio mortui, et hujusmodi. Illa vero dicuntur praeter naturam fieri in quae quidem natura potest quantum ad substantiam facti, sed tamen praeter operationem naturae fiunt jussu divino. [...] Contra naturam autem dicitur fierit, quando in re est aliquid contrarium ei quod fit; sicut si grave sursum moveretur, et quod virgo peperit, vel aliquid hujusmodi; ita quod miraculose sequatur actus manente contraria natura, quae scilicet est principium contrarii actus" (https://aquinas.cc/la/en/~Sent.II.D18.Q1.A3).

For further definitions of miracles in Aquinas see: Aquinas, *Summa theologica*, 1a q.110, art. 4: "miraculum proprie dicitur, cum aliquid fit praeter ordinem naturae. Sed non sufficit ad rationem miraculi si aliquid fiat praeter ordinem naturae alicuius particularis, quia sic, cum aliquis proiicit lapidem sursum, miraculum faceret, cum hoc sit praeter ordinem naturae lapidis. Ex hoc ergo aliquid dicitur esse miraculum, quod fit praeter ordinem totius naturae creatae. Hoc autem non potest facere nisi Deus, quia quidquid facit angelus, vel quaecumque alia creatura, propria virtute, hoc fit secundum ordinem naturae creatae; et sic non est miraculum. Unde relinquitur quod solus Deus miracula facere possit" (https://aquinas.cc/la/en/~ST.I.Q110.A4.SC).

For additional details on the scholastic debate on the natural and the miraculous see: Bartlett, *Supernatural*; Le Goff, *Imagination*; Walker-Bynum, "Miracles"; and Daston, "Marvelous."

the natural and the supernatural blurred, prompting medieval scholars to grapple with the intricate interplay between the observable, the hidden, and the divine. This nuanced exploration within the scholastic tradition underscores the complex web of beliefs that shaped medieval perceptions of magic, science, and the boundaries of the natural. The acknowledgment of occult properties in nature and the recognition of demonic influence opened up avenues for both wonder and scepticism, laying the groundwork for a multifaceted understanding of the mysterious forces at play in the medieval cosmos.

Thus, for scholastic theologians, the supernatural, encompassing magic and wonders, was perceived as a concealed dimension of nature, occupying a liminal space between the natural and the divine. This blurred boundary between the natural and the miraculous, fostered the debate and interaction of alternative categories within medieval thought. Gervase of Tilbury, for example, identified these phenomena as unfamiliar and unusual, thus he characterized them as *inaudita*. This Latin term referred to elements in the world that elicited wonder due to the inversion of natural order, our ignorance of the cause, and the unexpected nature of unfamiliar circumstances.[3] Within Gervase's framework, miracles were considered beyond nature, exclusively attributed to divine power, while marvels extended beyond human understanding, even when rooted in the natural world. These examples underscore the challenge faced not only by medieval thinkers but also by modern scholars when attempting to delineate the boundary between the natural and the supernatural, the miraculous, the wondrous and the magical.

Nonetheless, an intriguing proposition emerges from this framework—one that situates the magical and the wondrous within nature, albeit concealed, inhabiting the liminal space between the natural and the divine. This departure from earlier perspectives, such as Augustine's, marks a notable evolution in thought. Augustine, in contrast, regarded all of nature as a miracle, viewing wonders and miracles within it as manifestations and observable proof of God's magnificence and power.[4] The departure from Augustine's viewpoint reflects a nuanced shift in medieval thought, challenging the perception that the miraculous, the wondrous, and the magical are solely external interventions into the natural order. Instead, this perspective suggests an integration of the extraordinary within the natural world, prompting a re-evaluation of the boundaries between the divine, the natural, and the supernatural. Such evolving perspectives contribute to the intricate tapestry of medieval intellectual history, revealing the dynamic nature of thought during this period.

---

3 Gervase of Tilbury, *Otia Imperialia*, 3. Pref: "Que inaudita precipiuntur amplectimur, tum ex mutatione cursus naturalis quam admiramur, tum ex ignorancia cause cuius ratio nobis est imperscrutabilis, tum ex assuetudine nostra quam in aliis uariari sine cognitione iudicii iusti cernimus. Ex his, duo proueniunt: miracula et mirabilia, cum utrorumque finis sit admiratio. Porro miracula dicimus usitatius que preter naturam diuine uirtuti ascribimus [...}". Walker Bynum, "Miracles"; Bartlett, *Supernatural*.

4 Augustine, *De civitate Dei*, bk. 21, chap. 7: "cum sit omnibus quibus plenus est procul dubio maius et excellentius etiam mundus ipse miraculum?" (https://www.augustinus.it/latino/cdd/index2.htm). See also Daston, "Marvelous."

The proposed liminal space between the natural and the supernatural thus emerges as a dynamic realm defined in the interstice between God and His creation, shaping the landscape of both the natural and the supernatural. Within this liminal space, hidden properties in nature and demonic manipulation could give rise to phenomena that were wondrous to human eyes, evoking awe, and amazement. This liminal space also encapsulates the tension between the licit and the illicit, the acceptable and the unacceptable, in the context of human endeavours to access the powers inherent in God's creation.

This volume endeavours to explore this intricate liminal space, delving into the nuanced boundaries between the natural and the supernatural, the natural and the demonic, the scientific and the magical. Moreover, it seeks to unravel the intersections of the superstitious and the scientific, as well as the superstitious and the magical. Through a multidimensional exploration of these themes, the volume aims to contribute to a richer understanding of the complexities inherent in medieval perspectives on magic, science, and the intricate boundaries that define the natural world and its supernatural dimensions. As such, our endeavour transcends the mere examination of delineations; instead, it delves deep into the intricate interactions that shaped the intellectual landscape of the Middle Ages. Each contribution to this volume unfolds a nuanced exploration, unveiling the multifaceted relationships between magic, science, and the natural world. Boundaries shifted, and categories expanded, contracted, and were redefined—echoing Bartlett's suggestion that they were "fluid, potentially contradictory, and often indeed unexamined."[5] Beyond delineating boundaries, these essays navigate the dynamic interplay where the marvellous, the scientific, and the magical converge, unravelling the complex tapestry woven by medieval thinkers.

Consequently, unveiling the intricate boundaries between the licit and the illicit, the acceptable and the unacceptable, a collection of papers collectively navigate various juxtapositions, forming a diverse tableau where science, magic, superstition, religion, medicine, and the demonic converge and intertwine. Nuanced insights offer a deeper understanding of the complexities inherent in medieval perspectives. The subsequent contributions delve into specific juxtapositions, each shedding light on the dynamic intersections of medieval intellectual history. Thus, they trace a thematic progression exploring the relationships between science and magic, superstition and science, religion, medicine, and magic, the natural and demonic, and superstition and magic.

Three papers in particular examine in detail the cross-over between science and magic. Sebastià Giralt's chapter, "Magic and Science in the Middle Ages: The Building of the Boundaries Between Natural Magic and Necromancy, ca. 1230–1310," explores the liminal space between admissible and inadmissible magic in the thirteenth century. The focus is on discerning boundaries between magic and science through the lens of theologians. By concentrating on the theological discourse surrounding the soul, the utilization of magical figures, words, and characters, and the magic of images, Giralt scrutinises scholastic thinkers from the thirteenth to the early fourteenth century. The objective is to precisely define natural magic against necromancy and unravel the considerations of

5 Bartlett, *Supernatural*, 26.

licit and forbidden knowledge and occult practices within this context. Anne Lawrence-Mathers' chapter, "Astro-meteorology: Science or Divination?" examines the origins and ascent of weather forecasting through astrological techniques, termed "astro-meteorology." Lawrence-Mathers contends that certain forms of astrology were widely accepted, firmly rooted in medieval society, and considered valuable. Aligning with Giralt's exploration of natural magic as licit and beneficial, Lawrence-Mathers also probes the boundary between the licit and the illicit, between science and magic, particularly in the context of astrology. Lastly, Victoria Burns-Price's chapter, "The Boundaries of Magic and Medicine in Medieval Theology," navigates the intricate and evolving boundary between science and magic. The author elucidates instances, both formal and informal, where practices deemed legitimate by some in the realms of medicine or religion were considered unacceptable by others due to their perceived association with unknown forces. A key focus is on the changing definitions of magic and medicine over time, particularly within canon law, which outlines the theoretical and practical stance of the Church.

Janet Walls examines the interplay between superstition and science in her chapter, "Late-Medieval Brontologies: Popular Superstition or Astrological Medical Guide." She delves into brontologies, focusing on the use of thunder events for prognostication. Brontology consisted of the rules for interpreting thunderstorms as omens of future events, intended for application to communities rather than individuals. The anticipated events primarily pertained to weather, crop outcomes, the spread of illnesses, and the likelihood of wars, although there is evidence to suggest that the texts were also utilized by physicians. Despite challenging times with weather, pandemics, and political unrest, brontologies gained popularity, particularly among medical practitioners in the fourteenth and fifteenth centuries. Walls investigates their contexts in late-medieval England and their insights into the perceived relationship between human health and the natural world.

In a parallel exploration centred on weather and superstition, Carolina Escobar-Vargas examines intricate perceptions of weather manipulation through magic in the Middle Ages, unravelling the multifaceted attitudes that ranged from acceptance to disbelief and outright condemnation. Exploring the theological connection between the concept of demons and their potential influence on weather patterns, the paper raises crucial questions about the feasibility of humans manipulating or propitiating demons to control the weather. Escobar-Vargas navigates the complex interplay between theological considerations, human agency, and potential deception by demons. By examining the shifting attitudes towards weather magic, the article sheds light on dynamic and evolving perspectives on weather magic during the medieval period. The exploration of magical control of the weather becomes a nuanced journey through the intersections of belief, scepticism, and condemnation in medieval thought.

Probing the boundary between the natural and the supernatural, Claire Burridge's chapter, "Rhythms of the (Super)natural World: Timing Instructions in Early Medieval Medical Recipes," explores the interplay of religion, medicine, and magic. Burridge explores the intricate relationship between seasonality and herbal medicine, examining how collection instructions connect natural and supernatural realms through ancient taboos and rituals. This chapter examines early medieval perspectives on timing instructions for picking herbs, comparing them with classical and late antique medical recipes. Burridge contends that the integration of Christian and non-Christian timing instructions reveals a blurred distinction between "natural" and "supernatural" time, showcasing the dynamic influence of the monastic context on medical knowledge evolution in the early medieval West.

Focusing on the opposition between the natural and the demonic, Joanne Edge's chapter, titled "Between Natural and Demonic? Onomantic Divination in the Later Middle Ages," stands as a nuanced exploration of the late medieval perspective on onomancy. Aligning with the contributions of Giralt and Lawrence-Mathers in this volume, in this study, Edge brings to light the potential acceptability of onomancy by scrutinizing three pivotal factors. Firstly, the chapter delves into the historical intertwining of magic and divination within the Christian tradition's condemnatory discourse. Secondly, it engages with the lively debates in natural philosophical and theological circles concerning the problem of universals. Thirdly, it investigates the tentative creation of the category of natural magic and the rehabilitation of medical astrology in the thirteenth century. While not universally embraced, Edge argues that the introduction of subtleties in natural philosophical discourse during this period allowed for the interpretation of onomancy as a potentially acceptable practice. The chapter prominently positions the opposition of the natural to the demonic, emphasizing the complex dynamics shaping medieval perspectives on divination.

As we embark on the exploration of further dimensions within this volume, it becomes evident that our inquiry extends beyond mere delineations and boundaries. The ensuing papers delve into intricate interactions, probing the dynamic relationships between religion and nature, the interplay of nature and science, and the nuanced connections between history and the supernatural. Moreover, these contributions navigate the terrain of knowledge transmission, offering additional insights into the boundaries of the licit and the illicit. The overarching theme that emerges is one of fluidity—a fluidity of knowledge serving as a means to interact with God's creation.

In Judith Collard's thought-provoking contribution to this volume, titled "Matthew Paris, William of Conches, and the Use of Diagrams to Observe the World," a fascinating exploration unfolds, shedding light on the intricate relationship between visual representation, knowledge, and the divine in medieval thought. Collard brings forth a compelling perspective, emphasising the fluidity of knowledge as a means to interact with God's creation, with a specific focus on diagrams as a vehicle for comprehending God through nature. Collard's exploration illuminates the distinct nature of these diagrams, which operate in unconventional ways compared to traditional notions of the pictorial. Acting as intermediaries between text and image, they become a medium of thinking, aiding in the clarification of complexities. In this context, the natural world is not only observed but actively explored through visual aids. Collard's contribution invites an immersion into the fascinating intersection of visual representation, medieval intellect, and the fluidity of knowledge in the pursuit of understanding God's creation.

Caroline Bourne's chapter, "Time and Tide: The Creation of a Sea Travel Network in the Severn Region in the Early Middle Ages," intricately explores the interaction between religion and nature, focusing on a specific body of water: the Bristol Channel and the Severn area. The paper unveils the religious appropriation of nature in South Wales, delving into the intriguing testing of the saintly through the natural. Within this exploration, Bourne navigates the blurred boundaries where nature becomes a testing ground for the divine, employing signifiers and seeking the miraculous. The study unfolds a captivating narrative of how religious communities in the early Middle Ages actively engaged in deciphering the will of God through their interactions with the forces of nature.

Examining the interaction between nature and science, Anne Jeavons' contribution, titled "Natural and Non-Natural: Weather, Seasons, and Place in the Medical Recommendations of Constantine of Africa," explores specific questions on human health in the medieval period. Jeavons examines the medical insights of Constantine of Africa, a medical expert, translator, and monk, active in the eleventh century, shedding light on his significant contributions to the study of medicine in the Latin West. The paper focuses on Constantine's introduction of the concepts of naturals, non-naturals, and contra-naturals as pivotal elements influencing theoretical medicine in the period. It emphasizes the boundaries of health, considering the human body as an integral part of nature.

Victoria Flood's contribution, titled "Wonder and Wonderworking in Middle English Romance: The Prose Merlin," delves into the intricate relationship between history and the supernatural. The study centres on the Middle English Prose Merlin, situated within the broader context of Latin and French Merlinian writing traditions. Surviving in a mid-fifteenth-century manuscript, this work is a close translation of the Merlin section from the Old French Vulgate Cycle. Flood's exploration focuses on the construction of wonder and its interplay with perceptions of history and fiction in depictions of Merlin, which she labels as prophet and wonderworker. The Prose Merlin, considered one of the earliest English prose romances, blurs the boundaries between romance and history, reflecting the multi-generic nature of Arthurian literature. Flood's analysis highlights the historiographical nuances surrounding Merlin's historicity.

Further exploring interactions between admissible scientific knowledge and the medieval Latin tradition "Astral Forces and Arthurian Dragons in Geoffrey of Monmouth's *Historia regum Britanniae*," by Humma Mouzam, explores the influence of Arabic and Syriac astronomy and astrology on Geoffrey of Monmouth's *Historia regum Britanniae* (ca. 1136/1138). Focusing on the dragon as a symbol, Mouzam delves into Geoffrey's incorporation of astrological and astronomical elements, revealing a unique blend of scientific concepts and British legendary history.

In "Alchemical Poetry, Alchemical Practice," Zachary Matus explores the interaction between wonder and science through language. Focusing on medieval alchemical poetry, Matus argues that these verses provide valuable insights into how early alchemical authors conceptualized their craft, emphasizing the role of poetry in conveying the experiences of alchemists. The chapter highlights the boundary between the empirical limitations of alchemy and the expressive power of poetic language to capture its essence.

Helen Parish's concluding chapter in this volume, titled "Encountering the Wonder in Nature: The Science of the Sacred in the Early Modern Construction of the Natural World," explores the nuanced boundaries between the marvellous, the natural, and the supernatural in the early modern period. Focusing on Olaus Magnus' *Description of the Northern Peoples* and Edward Topsell's *History of Four-footed Beasts and Serpents*, Parish delves into the dominance of wonders and marvels in these early modern narratives. She notes that it is possible to "chart the evolution of ideas and attitudes, and the emergence of a syncretic approach where multiple interpretations could coexist on a single page." The chapter examines the early modern lexicon of the wondrous, encompassing miracles, portents, prodigies, and natural marvels, reflecting the fluidity and complexity of natural philosophy. Descriptions of ocean wonders highlight a polyvalent approach where physical, mental, and spiritual encounters coexist within natural histories. This volume collectively explores intricate boundaries and dynamic interactions that shaped medieval perspectives on the natural, supernatural, demonic, divine, and the wondrous, challenging simplistic narratives of separation between medieval and early modern periods. Parish's conclusion underscores the permeability of these boundaries, rejecting a linear progression towards a modern scientific worldview and emphasizing the multiplicity of meanings in the interpretation of wonders.

In these introductory remarks, we initiate our exploration by underscoring the fluid and dynamic nature of categories that shaped the medieval intellectual landscape. The intricate interplay between the natural and the supernatural takes centre stage, echoing past attempts at categorization by scholars such as Jacques Le Goff and Robert Bartlett. While these frameworks lay the groundwork for discussion, it is essential to recognize the rich diversity of beliefs and interpretations that defined medieval thought. Thus, we too are exploring boundaries. The focus sharpens on challenging concepts, including miracles and concealed causes within the fabric of nature. The exploration of the liminal space between the natural and the supernatural emerges as a recurring theme, shaping the landscape of both realms. This liminality, exemplified by occult properties in nature and demonic manipulation, gives rise to wondrous phenomena that evoke awe and amazement.

The subsequent papers contribute to the multifaceted understanding of medieval perspectives. They navigate the intersections of science and magic, superstition and science, religion, medicine, and magic, the natural and demonic, and superstition and magic. The examination of onomancy, weather manipulation, and medical recommendations showcases the complex dynamics shaping medieval perspectives on divination, human health, and the supernatural. As the inquiry extends beyond delineations and boundaries, the papers delve into intricate interactions, probing the dynamic relationships between religion and nature, the interplay of nature and science, and the nuanced connections between history and the supernatural. Each contribution unfolds a nuanced exploration, unveiling the multifaceted relationships between magic, science, and the natural world. Beyond delineating boundaries, these essays navigate the dynamic interplay where the marvellous, the scientific, and the magical converge, revealing the intricate threads woven through the fabric of medieval thought.

Bibliography

Primary Sources

Augustine. *De civitate Dei Libri XXII*. Edited by Bernard Dombart and Alfons Kalb. Stuttgart: Teubner, 1993.

Gervase of Tilbury. *Otia Imperialia*. Edited by S. E. Banks and J. W. Binns. Oxford: Clarendon, 2002.

Thomas Aquinas. *Scriptum Super Sententiis*. Edited by The Aquinas Institute. https://aquinas.cc/la/en/~Sent.I.

——. *Summa theologiae*. Translated by Fathers of the English Dominican Province. New York: Benziger, 1947–48. The Aquinas Institute. https://aquinas.cc/la/en/~ST.I.

Secondary Sources

Bartlett, Robert. *The Natural and the Supernatural in the Middle Ages*. Cambridge: Cambridge University Press, 2008.

Daston, Lorraine. "Marvelous Facts and Miraculous Evidence in Early Modern Europe." *Critical Inquiry* 18 (1991): 93–124.

Daston, Lorraine and Katharine Park. *Wonders and the Order of Nature, 1150–1750*. New York: Zone, 1998.

Le Goff, Jacques. *The Medieval Imagination*. Chicago: University of Chicago Press, 1988.

Walker Bynum, Caroline. "Miracles and Marvels: The Limits of Alterity" In *Vita Religiosa im Mittelalter. Festschrift für Kaspar Elm*, edited by Franz J. Felten and Nikolas Jaspert, 799–814. Berlin: Duncker und Humblot, 1999.

RHYTHMS OF THE (SUPER)NATURAL WORLD

TIMING INSTRUCTIONS IN EARLY MEDIEVAL MEDICAL RECIPES

CLAIRE BURRIDGE

> "You gather [betony] in its season—it is the month of August, when the other herbs begin to ripen—with [its] seed and roots, without iron. And after shaking it, so that the earth does not stick to it, you dry [it] in the shade and thus grind [it] with its roots through an aromatic sieve. When you want to use [it], [it is] finely ground into a powder. In this way, you use [it]."[1]

SO ENDS THE introduction to the late antique herbal *De herba vettonica liber*, a collection of forty-seven simple recipes in which betony, *Stachys officinalis*, is the main ingredient. The instructions for collecting this herb illustrate the innate relationship between seasonality and herbal medicine. In plant-based pharmacy, just as with agriculture, the rhythms of the natural world dictate when certain plants and plant products are ready to be harvested and used. As this passage reveals, however, other factors could also influence the collection process. After addressing the time of year to gather betony, the author of *De herba vettonica liber* states that iron is not to be used when harvesting it (i.e., to avoid digging up the roots or removing its leaves, seeds, etc., with an iron implement). The inclusion of such instructions transports the reader from the natural world of growing seasons to a supernatural realm of ancient taboos and rituals.[2]

Perhaps unsurprisingly, the individual recipes of *De herba vettonica liber* present no further information regarding ingredient collection since the gathering of betony, the central ingredient in the following recipes, has been covered in the introduction.

---

1 Pseudo-Antonius Musa, "De herba vettonica liber," ed. Howald and Sigerist, 4: "Hanc autem suo tempore colliges, id est mense Augusto, cum ceterae herbae maturescere incipiunt, cum semine et radicibus, sine ferro, eamque excussam, ne terra ei inhaereat, in umbra arefacies atque ita teres cum radicibus suis cribro aromatico; mollissime in puluerem redacta cum uolueris uti, sic uteris."

2 On iron taboos, see Luck, *Arcana Mundi*, 35, 219.

Claire Burridge is a Senior Researcher at the University of Oslo. Her first book, *Carolingian Medical Knowledge and Practice, c. 775–900: New Approaches to Recipe Literature*, has recently been published and is available open access. My first thanks go to this volume's editors, not only for all the work that went into producing this book but also for their helpful comments on earlier drafts. I should also like to thank the anonymous reviewers for their generous and useful feedback, and Bram van den Berg, who involved me in this project initially and has helped me to reflect on the intersections of medicine, prognostics, and the supernatural.

Recipes found in other classical and late antique pharmaceutical writings, however, provide a wide range of instructions relating to the appropriate time for collecting herbal ingredients. While some of these texts offer parallels to the natural, seasonal timing instructions of *De herba vettonica liber*, many root their information regarding when to gather plants or parts of plants in other types of time. In these cases, recipes might name specific days of the week or phases of the moon when an ingredient should be collected. Timing instructions based on the lunar cycle, certain days of the week or dates during the year, and other preternatural features appear to have no grounding in seasonality and instead can be linked to ancient beliefs and ritual practices. Distinctions between natural and supernatural time, however, are often blurred and combined in these instructions, revealing the complex amalgamation of influences that shaped classical and late antique pharmacy.

Many of these (late) ancient texts were actively copied and excerpted in the early medieval West, providing the fundamental building blocks on which pharmaceutical writings were constructed during this period. The scribes working with these texts would have approached the material with a different perspective—a Christian mental framework—and their scribal activities often took place within an explicitly Christian environment: monastic centres of manuscript production. How did these individuals perceive, engage with, and respond to the various kinds of timing instructions presented in pre-Christian texts? Given the multiple modes of temporality invoked in these instructions, including those linked to supernatural forces that might conflict with Christian teachings, it seems possible that early medieval compilers may have adapted their compositions, adjusting the information presented in their exemplars to suit their beliefs. Do early medieval recipes provide evidence of such developments?

The polemical treatises penned by certain late antique and early medieval theologians on the dangers of the continuation of pre-Christian rituals among common people, as well as the development of unorthodox beliefs at any level of society, suggest that much of the information contained within timing instructions would have been understood as crossing the threshold between licit and illicit knowledge.[3] While seasonal timing instructions aligning with agricultural cycles might not have been a cause for concern, were non-Christian, supernatural timing rituals excised from early medieval recipe collections? On the other hand, do timing instructions linked to the Christian calendar appear alongside or in place of such information? Or rather, do the texts document a continued fluidity in which natural and supernatural time, Christian or otherwise, can be found in recipe instructions? As Peregrine Horden has pointed out, in early medieval

3 Consider, for example, Isidore's comments on superstitious beliefs related to astronomy in Book 3, "Mathematics," of his highly influential *Etymologies*; Isidore of Seville, *Etymologiarum*, ed. Lindsay, 3.27 and 3.71. (Note that he discusses the etymology of "superstitio" in Book 8; "The Church and Sects," see bk. 8, chap. 3, §§6–7.) For an English translation, see Isidore of Seville, *Etymologies*, trans. Barney et al. Hrabanus Maurus, Agobard of Lyon, and other Carolingian intellectuals expressed especially strong views on orthodoxy and their concerns regarding popular beliefs; see, for example, Agobard of Lyon, "Liber contra insulsam," ed. Van Acker, 3–15. For further contextualization, see Dutton, *Charlemagne's Mustache*, 169–88; and Filotas, *Pagan Survivals*.

medicine, "the real contrast was less between incompatible systems of ideas—religion, medicine, magic—or between the orthodox and the deviant, than between different authorities."[4] The following chapter thus seeks to investigate the complex interface of "religion, medicine, [and] magic" through the lens of timing instructions for the collection of herbal ingredients, presenting the first systematic review of this material.

By comparing early medieval timing instructions to those found in classical and late antique recipes, I identify not only continuities in these instructions with respect to both natural and supernatural timing rituals, but also a significant new development, namely introduction of Christian elements. I argue that this paradox, i.e., the continued copying of non-Christian, supernaturally-inflected timing instructions alongside the deployment of those based on the Christian calendar and other liturgical rituals, reveals neither conflicting evidence nor a drive to replace non-Christian material with sanctified content. Rather, these findings illustrate the lack of a clear distinction between "natural" and "supernatural" time whilst simultaneously highlighting the influence of the monastic context on the evolution of medical knowledge, the relationship between physical and spiritual health, and the dynamic points of intersection across multiple fields of learning.

My research questions and resulting arguments build on, and seek to contribute to, two related areas of scholarship that have been growing in recent years: first, work on computus and calendrical texts and, second, studies exploring the intersections of medicine and the Church and the relationship between healing body and soul. The analysis draws on recipes found outside direct copies of classical and late antique recipe collections, representing a traditionally overlooked body of evidence that must be considered alongside the texts more clearly descended from the (late) ancient corpus of medical writings. This chapter begins with a brief sketch of the two research areas named above and an overview of the manuscript evidence to contextualize the following analyses and provide its methodological framework. I then turn to the variety of timing instructions found in classical and late antique recipes before reviewing the sample of early medieval material, demonstrating how timing instructions build on earlier precedents while concurrently moving in new directions. Finally, I demonstrate the significance of this comparative study for understanding the evolution of recipe literature in the early medieval West and the importance of situating this analysis within the monastic environments in which the manuscripts were produced.

Research Background and Framework

The study of computus and related calendrical writings, tables, and diagrams has greatly expanded in the past few decades, pioneered especially by Faith Wallis and Dáibhí Ó Cróinín and continued by Jacopo Bisagni, Philipp Nothaft, and Immo Warntjes, among others.[5]

---

4 Horden, "What's Wrong with Early Medieval Medicine?," 8.

5 See, for example, Wallis, "The Church, the World and the Time," 15–29; Wallis, "Medicine in Medieval Calendar Manuscripts," 105–43; McCarthy and Ó Cróinín, "Easter Table Rediscovered," 227–42; Warntjes and Ó Cróinín, eds., *Late Antique Calendrical Thought*; Bisagni, "Newly-Discovered Irish,"

Medical texts have long been acknowledged as part of "a halo of non-computistical materials" that often circulated alongside computistical and calendrical writings.[6] Indeed, the frequent appearance of *lunaria* (lists of prognostications for each day of the lunar month), month-based *regimina* (texts describing health-related activities, such as eating certain foods or bloodletting, that should be performed or avoided each month), and Egyptian Days (days thought to be unlucky, especially with respect to bloodletting) reveal the extent to which medical knowledge depended on lunar, solar, and seasonal calendars and calculations.[7] Yet, despite this acknowledgement of the centrality of calendrical thinking to medical knowledge, questions of time have rarely been explored in medical texts that are not structured around a calendar (whether lunar, solar, or seasonal). Timing instructions in recipes, therefore, have been largely passed over in the scholarship so far.[8] The present study aims to integrate these less well studied instances of calendrically orientated thinking into wider conversations concerning computus, calendars, and medicine.

Secondly, a number of recent studies have refocused attention on the dynamic, evolving inter-relationship between medicine and the Church, the overlapping treatment of bodily and spiritual health, and the connection(s) between healing and salvation in late Antiquity and the early Middle Ages.[9] This work has productively expanded on Horden's re-evaluation of early medieval medicine, not simply blurring the boundaries between "medicine" and "religion," but taking a more holistic approach that treats the evidence in context and "respects local definitions and categories."[10] As Meg Leja, Carine van Rhijn, and others have shown, spiritual and corporeal health were not in opposition; instead, medicine often operated on both body and soul.[11]

13–34; Bisagni and Warntjes, "Early Old Irish," 77–105; and Warntjes, *The Munich Computus*. For a wider chronological perspective as well as more focused studies of the central and later Middle Ages, see especially the work of Philipp Nothaft, such as Nothaft, *Scandalous Error*; Nothaft, "Reception and Application of Arabic Science," 35–60; and Nothaft, "Roger of Hereford," 27–43.

6 Wallis, "Medicine in Medieval Calendar Manuscripts," 107.

7 For a sense of the numbers of surviving examples of these types of texts, see Beccaria, *I codici*; Sabbah, Corsetti, and Fischer, *Bibliographie des textes médicaux latins*; and Fischer, *Bibliographie des textes médicaux latins*. On *lunaria*, see Weisser, "Das Krankheitslunar aus medizinhistorischer Sicht," 390–400. On monthly *regimina*, see Groenke, "Die frühmittelalterlichen Lateinischen Monatskalendarien." On Egyptian Days, see Skemer, "*Armis Gunfe*," 75–106. On prognostics more generally, see Heiduk, Herbers, and Lehner, *Prognostication in the Medieval World*.

8 Ernest Wickersheimer provides a notable exception, but his work on this area in the first half of the twentieth century can be updated in the light of new developments in the study of early medieval computus, medical texts, and manuscripts. See, for example, Wickersheimer, "Epistola Ypocratis," 145–52; Wickersheimer, "Nouveaux textes médiévaux," 342–55.

9 Recent work on this topic includes Leja, *Embodying the Soul*; Leja, "Sacred Art," 1–34; van Rhijn, *Leading the Way to Heaven*; Zecher, *Spiritual Direction*; and Burridge, "Healing Body," 46–67.

10 Horden, "What's Wrong with Early Medieval Medicine?," 8.

11 See especially Leja, *Embodying the Soul*, and, more specifically on the presence of medical advice within priests' handbooks, see van Rhijn, *Leading the Way to Heaven*.

Although there is no doubt that spiritual and bodily health and healing were deeply entangled, the writings of a number of leading Carolingian intellectuals, such as Hrabanus Maurus and Agobard of Lyon, document serious anxieties regarding the continuation of pre-Christian beliefs and rituals in opposition to Christian teachings.[12] Given the strident articulation of these concerns, if only among a subset of theologians, it is essential to analyse recipes on a granular level to explore whether all aspects of the medical knowledge inherited from pre-Christian sources was equally accepted and copied. That is, how were potentially illicit elements handled at the level of individual recipes and to what extent were such features recorded in new compilations? Instructions for the proper time to collect herbal ingredients present an ideal case study for investigating these questions. By directing attention to the recipe literature and the modes of temporality seen within individual recipes, the present study thus aims to expand the current discourses connecting body and soul, natural and supernatural, as well as Church teachings and medical knowledge in a new direction.

Before reviewing the manuscript evidence, it must be noted that scholars of Old English medical texts have often led the way in re-evaluating the written record in the light of its cultural context, and especially with respect to the supernatural and questions of "magic" and "superstition."[13] Early Insular "charms" involving plants, for example, have been studied by Karen Louise Jolly and Debby Banham, and recently revisited by Ciaran Arthur.[14] Despite their differences in language, it appears that the Old English texts share many sources with the continental manuscripts.[15] While the present study does not have the space to address these connections, a comparative study of herbal recipes and performative rituals from both linguistic traditions is a major desiderata.[16]

Returning to continental Europe, it is important to outline the recipe literature and manuscript evidence under analysis. Although the field of early medieval medicine has traditionally focused on Carolingian copies of classical and late antique texts, many manuscripts preserve recipes outside of this corpus, ranging from new compilations containing hundreds of recipes and related writings (including some of the calendrical material, such as dietary *regimina*, mentioned above) to individual recipes added to flyleaves or other marginal spaces. While these recipes are intimately connected with classical and late antique sources, crucially, they not only represent new combinations of earlier texts but also bear witness to the integration of non-classical influences, such as eastern pharmaceutical information unrecorded in ancient western medical

---

12 Leja, *Embodying the Soul*, 112–21. See also n. 3 above.

13 See, for example, Meaney, "Practice of Medicine," 221–37; Meaney, "Extra-Medical Elements," 41–56; Van Arsdall, "Challenging the 'Eye of Newt' Image," 195–206.

14 Jolly, *Popular Religion*; Banham, "Staff of Life," 279–318; and Arthur, *"Charms."* Much work has also explored charms in later medieval England, including Olsan, "Charms and Prayers," 343–66 and Olsan, "Corpus of Charms," 214–37.

15 Doyle, *Reception of Latin Medicine*; Cameron, *Anglo-Saxon Medicine*.

16 Indeed, although Peter Murray Jones and Lea T. Olsan note the distinctive nature of "magic in Anglo-Saxon medicine," it appears that there may be more parallels than have previously been acknowledged; Jones and Olsan, "Medicine and Magic," 300–301.

writings.[17] Given that early medieval recipe collections, and marginal added recipes have both been shown to incorporate elements outside the classical canon of medicine, when investigating early medieval responses to classical and late antique traditions, it is necessary to concentrate on these types of texts as opposed to Carolingian copies of earlier sources.[18]

The present study is therefore built on a corpus of approximately six thousand medical recipes found in forty-six manuscripts produced between the late eighth and eleventh centuries in writing centres around western continental Europe.[19] While some of the manuscripts contain only a handful of treatments (and tend to be additions to these codices—codices in which the primary focus is often unrelated to health and medicine), several contain hundreds of prescriptions gathered into recipe collections modelled on classical and late antique texts. The range of manuscripts and codicological environments in which recipes are located provides a representative sample as well as an opportunity to consider how recipes' manuscript contexts can offer further information regarding the transmission of medical knowledge.

Recipe Instructions in Classical and Late Antique Texts Relating to the Timing of Ingredient Collection

As noted above, classical and late antique medical recipes present a wide range of instructions concerning the appropriate time to gather ingredients. That being said, it must also be recognized that, although such instructions appear across many different (late) ancient sources, they do not occur in all texts nor are they included with great frequency. In some recipes, the specifics of timing may have been seen as less important, while in others, as is the case with the recipes of *De herba vettonica liber*, a single instruction could have applied to multiple recipes. Moreover, this relative rarity, which is replicated by early medieval recipes, marks timing instructions as particularly notable: since

17 On early medieval medical manuscripts, see Wallis, "Experience of the Book," 101–26. On the introduction of new influences, see Riddle, "Introduction and Use of Eastern Drugs," 185–98; McCormick, *Origins of the European Economy*; Burridge, "Incense in Medicine," 219–55. While some editions of anonymous recipe collections have been published, an enormous amount of material remains unpublished; the handful of landmark editions of early medieval recipe collections includes *Studien und Texte*, ed. Sigerist; *Frühmittelalterliche Rezeptarien*, ed. Jörimann; *Vademecum eines frühmittelalterlichen Arztes*, ed. and trans. Köpp; *Das Lorscher Arzneibuch*, ed. and trans. Stoll; and *Der St. Galler Botanicus*, ed. and trans. Niederer.

18 "Copies" of earlier texts were not, of course, entirely stable, but they do not display the same degree of external influences, such as the introduction of sacred Christian ingredients (e.g., holy water) as *materia medica*; Burridge, "Healing Body."

19 All transcriptions of early medieval recipes are my own, though transcriptions of four of the recipe collections under consideration have been published previously; see *Studien und Texte*, ed. Sigerist, 78–99; *Frühmittelalterliche Rezeptarien*, ed. Jörimann, 37–61; and *Vademecum eines frühmittelalterlichen Arztes*, ed. and trans. Köpp. Editions of the previously unpublished material are in preparation. Note: where I have supplied letters due to an abbreviation in the manuscript, I have indicated this by underlining the letters I have added; deleted material is indicated by parentheses and inserted material by slashes.

they are not especially common and are unevenly distributed, they stand out as special features. In other words, most recipes do not require that their *materia medica* are gathered at a particular time (or at least this was not recorded), but some recipes define a specific time as the correct or optimal period or moment for ingredient collection. In these cases, the treatment's perceived therapeutic efficacy often appears to depend on following these instructions. Despite the rarity of timing instructions, given the substantial corpus of classical and late antique pharmaceutical writings, recipes containing information on the time to harvest ingredients still provide a significant body of material when taken collectively, and the following section can offer only a brief overview.

Some classical and late antique timing instructions record advice that, like the seasonal information recorded in *De herba vettonica liber*, advocates for collection times based on natural phenomena. In the introduction to the monumental *De materia medica*, for example, Dioscorides emphasizes the importance of the "timely collection of each drug" since "whether drugs are strong or weak depends strictly on whether the collection was made at the right time."[20] He notes that "clear weather" is essential and that the effects of recent weather must be taken into account when planning when to collect ingredients. Dioscorides also reminds his readers that "plants often reach their peak either sooner or later, depending on the particular nature of the site and on climatic conditions," reflecting the local environment's role in determining the proper time at which ingredients should be collected.[21]

Other texts, such as *The Alphabet of Galen*, also occasionally provide instructions based on seasonality. The neighbouring entries for opopanax (201) and Mecca balsam (202), for instance, both describe the best season for collecting these products: opopanax should be dug up in the middle of summer whereas the sap of Mecca balsam "is collected from spring right up to autumn."[22] On the other hand, Marcellus of Bordeaux, a late-antique Gallo-Roman statesman, returns to monthly harvesting advice and, paralleling *De herba vettonica liber*, recommends that betony should be collected in August in a recipe within his chapter on stomach complaints.[23] In the chapter on kidney, bladder, and various urinary conditions, Marcellus records a treatment for kidney stones that uses ash seeds; he instructs that these should be collected immediately before the Ides of November.[24] Since ash fruits develop in late summer and autumn and then usually remain on the tree for several months (falling off in winter and early spring), it makes sense to pick the seeds at this time of year. The precise specificity in timing, however,

20 Dioscorides, *De materia medica*, ed. Wellmann, 1.6. For an English translation, see Dioscorides, *De materia medica*, trans. Beck.

21 Dioscorides, *De materia medica*, ed. Wellmann, 1.6–7.

22 *Alphabet of Galen*, ed. and trans. Everett, nos. 201 and 202, pp. 298–99. On the collection of sap: "Huius ergo arboris lachryma colligitur a uerno usque ad autumnum."

23 Marcellus of Bordeaux, *De medicamentis liber*, ed. Liechtenhan and Niedermann, trans. Kollesch and Nickel, 20.106, at 1:358. See also Stannard, "Marcellus of Bordeaux," 47–53.

24 Marcellus of Bordeaux, *De medicamentis liber*, 26.28, at 2:432: "Mense Nouembri ante Idus easdem semen fraxini colliges et in tepido furno siccabis, die postera siccatum tundes et cribrabis et repones et ex eo dabis calculoso ad diem cum uino uetere bibendam ligulam unam."

blurs natural and supernatural time: by defining the moment of collection as the period immediately before the Ides of November, an element of more calendrically-focused time enters the recipe's instructions.

Indeed, Marcellus incorporates many further examples of timing advice that do not depend on seasonality but are based on other natural phenomena, including lunar cycles; calendrical time, such as days of the week; or combinations of multiple modes of time. In a treatment for cough, for example, he states that the herb called "calliomarcus" by local Gallic communities and "equi ungula" in Latin ("horse hoof") should be collected when the moon is waning, the tide is receding, and on a Thursday.[25] In a later recipe for hip and other joint pain, Marcellus provides a fairly detailed description of the plant known in Latin as "cytisus." On the proper time to collect this shrub, which he specifically notes is evergreen, he states that, like the preceding example, it should occur when the moon is waning, the tide is receding, and on a Thursday, while also adding an extra note that the ritual should take place before breakfast.[26] Similar instructions regarding different herbs ("brittanice" and cinquefoil) appear in two other recipes for hip pain.[27]

Although the above examples do not have direct parallels to recipes in the pharmaceutical sections of Pliny's *Natural History*, this earlier encyclopaedic work contains many additional cases of collection instructions combining the natural rhythms of time with supernatural temporal rituals. On collecting grapes (though not specifically targeting their application in medicine), Pliny writes that, according to his sources, "grapes should be picked early for the purpose of storage, when the moon is waning, after nine o'clock in the morning, in fine weather or with a dry wind blowing."[28] Notably, when describing minor farm activities, Pliny does, in fact, provide an explanation regarding the involvement of lunar cycles in timing the collection of plant products: "all cutting, gathering and trimming is done with less injury to the trees and plants when the moon is waning than when it is waxing."[29]

Sunrise, too, is mentioned with some frequency in Pliny's timing instructions. Concerning the plant called "cat's-eye" by the Romans, he reports that "some instruct the diggers to say nothing until they have saluted it before sunrise, and then to gather it and extract the juice, for so they say its efficacy is at its greatest."[30] On mulberries, Pliny notes

25 Marcellus of Bordeaux, *De medicamentis liber*, 16.101, at 1:292: "Ad tussem remedium efficax: Herba, quae Gallice calliomarcus, Latine equi ungula uocatur, collecta luna uetere liduna die Iouis [...]."

26 Marcellus of Bordeaux, *De medicamentis liber*, 25.11, at 2:416: "Frutectum ipsum semper uirens aestate atque hieme colligitur die Iouis luna uetere liduna ante prandium [...]."

27 Marcellus of Bordeaux, *De medicamentis liber*, 25.13, at 2:418; 25.46, at 2:426.

28 Pliny, *Natural History*, 15.62, trans. Rackham, Jones and Eichholz, 330–31: "E proximis auctoribus quidam altius curam repetunt, deputarique statim poma ac vites ad hunc usum praecipiunt decrescente luna, post horam diei tertiam, caelo sereno aut siccis ventis."

29 Pliny, *Natural History*, trans. Rackham, Jones and Eichholz, 18.321, pp. 390–91: "Omnia quae caeduntur, carpuntur, tondentur innocentius descrescente luna quam crescente fiunt."

30 Pliny, *Natural History*, trans. Rackham, Jones and Eichholz, 25.145, pp. 238–39: "Praecipiunt aliqui effossuris ante solis ortum priusquam quicquam aliud loquantur, salutare eam, sublatam exprimere, ita praecipuas esse vires."

that "it is a remarkable fact [...] that when doctors require its juice they strike it with a stone two hours after sunrise in spring."[31] Many of the treatments recorded by Pliny involve multiple layers of ritual preparations, and the time at which the plant or plant product should be collected represents just one element within a much more complex process. For example, he notes that "any plant whatsoever, gathered before sunrise out of streams or rivers, provided that nobody sees the gatherer, if it is tied as an amulet to the left arm, is said to keep away tertian agues, provided that the patient does not know what is going on."[32] Many of these types of instructions were continued by Pliny's late antique descendants, such as the *Medicina Plinii.* In the chapter on tertian fevers, the *Medicina Plinii* records a treatment corresponding to Pliny's instructions: "a plant which grows in rivers or streams is tied on the [patient's] left arm without their knowledge; it disperses tertian fevers. It ought to be gathered before sunrise in such a way that no one sees him who collects it."[33]

This brief overview offers but a glimpse into the ways in which classical and late antique medical recipes, from both Greek and Latin traditions, describe when plants and plant products should be collected. In many cases, rhythms of the natural world sit alongside supernatural rituals. Overall, a diverse array of timing instructions can be found in these sources with practices repeated across multiple texts. So, to what extent do early medieval recipes continue these traditions?

Recipe Instructions in Early Medieval Manuscripts Relating to the Timing of Ingredient Collection

Of the forty-six manuscripts that contributed recipes to the sample under analysis in this study, eleven contained recipes with instructions regarding the collection of herbal ingredients.[34] In most cases, these examples are located within large recipe collections, paralleling the way in which such instructions are scattered throughout classical and late antique texts. There are, however, two exceptions: single instances of collection

---

31 Pliny, *Natural History*, trans. Rackham, Jones and Eichholz, 16.182, pp. 504–5: "mirum, is in moro medicis sucum quaerentibus vere hora diei secunda lapide incussus manat."

32 Pliny, *Natural History*, trans. Rackham, Jones and Eichholz, 24.170, pp. 120–21: "Herba quaecumque e rivis aut fluminibus ante solis ortum collecta ita ut nemo colligentem videat adalligata laevo bracchio ita ut aeger quid sit illud ignoret tertianas arcere traditur."

33 *Plinii Secundi Iunioris*, ed. Önnerfors, 3.16.4: "herba quae in fluminibus aut riuis nascitur adalligatur in laeuo brachio quid sit nescienti, tertianas discutit: legi debebit ante solis ortum sic ut eum qui colligit nemo uideat." I have lightly modified Lily Hunt's translation of this passage; see *The* Medicina Plinii, trans. Hunt, 86–87.

34 The eleven manuscripts are as follows: Cambridge, University Library, Gg.5.35 (two out of 103); Melk, Benediktinerstift, MS 412 (370, G 32) (one out of thirty); Paris, Bibliothèque nationale de France, lat. 6862 (one out of 214); lat. 9332 (two out of nine); lat. 11218 (four out of 793); St. Gallen, Stiftsbibliothek, MS (Cod. Sang.) 44 (eighteen out of 917); Cod. Sang. 751 (fifteen out of 1185); Cod. Sang. 759 (eight out of 451); Cod. Sang. 899 (one out of forty-two); Vatican City, Biblioteca Apostolica Vaticana, Pal. lat. 1088 (six examples out of 835 recipes); and Reg. lat. 1143 (six out of 312). See the bibliography for a list of all manuscripts under analysis.

instructions can be found in the recipes added to Paris, Bibliothèque nationale de France (hereafter BnF), lat. 6862 and Melk, Benediktinerstift, MS 412 (370, G 32).[35] While Paris, BnF, lat. 6862 is a medical manuscript in which extra recipes have been added, the recipes in Melk, Benediktinerstift, MS 412 (370, G 32) were inserted into a codex that primarily contains works by Bede and other material related to his writings, such as computistical texts—the manuscript thus fits with Faith Wallis's observation that medical recipes are "the most common kind of adventitious marginal addition to a computus manuscript."[36] The potential significance of these different codicological contexts will be considered further below.

While recipes include simple commands to gather the *materia medica* needed to prepare a treatment with some regularity, the addition of extra information concerning the collection *process* is rarer, aligning with the classical and late antique recipes surveyed above. Of the roughly six thousand recipes under analysis, only sixty-four provide specific instructions for the collection process. Within these sixty-four recipes, forty-four include instructions related to the timing of ingredient collection. As above, although the appearance of timing instructions in less than one percent of the sampled recipes may seem somewhat inconsequential, I argue that their inclusion in the written record is highly significant precisely because they are unusual as well as eye-catching given the nature of the information they present.

Of the forty-four recipes with timing instructions, twenty-two appear to be directly connected to seasonality and the maturation of the plant or plant product. In all twenty-two cases, a month (or, occasionally, a period within a month) is specified as the time to harvest the item in question, and this advice seems directly related to its maturation and life cycle.[37] In St. Gallen, Stiftsbibliothek, MS (Cod. Sang.) 44, for example, a recipe for "oleum cissimum" based on ivy berries, "bacis edere," states that these should be collected in the month of January.[38] These instructions fit with the time of year when ivy berries are in season. Turning to the summer months, in a recipe for dropsy in BnF, lat. 9332, centaury is said to be collected in July, while a potion in Cod. Sang. 44, notes that

35 On Paris, Bibliothèque nationale de France, lat. 6862, see Beccaria, *I codici*, no. 24, pp. 143–45; Wickersheimer, *Les manuscrits*, no. 61, pp. 67–70; and Bischoff, *Katalog*, 3:119, no. 4417. On Melk, Benediktinerstift, MS 412 (370, G 32), see Glaßner, *Inventar*, 191–93; Bischoff, *Katalog*, 2:180, no. 2739.

36 Wallis, "Medicine in Medieval Calendar Manuscripts," 126.

37 It must be noted that by considering months as representative of natural timing, this study differs from Faith Wallis's interpretation of months as representative of more arbitrary, calendrical time, not unlike days of the week.

38 St. Gallen, Stiftsbibliothek, Cod. Sang. 44, pp. 259–60. My transcription of the recipe is as follows: "Oleum cissimum hoc est de bacis edere . ianuario mense . cum ceperint edere grana gcrescere [*sic*] colligis ea . et tertia die miscis inde in frixoria uncias iii . oleo libras . iii . quoquis ad medium tollis desuper igne et colas et addis ibi de ipsis bacis uncias i semis . tritis reponis uteris eum ad eos qui non dormiunt caput inunguis . et mox dormit . et dolorem capitis tollit quia narcorticum est sonitum aurium si tepidum . mittatur emendat . est enim eius uirtus mediocriter calida." Cf. *Studien und Texte*, ed. Sigerist, 99. On Cod. Sang. 44, see Beccaria, *I codici*, no. 129, pp. 364–68; Bischoff, *Katalog*, 3:301–2, nos. 5529a and 5530.

basil should be gathered in September. Indeed, most of the months specified occur in summer and early autumn, the primary harvest season: July is named in five recipes, August in six, and September in seven, though several of these individual recipes reappear across different manuscripts.[39] While this might inflate the total number of recipes with monthly timing instructions, it illustrates the movement of knowledge between different centres of manuscript production and the use of shared traditions and perhaps even specific exemplars when compiling new collections of recipes. Notably, in treatments that appear to involve the supernatural in other ways (e.g., the fumigation is a treatment against worms caused by evil things, "contra uermes qui maleficio dominantur"), the months specified for harvesting ingredients seem strongly rooted in seasonality and natural time.

Just as in the classical and late antique material, natural rhythms unrelated to seasonality are also invoked in early medieval recipes. The daily movements of the sun and moon as well as the lunar cycle are mentioned in twenty-two recipes. In one instance, found in St. Gallen, Stiftsbibliothek, MS (Cod. Sang.) 751, both the sun and moon are used to define the appropriate time to collect an ingredient: verbena should be collected before sunrise *and* with setting moon (the instructions also involve several other timing elements addressed in more detail below).[40] More frequently, however, either the sun (six recipes) or the moon (fifteen recipes) are mentioned separately, though the recipes may include additional temporal rhythms and rituals beyond solar and lunar cycles.

Within this recipe sample, references to the sun always stipulate that the collection must occur before sunrise, such as a treatment for haemorrhoids found in Vatican City, Biblioteca Apostolica Vaticana (hereafter BAV), Pal. lat. 1088.[41] In this case, several

---

39 July: Vatican City, Biblioteca Apostolica Vaticana, Reg. lat. 1143, fol. 196r ("Opio comodo facis"); Paris, Bibliothèque nationale de France, lat. 9332, fol. 233v ("Ad idropicus"); Melk, Benediktinerstift, MS 412 (370, G 32), p. 33 (untitled section on a herb called "priapus" (i.e., *priapiscus*, orchid) preceding several recipes that use this herb); St. Gallen, Stiftsbibliothek, Cod. Sang. 751, p. 416 ("Satirion"); Cod. Sang. 759, p. 45 ("Opio quomodo facias"). August: Vatican City, Biblioteca Apostolica Vaticana, Reg. lat. 1143, fols. 196v–197r ("Comodo diagridia facere debes"); St. Gallen, Stiftsbibliothek, Cod. Sang. 44, pp. 344–45 (second entry under "Ad cancoris occidendum"); Cod. Sang. 751, p. 408 (untitled recipe relating to stomach pain); Cod. Sang. 759, p. 45 ("Quomodo dagridium facere"), p. 46 ("Alio modo ad scamonia faciendo"), and p. 90 (second entry under "Ad canis rapidi morsum"). September: Vatican City, Biblioteca Apostolica Vaticana, Reg. lat. 1143, fol. 196v ("Licio comodo facies" and "Agasicia comodo facis"); St. Gallen, Stiftsbibliothek, Cod. Sang. 44, p. 344 (fourth entry under "Remedium ad ficum") and p. 350 (second entry under "Suffumicatio contra uermes qui maleficio dominantur"); Cod. Sang. 751, p. 418 ("Quomodo facis licio"); Cod. Sang. 759, p. 45 ("Litio quomodo facies" and "Agatia quomodo facies").

40 St. Gallen, Stiftsbibliothek, Cod. Sang. 751, p. 392. My transcription: "De birbina dicitur hoc est erba sanguinaria ipsa collegis in mense madio die iouis luna decurrente ante sole leuante […]." On the interpretation of "decurrente," see n. 43 below.

41 Vatican City, Biblioteca Apostolica Vaticana, Pal. lat. 1088, fol. 65v. My transcription: "Ad ficum rem probatam . Plantingine manipulos . iii . Milfolio manipulos . iii . Sagitolada manipulos . iii . Mentastro manipulos . iii . costo denarios . vi . Grano mastice denarium . i . Elna radices . Piper grana xc . uino staupos . viiii . Mel quod sufficit . Bibatur luna crescente . et decrescente . et iste erbe colligantur ante solis ortum."

different herbs, including handfuls of plantain, milfoil, and wild mint, are to be collected before sunrise and mixed with a number of other ingredients, including grains of mastic and pepper, nine cups of wine, and "a sufficient amount" of honey. The recipe also states that the patient should drink the resulting potion with either a waxing or waning moon, thereby integrating the lunar cycle into a different stage of the treatment process.

In contrast to the consistency of sun-based collection times, instructions for the timing of plant collection concerning the moon are more variable: recipes advise harvesting the plant in question when the moon is full ("plena"), waning ("descrescente" or "uetere"), waxing ("crescente"), or setting ("decurrente").[42] Although, as seen above, the terms "crescente" and "descrescente" sometimes appear in recipes to provide guidance on the timing of other aspects of the treatment process, with respect to ingredient collection, each term occurs only once within the sample. Regarding the former, in a potion intended to alleviate spleen complaints in Paris, BnF, lat. 11218, the roots of "epuli" (perhaps *ebulus*, danewort or dwarf elder) are to be collected with, confusingly, a full waning moon ("luna plena descrescente").[43] On the other hand, a waxing moon is specified in the second entry within a series of recipes intended to encourage arousal and virility ("Ad excitandum libidinem") in St. Gallen, Stiftsbibliothek, Cod. Sang. 751; this recipe adds the extra detail that the herb ought to be picked using the thumb and ring finger.[44]

While the words "crescent" and "descrescente" are infrequently paired with instructions relating to the timing of ingredient collection, the phrase "luna uetere" appears in nine recipes. Intriguingly, all nine of these "old moon" examples can be found in Cod. Sang. 44, suggesting the circulation of a particular tradition and/or standard phraseology within the centre that produced this codex.[45] More specifically, these recipes are located between p. 340 and p. 352, and, looking more closely at the structure of this manuscript, it becomes apparent that the recipes using this expression are thus not only found within the same codex but are also located within the same recipe collection within the codex. This complex, composite manuscript contains three large early medieval recipe collections and all examples of the "luna uetere" construction used to define the time at which a herbal ingredient should be collected can be found in the

---

42 I have interpreted the term "decurrente" as "setting," distinguishing it from "decrescente" (waning), since it comes from the verb "decurro," but I think it could be understood as a synonym for "descrescente."

43 Paris, BnF, lat. 11218, fol. 74v. My transcription: "Pucio ad splen radicis epuli candedas siccas collegis in luna plena decrescente et dabis cocliarium . unum plenum puluer cum uino ueteri."

44 St. Gallen, Stiftsbibliothek, Cod. Sang. 751, p. 412. My transcription: "Ad excitandum libidinem [...]. Item si quis autem perpetuu intermis ad cupidinis bella festinat magnum uenerem fisicorum ei est reddenda est uerilitate . Herbam dicitur quae in ribulis perennibus ita ut defluentium unda mergatur et modo subleuete ter(e)\i/gat caput anc luna crescente digito police et medicinale collegis . et contritam accipies ieiunus in potu."

45 St. Gallen, Stiftsbibliothek, Cod. Sang. 44; the nine recipes can be found on pp. 340–41, 344, 346–48, and 352.

middle compilation.[46] For example, on p. 341, a treatment for ear problems and deafness recommends that ash, though the part of the tree is not specified, should be collected on a Thursday with a waning moon.[47] The construction "die iouis luna uetere" occurs on a number of occasions in Marcellus's *De medicamentis liber* and may suggest that this source left a strong imprint on this particular recipe collection within Cod. Sang. 44. Furthermore, though the individual recipes appear to be otherwise unrelated, it may be worth remembering that Marcellus provided temporal instructions with respect to the collection of ash seeds, noting that they should be collected immediately before the ides of November.[48]

Although timing instructions that feature the moon and/or sun sometimes appear alone, they are frequently paired with at least one additional temporal instruction, such as a particular day of the week, as illustrated by the previous example. Consistent with the classical and late antique recipe literature, Thursdays, "die iouis," are named most often, appearing in twelve recipes. In fact, within this sample, days of the week never occur singly. Rather, they are also paired with further details regarding the timing of ingredient collection: eleven of the twelve recipes that feature Thursdays also include lunar instructions, such as the example given above as well as all others with the phrase "luna uetere" and two recipes with a setting moon ("decurrente") in Cod. Sang. 751.[49] Exceptionally, the potion intended to expel worms in Cod. Sang. 44 both broadens and narrows the temporal window for ingredient collection, specifying, on the one hand, that "herba basilerica" can be collected on Tuesdays, Thursdays, or Saturdays but, on the other hand, only in the month of September and with the setting moon.[50]

Individual days of the year appear very rarely. In one case from BAV, Reg. lat. 1143, the day before the Kalends of July is listed as the day on which squill should be col-

46 The different collections can be found on pp. 228–60, 337–54, and 354–68.

47 St. Gallen, Stiftsbibliothek, Cod. Sang. 44, p. 341. My transcription: "Ad grauitatem auris . uel ad surdo . die iouis uetere luna colligis tres fraxanos mittis eos in igne aqua quae de ipsos exit collige . et misce ius melle atico et barba iouis . cum folia persici . ius miscis in unum corpus . per taratroliola in aurem mittatur . cum celedoniae ius quamuis quo surdum audire facias."

48 See n. 24 above.

49 For the examples in St. Gallen, Stiftsbibliothek, Cod. Sang. 44, see n. 45 above. The two recipes in St. Gallen, Stiftsbibliothek, Cod. Sang. 751 can be found on pp. 383 and 392; the latter example extends the instructions given in n. 40. The instructions continue as follows: "De birbina dicitur hoc est erba sanguinaria ipsa collegis in mense madio die iouis luna decurrente ante sole leuante cum oratione dominica et nullum ferrum super te non habeas [...]."

50 St. Gallen, Stiftsbibliothek, Cod. Sang. 44, p. 350. My transcription: "Potio bibenda contra ipsos uermes eiciendos . aut quacumque maleficio in se habuerit Herba basilerica quae nascitur per montes . in loca arida ubi petras minutas sunt . folia simili porro . radix eius crispa . et fistolas . colligis eam mense septembri luna decurrente die martis aut iouis . aut sabbati . herba ipsa teris diligenter . miscis cum nouella ceruisia calice pleno das ei ieiuno bibere . et ante die abstineat se a cibo . die iouis luna uetere debet bibere . si uermes ipsa die iactauerit . priusquam manducet calido bibat aut exouera ."

lected.[51] Unusually, the recipe continues with further temporal instructions regarding the preparation of the squill-based potion that are also linked to calendrical time: having been mixed with vinegar and wine, the potion should be suspended in the sun and moon for thirty days, from the Kalends of July to the Kalends of August. One of the very few other examples within the sample that invokes a specific day of the year for collecting herbal ingredients is found in Cod. Sang. 44. In this treatment for demon possession, the "herb that is called paniscardi" should be collected on Easter and then put on the altar where mass is said that day.[52] The recipe explicitly emphasizes Easter as the chosen day, writing that the herb should be collected on "the day of the resurrection of the Lord" and then reiterating that "this is Easter": "dies resurrectionis domini. Hoc est prima pascha."

Significantly, although the Christian calendar does not appear frequently in recipes as a type of time delineating when ingredients should be collected, in five recipes that include ingredient collection timing instructions, other Christian rituals are also listed as part of the collection process. In a treatment for fevers found in Paris, BnF, lat. 6862, for example, the gathering of sage leaves should happen not only before sunrise but also while facing east and reciting the Lord's Prayer.[53] The recipe appears to draw on the perceived potency of number symbolism and repetition, specifying that 150 sage leaves should be collected, the Lord's Prayer should be said 150 times, and 150 pepper grains should be added to the potion.

While the example in BnF, lat. 6862 only brings together two types of collection instructions, the information recorded in Cod. Sang. 751 regarding the gathering of verbena, mentioned above, combines multiple layers of instruction that create a highly complex process: verbena ought to be collected in the month of May, on a Thursday, with a setting moon, before sunrise, without iron, and whilst saying the Lord's Prayer.[54] Instructions to collect herbs without iron, a feature that was noted in the opening example, also occur in two other recipes. First, the recipe in Cod. Sang. 44 highlighted above that named Easter as the day to gather "paniscardi" included this prohibition against iron, while the other example, found in a treatment in Cod. Sang. 751, is located within a

51 Vatican City, BAV, Reg. lat. 1143, fols. 154v–155r. My transcription: "Confectio acetii scilletici pridiae calendarum iuliarum collegis scilla et tollis ei corticem omnem quae dura fuerit una cum foliis et radicebus et quod est obitum ipsius scille incidetis tesselatim menutum uncias viii et mittis in sextaria duo aceto obtimi et uino ueteri duo sextarios in uaso uetereo et suspendis sub diuo signato et bene claudis nec uentum admittat et suspendis in sole et luna ex dię kalendas iulias . usque in dię kalendas augustas deinde conpleti diebus xxx [...]."

52 St. Gallen, Stiftsbibliothek, Cod. Sang. 44, pp. 346–47. My transcription: "Remedium ad inmissiones diaboli . Herba quae dicitur paniscardi dies resurrectionis domini . hoc est prima pa\s/cha colligis ipsum cardo sine ferro uerticulo habet in suma radice et sit in altario . ubi ipsa die missa dicitur . et postea cui necesse fuerit . in aqua . aut in uino bibat . sanat."

53 Paris, BnF, lat. 6862, fol. 10v. My transcription: "Potio Ad frigoras . Saluia folia integra . ante solis ortum contra orientem colligis . folia cl . et dicis oratione dominica . cl uices . et addis piper grana cl . et distemperas cum uino calicem i . et dabis bibere . ieiuno ante accessam . hoc per triduum facis . et liberabitur."

54 See nn. 40 and 49 above.

section of recipes excerpted from *De herba vettonica liber* and thus relates to the instructions given in this text's introduction.[55]

Finally, having now considered two recipes in which extra information regarding the collection of ingredients (i.e., information not linked to the timing of this process) that circulated *alongside* timing details, what types of information were included in instructions regarding the collection of ingredients that do *not* refer to the timing of this process? In all twenty recipes within the sample that provide specifications on the process of collecting ingredients *without* temporal guidance, the reader is instructed to collect the plant or plant product while saying the Lord's Prayer, making the sign of the cross, or both together. Five recipes in Vatican City, BAV, Pal. lat. 1088, for example, state that the herbal ingredients should be collected with the Lord's Prayer, providing no further details with respect to the collection process.[56] A treatment for madness and epilepsy ("Ad lunaticos et cadiuos") on fol. 33v exemplifies this trend, recording that ribwort, mistletoe from oak, agrimony, and milfoil should be gathered with this prayer.[57] A nearly identical recipe occurs in Cod. Sang. 44, though with the added information that the patient should drink the potion for four lunar cycles.[58] Notably, in both cases, the herbal mixture is liquefied by the addition of holy water (*aqua benedicta*), extending the treatment's incorporation of Christian elements to the *materia medica* itself.

This review of the ways in which instructions for collecting ingredients integrate temporal guidance highlights the diversity of information contained in early medieval recipes. Not unlike the instructions seen in classical and late antique texts, multiple kinds of time appear, whether singly or in combination, throughout the prescriptions within the present analysis. Indeed, even though exact parallels remain relatively rare, the overall similarities in timing instructions between early medieval recipes and (late) ancient material is striking. Although temporal information based on the Christian calendar was identified, the introduction of such timing instructions does not appear to have been a widespread phenomenon. Christian rituals unrelated to timing, however, do appear with relative frequency within instructions relating to the process of collecting herbal ingredients. These findings have important implications for understanding the development of medical knowledge and its place in society within early medieval Europe, the final topic considered in this chapter.

55 On the first example, see n. 52 above; on the second, see St. Gallen, Stiftsbibliothek, Cod. Sang. 751, p. 408.

56 The five recipes in Vatican City, BAV, Pal. lat. 1088 can be found on fols. 33v, 47v, 61r, and 62r.

57 Vatican City, BAV, Pal. lat. 1088, fol. 33v. My transcription: "Ad lunaticos et cadiuos . erba lantiolata uisco roboreo agrimonia millefolia ista omnia cum oratione dominica collegis . et per tres lunationes dabis bibere cum aqua benedicta."

58 St. Gallen, Stiftsbibliothek, Cod. Sang. 44, p. 358. My transcription: "AD LUNATICOS . ET CADIUOS . Herba lanciolata . uiscu . ruborio agrimonia . milfolio . ista . omnia cum oratione dominica colligis. et per quattuor lunaciones das bibere ieiuno cum aqua benedicta."

Contextualizing Early Medieval Recipe Instructions Relating to the Timing of Ingredient Collection

The instructions surveyed above offer significant insights into the transmission and perception of medicine in the Carolingian world. The extensive continuities between the information recorded in classical and late antique recipes and the content of early medieval prescriptions reflects the magnitude of the former's long-term influence. These (late) ancient texts remained the fundamental building blocks of medical writing over the following centuries, and early medieval compilers drew heavily on these sources when creating new compositions. Yet, alongside this strong continuity, the early medieval recipe literature testifies to the evolution of healing practices and the fusion of classical knowledge with a new system of belief. Although, by the Carolingian period, Christian approaches to medicine were not a new phenomenon and had long been documented in non-medical writings, the recording of liturgical rituals within medical texts—texts largely based on pre-Christian sources—first appears during this time.[59]

With respect to ingredient collection, the recipes sampled in this study provide few examples of timing instructions based on the Christian calendar; instead, however, they showcase that prayers and performative rituals were introduced to the collection process. Significantly, such instructions, although they are sometimes found alongside timing and other information rooted in non-Christian sources (e.g., using the lunar cycle to guide the time of collection or prohibiting the use of iron implements), often occur in recipes that have no other ritualistic elements. This finding suggests that Christian features were not added to recipes in an attempt to sacralize pre-Christian knowledge perceived as dangerous and unorthodox. Likewise, given the degree to which non-Christian timing instructions continued to appear in early medieval recipes, it cannot be said that explicitly Christian elements replaced this potentially illicit information. Overall, just as Ciaran Arthur has compellingly argued in relation to Old English "charms," non-Christian rituals concerning the time to collect herbal ingredients should not be interpreted "as remnants of heathen religion or heterodox blends of Christianity and paganism."[60] Rather, the coexistence of Christian and non-Christian material (and, relatedly, natural and supernatural timing instructions) reflects the general impact of the environment in which these texts were produced.

As Horden points out, few early medieval individuals would have "disputed that ritual words and gestures had power over invisible forces. That was seen by most Christians in the mass. The question was: whose words, which forces?"[61] Timing instructions offer an ideal case study to explore this perceived authority in relation to orthodoxy. According to the polemical treatises of certain Carolingian theologians, it would seem that much of the ritualistic material included within the recipe literature should have

---

59 For earlier evidence of a Christian healthscape, see, for example, Gregory of Tours, *History of the Franks*, trans. Thorpe; Knipp, "Chapel of the Physicians," 1–23; Ferngren, *Medicine and Health Care*. On the wider range of Christian elements in recipes, see Burridge, "Healing Body."

60 Arthur, *"Charms,"* 215.

61 Horden, "What's Wrong with Early Medieval Medicine?," 8.

registered as illicit, pre-Christian knowledge among the scribes copying and compiling medical texts. Yet, to a monk well-versed in computistical texts and tables, would collecting an ingredient in relation to the phase of the moon have seemed inappropriate or dangerously heterodox? Given the various fields of learning that were enmeshed within monastic communities (which, crucially, are the very locations in which many surviving medical manuscripts were produced), such environments would seem to present the perfect conditions for maintaining diverse and divergent traditions of knowledge.[62] By zooming in on the manuscript evidence and considering how such potentially illicit material is presented in practice, it becomes possible to look beyond the treatises of thunderous theologians and investigate the transmission of knowledge on the ground.

A manuscript-based approach, moreover, enables highly localized studies of knowledge transfer, concentrating on specific centres, compilers, and codices. This level of analysis reinforces the fact that individual communities had access to different sources, experienced varying degrees of connectivity with other intellectual centres, and may have preserved or developed distinct traditions within the wider, shared framework of early medieval intellectual culture. Consider the example of Cod. Sang. 44 highlighted above. This manuscript contains a wide array of medical writings, including three different early medieval recipe collections. One of these collections repeatedly uses the phrase "die iouis luna uetere," terminology unique to this particular collection of recipes, at least within the sample of recipes under analysis. These examples of individuality among manuscripts and their constituent parts emphasize the complex processes of knowledge transmission and adaptation that underpinned the development of recipe collections. What sources were used to produce *this* collection in Cod. Sang. 44 and how did they differ from those of its neighbouring texts? By identifying patterns within and between codices, it may be possible to detect more relationships between texts, manuscripts, and writing centres, further enriching and deepening our understanding of how medical knowledge evolved during this period.

Conclusion

By reopening the study of how instructions for collecting herbal ingredients deploy different types of time, whether natural, supernatural, or both, this chapter seeks to provide a fresh perspective on the written record of early medieval medicine. It points to how a granular approach can be used to interrogate and inform major questions concerning the inter-relationship between medicine and the Church, the perceptions of licit and illicit knowledge, and the ways in which cultures of healing were actively documented during this period. More specifically, this contribution has offered a look at calendrical thinking through the lens of recipe literature, centring the medical material rather than approaching it as an appendage to calendrical content. In doing so, the present study adds another layer to the ongoing discourse on the relationship between spiritual and bodily health and healing in the early Middle Ages by identifying and examining continu-

62 On the production environments of medical manuscripts, see Glaze, "Perforated Wall."

ities with pre-Christian traditions alongside the introduction of liturgical rituals within medical writings. Much work remains to be done, and to expand this research further it will be crucial to connect continental material with the Old English corpus of medical texts, investigate instructions in recipes beyond ingredient collection (namely, during the preparation and administration of a treatment), and compare pharmaceutical recipes with performative rituals (e.g., "charms") in the context of healing. Ultimately, timing instructions for ingredient collection present a valuable case study that can help to trace the evolution of early medieval medicine on the ground while exploring the influence of the monastic environment in concert with classical and late antique medical traditions.

Bibliography

Manuscripts Consulted

*Entries marked * indicate the manuscripts in which recipes with instructions for the collection of herbal ingredients were found.*

Angers, Bibliothèque municipale, MS 275.
Arras, Bibliothèque municipale, MS 0636 (0709).
Autun, Bibliothèque municipale, MS S 37.
Bern, Burgerbibliothek, MS 109.
Bern, Burgerbibliothek, MS 224.
Bern, Burgerbibliothek, MS 318.
Brussels, Koninklijke Bibliotheek van België, MS 3701-15.
Brussels, Koninklijke Bibliotheek van België, MS 5325-27.
Brussels, Koninklijke Bibliotheek van België, MS 5649-67.
Cambridge, University Library, Gg.5.35.*
Cambridge, Corpus Christi College, MS 223.
Einsiedeln, Stiftsbibliothek, MS 263.
Einsiedeln, Stiftsbibliothek, MS 321(647).
Karlsruhe, Badische Landesbibliothek, Aug. perg. 172.
Laon, Bibliothèque municipale, MS 199.
London, British Library, Harley MS 2735.
Melk, Benediktinerstift, MS 412 (370, G 32).*
Paris, Bibliothèque nationale de France, lat. 2849A.
Paris, Bibliothèque nationale de France, lat. 2858.
Paris, Bibliothèque nationale de France, lat. 4627.
Paris, Bibliothèque nationale de France, lat. 5543.
Paris, Bibliothèque nationale de France, lat. 6862.*
Paris, Bibliothèque nationale de France, lat. 6882A.
Paris, Bibliothèque nationale de France, lat. 7021.
Paris, Bibliothèque nationale de France, lat. 9332.*
Paris, Bibliothèque nationale de France, lat. 11218.*
Paris, Bibliothèque nationale de France, lat. 11219.
Paris, Bibliothèque nationale de France, lat. 13955.
St. Gallen, Stiftsbibliothek, Cod. Sang. 44.*

St. Gallen, Stiftsbibliothek, Cod. Sang. 217.
St. Gallen, Stiftsbibliothek, Cod. Sang. 397.
St. Gallen, Stiftsbibliothek, Cod. Sang. 550.
St. Gallen, Stiftsbibliothek, Cod. Sang. 751.*
St. Gallen, Stiftsbibliothek, Cod. Sang. 752.
St. Gallen, Stiftsbibliothek, Cod. Sang. 759.*
St. Gallen, Stiftsbibliothek, Cod. Sang. 761.
St. Gallen, Stiftsbibliothek, Cod. Sang. 878.
St. Gallen, Stiftsbibliothek, Cod. Sang. 899.*
St. Gallen, Stiftsbibliothek, Cod. Sang. 1396.
Stuttgart, Württembergische Landesbibliothek, MS HB XI 8.
Vatican City, Biblioteca Apostolica Vaticana, Pal. lat. 187.
Vatican City, Biblioteca Apostolica Vaticana, Pal. lat. 1088.*
Vatican City, Biblioteca Apostolica Vaticana, Reg. lat. 598.
Vatican City, Biblioteca Apostolica Vaticana, Reg. lat. 1143.*
Vatican City, Biblioteca Apostolica Vaticana, Vat. lat. 5951.
Vienna, Österreichische Nationalbibliothek, MS 1761.
Wolfenbüttel, Herzog August Bibliothek, MS 56. 18. Aug. 8.
Wrocław, Biblioteka Uniwersytecka, MS III. F. 19.
Würzburg, Universitätsbibliothek, M. p. th. f. 146.

Primary Sources

Agobard of Lyon. "Liber contra insulsam uulgi opinionem de grandine et tonitruis." In *Agobardi Lugdunensis Opera Omnia*. Edited by L. Van Acker, 3–15. Corpus Christianorum: Continuatio Mediaevalis 52. Turnhout: Brepols, 1981.

The Alphabet of Galen: Pharmacy from Antiquity to the Middle Ages. Edited and translated by Nicholas Everett. Toronto: University of Toronto Press, 2012.

Dioscorides. *De materia medica*. Translated by Lily Y. Beck, 4th ed. Hildesheim: Olms, 2005.

———. *De materia medica libri quinque*. Edited by Max Wellmann. 3 vols. Berlin: Weidmann, 1906–1914.

Frühmittelalterliche Rezeptarien. Edited by Julius Jörimann. Zurich: Füssli, 1925.

Gregory of Tours. *The History of the Franks*. Translated by Lewis Thorpe. London: Penguin, 1974.

Isidore of Seville. *Etymologiarum sive originum, libri XX*. Edited by W. M. Lindsay. 2 vols. Oxford: Oxford University Press, 1911.

———. *The Etymologies of Isidore of Seville*. Edited and translated by Stephen A. Barney, W. J. Lewis, J. A. Beach, and Oliver Berghof. Cambridge: Cambridge University Press, 2006.

Das Lorscher Arzneibuch: Ein medizinisches Kompendium des 8. Jahrhunderts (Codex Bambergensis Medicinalis 1): Text, Übersetzung und Fachglossar. Edited and translated by Ulrich Stoll. Stuttgart: Steiner, 1992.

Marcellus of Bordeaux. *De medicamentis liber*. Edited by Eduard Liechtenhan and Maximilian Niedermann. Translated by Jutta Kollesch and Diethard Nickel. Corpus Medicorum Latinorum 5. 2 vols. Berlin: Akademie, 1968.

The Medicina Plinii*: Latin Text, Translation, and Commentary*. Translated by Yvette Hunt. Abingdon: Routledge, 2020.

Plinii Secundi Iunioris qui feruntur de medicina libri tres. Edited by Alf Önnerfors. Corpus Medicorum Latinorum 3. Berlin: Akademie, 1964.

Pliny the Elder. *Natural History*. Translated by H. Rackham, W. H. S. Jones, and D. E. Eichholz. 10 vols. Loeb Classical Library 330, 352–53, 370–71, 392–94, 418–19. Cambridge, MA: Harvard University Press, 1938–1963.

Pseudo-Antonius Musa. "De herba vettonica liber." In *Antonii Musa De herba vettonica liber, Pseudoapulei Herbarius, Anonymi De taxone liber, Sexti Placiti Liber medicinae ex animalibus, etc.* Edited by Ernest Howald and Henry E. Sigerist, 3–11. Corpus Medicorum Latinorum 4. Leipzig: Teubner, 1927.

Pseudo-Apuleius. "Herbarius." In *Antonii Musa De herba vettonica liber, Pseudoapulei Herbarius, Anonymi De taxone liber, Sexti Placiti Liber medicinae ex animalibus, etc.* Edited by Ernest Howald and Henry E. Sigerist, 15–225. Corpus Medicorum Latinorum 4. Leipzig: Teubner, 1927.

Der St. Galler Botanicus: Ein frühmittelalterliches Herbar: Kritische Edition, Übersetzung und Kommentar. Edited and translated by Monica Niederer. Bern: Lang, 2005.

Studien und Texte zur frühmittelalterlichen Rezeptliteratur. Edited by Henry E. Sigerist. Leipzig: Barth, 1923.

Vademecum eines frühmittelalterlichen Arztes: Die gefaltete lateinische Handschrift medizinischen Inhalts im Codex 217 und der Fragmentensammlung 1396 der Stiftsbibliothek in St. Gallen. Edited and translated by Peter Köpp. Aarau: Sauerländer, 1980.

Secondary Sources

Arthur, Ciaran. *"Charms," Liturgies, and Secret Rites in Early Medieval England*. Woodbridge: Boydell and Brewer, 2018.

Banham, Debby. "The Staff of Life: Cross and Blessings in Anglo-Saxon Cereal Production." In *Cross and Cruciform in the Anglo-Saxon World: Studies to Honour the Memory of Timothy Reuter*. Edited by Sarah Larratt Keefer, Karen Louise Jolly, and Catherine E. Karkov, 279–318. Morgantown: West Virginia University Press, 2010.

Beccaria, Augusto. *I codici di medicina del periodo presalernitano (secoli IX, X ed XI)*. Rome: Storia e Letteratura, 1956.

Bisagni, Jacopo. "The Newly-Discovered Irish and Breton *Computistica* in Città del Vaticano, BAV, MS Reg. Lat. 123." *Peritia* 28 (2017): 13–34.

Bisagni, Jacopo, and Immo Warntjes. "The Early Old Irish Material in the Newly Discovered *Computus Einsidlensis* (c. AD 700)." *Ériu* 58 (2008): 77–105.

Bischoff, Bernhard. *Katalog der festländischen Handschriften des neunten Jahrhunderts (mit Ausnahme der wisigotischen)*. 3 vols. Wiesbaden: Harrassowitz, 1998–2014.

Burridge, Claire. "Healing Body and Soul in Early Medieval Europe: Medical Remedies with Christian Elements." In *The Church in Sickness and in Health*. Edited by Charlotte Methuen and Andrew Spicer, 46–67. Studies in Church History 5. Cambridge: Cambridge University Press, 2022.

——. "Incense in Medicine: An Early Medieval Perspective." *Early Medieval Europe* 28 (2020): 219–55.

Cameron, Malcolm L. *Anglo-Saxon Medicine*. Cambridge: Cambridge University Press, 1993.

Doyle, Conan T. *The Reception of Latin Medicine in Anglo-Saxon England: Evidence from Old English Medical Texts*. York: York Medieval Press, forthcoming.

Dutton, Paul Edward. *Charlemagne's Mustache and Other Cultural Clusters of a Dark Age*. New York: Palgrave Macmillan, 2004.

Ferngren, Gary B. *Medicine and Health Care in Early Christianity*. Baltimore: Johns Hopkins University Press, 2009.

Filotas, Bernadette. *Pagan Survivals, Superstitions and Popular Cultures in Early Medieval Pastoral Literature*. Toronto: Pontifical Institute of Mediaeval Studies, 2005.

Fischer, Klaus-Dietrich. *Bibliographie des textes médicaux latins: Antiquité et haut Moyen Âge; Premier supplement, 1986–1999*. Saint-Étienne: Publications de l'Université de Saint-Étienne, 2000.

Glaßner, Christine. *Inventar der Handschriften des Benediktinerstiftes Melk, teil 1: Von den anfängen bis um ca. 1400*. Vienna: Verlag der Österreichischen Akademie der Wissenschaften, 2000.

Glaze, Florence Eliza. "The Perforated Wall: The Ownership and Circulation of Medical Books in Medieval Europe, ca. 800–1200." PhD diss., Duke University, 1999.

Groenke, Frank-Dieter. "Die frühmittelalterlichen Lateinischen Monatskalendarien: Text—Übersetzung—Kommentar." PhD diss., Institut für Geschichte der Medizin der Freien Universität Berlin, 1986.

Heiduk, Matthias, Klaus Herbers, and Hans-Christian Lehner, eds. *Prognostication in the Medieval World: A Handbook*. 2 vols. Berlin: De Gruyter, 2021.

Horden, Peregrine. "What's Wrong with Early Medieval Medicine?" *Social History of Medicine* 24 (2011): 5–25.

Jolly, Karen Louise. *Popular Religion in Late Saxon Religion: Elf Charms in Context*. Chapel Hill: University of North Carolina Press, 1996.

Jones, Peter Murray, and Lea T. Olsan. "Medicine and Magic." In *The Routledge History of Medieval Magic*. Edited by Sophie Page and Catherine Rider, 299–311. London: Routledge, 2019.

Knipp, David. "The Chapel of the Physicians at Santa Maria Antiqua." *Dumbarton Oaks Papers* 56 (2002): 1–23.

Leja, Meg. "The Sacred Art: Medicine in the Carolingian Renaissance." *Viator* 47 (2016): 1–34.

——. *Embodying the Soul: Medicine and Religion in Carolingian Europe*. Philadelphia: University of Pennsylvania Press, 2022.

Luck, Georg. Arcana Mundi*: Magic and the Occult in the Greek and Roman Worlds*. 2nd ed. Baltimore: Johns Hopkins University Press, 2006.

Meaney, Audrey L. "The Practice of Medicine in England about the Year 1000." *Social History of Medicine* 13 (2000): 221–37.

——. "Extra-Medical Elements in Anglo-Saxon Medicine." *Social History of Medicine* 24 (2011): 41–56.

McCarthy, Daniel P., and Dáibhí Ó Cróinín. "The 'Lost' Irish 84-Year Easter Table Rediscovered." *Peritia* 6–7 (1987–88): 227–42.

McCormick, Michael. *Origins of the European Economy: Communications and Commerce, AD 300–900*. Cambridge: Cambridge University Press, 2001.

Nothaft, Philipp. "The Reception and Application of Arabic Science in Twelfth-Century Computistics: New Evidence from Bavaria." *Journal for the History of Astronomy* 44 (2013): 35–60.

Nothaft, Philipp. *Scandalous Error: Calendar Reform and Calendrical Astronomy in Medieval Europe*. Oxford: Oxford University Press, 2018.

——. "Roger of Hereford and the Transformation of Computus in Twelfth-Century England." In *Medieval Science in the North: Travelling Wisdom, 1000–1500*. Edited by Christian Etheridge and Michele Campopiano, 27–43. Turnhout: Brepols, 2021.

Olsan, Lea T. "Charms and Prayers in Medieval Medical Theory and Practice." *Social History of Medicine* 16 (2003): 343–66.

——. "The Corpus of Charms in the Middle English Leechcraft Remedy Books." In *Charms, Charmers and Charming: International Research on Verbal Magic*. Edited by Jonathan Roper, 214–37. London: Palgrave Macmillan, 2009.

Rhijn, Carine van. *Leading the Way to Heaven: Pastoral Care and Salvation in the Carolingian Period*. London: Routledge, 2022.

Riddle, John M. "The Introduction and Use of Eastern Drugs in the Early Middle Ages." *Sudhoffs Archiv für Geschichte der Medizin und der Naturwissenschaften* 49 (1965): 185–98.

Sabbah, Guy, Pierre-Paul Corsetti, and Klaus-Dietrich Fischer. *Bibliographie des textes médicaux latins: Antiquité et haut Moyen Âge*. Saint-Étienne: Publications de l'Université de Saint-Étienne, 1987.

Skemer, Don C. "*Armis Gunfe*: Remembering Egyptian Days." *Traditio* 65 (2010): 75–106.

Stannard, Jerry. "Marcellus of Bordeaux and the Beginnings of Medieval *Materia Medica*." *Pharmacy in History* 15 (1973): 47–53.

Van Arsdall, Anne. "Challenging the 'Eye of Newt' Image of Medieval Medicine." In *The Medieval Hospital and Medical Practice*. Edited by Barbara S. Bowers, 195–206. Aldershot: Routledge, 2007.

Wallis, Faith. "The Church, the World and the Time: Prolegomena to a History of the Medieval '*Computus*'." In *Normes et pouvoir à la fin du Moyen Âge: Actes du Colloque "La recherche en études médiévales au Québec et en Ontario," 16–17 mai 1989, Montréal*. Edited by Marie-Claude Déprez-Masson, 15–29. Montréal: CERES, 1989.

——. "Medicine in Medieval Calendar Manuscripts." In *Manuscript Sources of Medieval Medicine: A Book of Essays*. Edited by Margaret R. Schleissner, 105–43. Abingdon: Routledge, 1995.

——. "The Experience of the Book: Manuscripts, Texts, and the Role of Epistemology in Early Medieval Medicine." In *Knowledge and the Scholarly Medical Traditions*. Edited by Don G. Bates, 101–26. Cambridge: Cambridge University Press, 1995.

Warntjes, Immo, and Dáibhí Ó Cróinín, eds. *Late Antique Calendrical Thought and Its Reception in the Early Middle Ages: Proceedings of the 3rd International Conference on the Science of Computus in Ireland and Europe, Galway, 16–18 July, 2010*. Turnhout: Brepols, 2018.

Warntjes, Immo. *The Munich Computus: Text and Translation: Irish Computistics between Isidore of Seville and the Venerable Bede and its Reception in Carolingian Times*. Stuttgart: Steiner, 2010.

Weisser, Christoph. "Das Krankheitslunar aus medizinhistorischer Sicht: Ein Beitrag zur iatromathematisch-astrologischen Fachliteratur des Mittelalters." *Sudhoffs Archiv* 65 (1981): 390–400.

Wickersheimer, Ernest. "Epistola Ypocratis ad Alexandrum de tempore herbarum." *Janus* 41 (1937): 145–52.

——. *Les manuscrits latins de médecine du haut Moyen Âge dans les bibliothèques de France*. Paris: Éditions du Centre National de la Recherche Scientifique, 1966.

——. "Nouveaux textes médiévaux sur le temps de cueillette des simples." *Archives internationals d'histoire des sciences* 3 (1949): 342–55.

Zecher, Jonathan. *Spiritual Direction as a Medical Art in Early Christian Monasticism*. Oxford: Oxford University Press, 2022.

TIME AND TIDE

THE CREATION OF A SEA TRAVEL NETWORK IN THE SEVERN REGION IN THE EARLY MIDDLE AGES

CAROLINE BOURNE

BODIES OF WATER provide clear distinctions between the modern countries of far northwestern Europe. The English Channel acts as a border between England and France, and further north, across the Irish Sea, Wales is separated from Ireland to the west and to the south, on the other side of the Bristol Channel and Severn Estuary is England. However, in the fifth and sixth centuries, far from being a prohibitive border, these bodies of water were the means through which these countries were connected. A key factor in this was the relatively short distances between countries, which meant that at the closest points, land across the water was visible. Such visibility brings other regions within the sphere of reference of those living around the nearest points. The faraway becomes known and with that, the potential for accessibility becomes a possibility. Evidence for the creation of a network of sea routes in the early medieval period is limited. However, the narratives contained within hagiographical material written many centuries later can provide an indication of how the early saints interacted with bodies of water.

In the case of the body of water that connects Wales to England, the development of the ways in which it was used for religious travel in this period can be assessed. Despite the hagiographies of saints being written centuries after their death and dedications to them not necessarily indicating a personal presence, a general picture can be formed if these are used in combination with place-name and archaeological evidence. This chapter will look at the Severn region during the fifth and sixth centuries, focusing on why this area became a centre for the development of Christianity, and what motivated people to travel for religious purposes. The way in which these religious travellers engaged with this body of water will first be explored, with the dangers posed by marine geography, weather, and tides influencing navigation and boat design. As Christianity developed, there was a change in the way that ecclesiastics interacted with the Severn region. During the sixth century a combination of climatic factors and changing religious motivations took effect. The development of this relationship with the Severn region will be examined, as the impetus for religious travel changed from individual spirituality to institutional endeavours.

Caroline Bourne is a doctoral research student with the Graduate Centre for Medieval Studies, University of Reading, working on the impact of the Normans on the Gower region of south Wales, in terms of secular power, ecclesiastical networks, and settlement. The author would like to thank the volume's editors, Anne Lawrence-Mathers and Carolina Escobar-Vargas, and the anonymous peer-reviewer for their support and feedback.

Wales is separated from the southwestern peninsula of England by the Bristol Channel, which opens out to the Atlantic below Ireland in the west and narrows as it merges with the estuary of the Severn to the east. The wide estuary is banked by extensive mudflats until it opens out into a deep channel to the west, where high cliffs dominate the coastlines. However, on the northern side of this "drowned valley," the cliffs are punctuated by river valleys, whose estuaries form wide bays, most noticeably by the Tawe, Loughor, and Tywi rivers.[1] This is not the case on the opposite coastline, but there are some estuaries situated on Devon's west coast.[2] On the English side of the Bristol Channel, cliffs dominate until the eastern lowland beaches of north Somerset. The Severn region is dominated by an extreme tidal range, with the vertical movement of the sea causing a significant difference in height between high and low tides, which occur at approximately six-hour intervals. This tidal range also results in a more powerful horizontal movement of the sea and these tidal streams create strong currents due to the funnelling of water in and out of a narrow channel. In order to understand why the Severn region was utilized for religious travel, the reasons why south Wales became the focus for Christianity must first be explored. There are two main practical reasons why south Wales became a centre for Christianity in Britain. Firstly, early in the fifth century, the turmoil on the Continent, with the struggle to maintain Roman control, meant that access to the southeast of Britain through short routes across the Channel, such as that from Dover to Calais, became less safe. Therefore, as safer routes were sought, this resulted in increased sea activity further west. That such a disruption of cultural contacts occurred between the Continent and the southeast of England can be illustrated from the fact that the reintroduction of Christianity via this route did not happen until almost a century later.[3] That Christianity spread along the western seaways in the post-Roman period was originally demonstrated by Nash-Williams through his work on inscribed stones.[4] But this in itself does not account for the concentration of Christian activity in the south Wales region, as this could have occurred at any point along this seaway from western Gaul to northern Scotland. Emrys Bowen argues that the reason south Wales became a focus for the development of Christianity was not solely due to the transmission of it through the western seaways. Firstly, existing Christianity in Britain during the Roman period was evident in the Severn-Cotswold region and the resulting Saxon pressure from the east during the fifth century caused this form of Romano-British Christianity to spread westwards into south Wales. Here, Romano-British Christianity fused with the form coming from Gaul via the seaways and the result was a focus in the development of the religion in that area.[5] Secondly, physical conditions in south Wales made it easier for Christianity to be spread across the region. People using these western seaways from Gaul were able to utilize the existing network of Roman roads in

1 North, *Evolution of the Bristol Channel*, 90.

2 North, *Evolution of the Bristol Channel*, 90.

3 Bede, *Ecclesiastical History*, ed. and trans. McClure and Collins, 37–38.

4 Nash-Williams, *Early Christian Monuments*.

5 Bowen, *Britain and the Western Seaways*, 71.

south Wales to take their religious ideals far inland. Elsewhere in Britain, these optimal conditions were not replicated.[6]

Another factor was the location in south Wales of one of the main saintly families. With the end of Roman rule in the fifth century, the power vacuum was filled by petty kingdoms, which made up the geographical region that is now Wales. Political marriages within areas of long-standing cultural affinities, resulted in the creation of a network of related kinship groups over a large geographical area, encompassing Brittany, south-western England, Ireland, Scotland, and Wales. The result of one of these marriages was Brychan, who was probably born in the first half of the fifth century and his importance is indicated by the fact that his kingdom, Brycheiniog, is thought to be derived from his name. His father's kingdom was in the mountainous region of mid-Wales and due to a political alliance, his mother was from Ireland. This meant that Irish culture was a prominent influence on Brychan's life and through this, he was exposed to Christian ideas. With the spread of religious ideals of monasticism focusing on living in isolation and missionary work, those who embraced this way of life in the middle of the fifth century were often considered to be saintly and Brychan's very large family were among the first to have such saints.

With such a strong focus on kinship and pedigree, the embracing of a celibate religious life was often incompatible with societal expectations. There are many cases of married saints who went on to produce saintly offspring, thus continuing the familial line. Some saints gave up their marriages to devote themselves to Christianity, whilst others rejected the idea of marriage altogether. Although avoiding marriage was clearly a factor for some, religious fervour was the main driving force. Although a greater number of saintly children have been attributed to Brychan than perhaps was the case, it is likely that those named were related to him in some way.[7] From those who have been attributed as children of Brychan, sixteen sons and ten daughters may have crossed the Bristol Channel from Wales to southwestern England, as suggested from hagiographical and dedication evidence. There is also a specific reference of this for his daughter, Ceinwen, as the *De Sancta Keyna* states that she desired to find a deserted place for contemplation and in order to achieve this, she crossed the Severn.[8] The journeys of this elite family and others in the region are known to us as they have been recorded. It is unknown how many ordinary people devoted themselves to God and travelled to find a place of solitude. However, the religious activities of both Brychan's family and others at the time were influential in the development of Christianity not only in Wales, but further afield.

With their Irish heritage, it would have been easier for Brychan's family to migrate westwards, taking the short sea journey to Ireland and being with relatives who could facilitate the establishment of religious settlements there. So why did they cross the Bristol Channel instead? Ralph Griffiths argues that the historical movement of peoples

6 Bowen, *Britain and the Western Seaways*, 74–75.

7 Baring-Gould and Fisher, *Lives of the British Saints*, 310–14.

8 *Nova Legenda Anglie*, ed. Horstman, 103.

went in a northerly direction as the Welsh coast provided sheltered harbours.[9] However, for these particular religious travellers, this may have been part of the reason why they went in the opposite direction. The foreboding cliffs on the opposite shore added to the physical trial in this test of faith. If a person survived the boat journey, they would face not only the difficulty of safely making it to land with few options of a safe haven, but they would be greeted with a seemingly impenetrable cliff face barring the way inland. The way in which these early Welsh ecclesiastics engaged with this marine environment was based on fear. It was a hostile environment and crossing it would be to place a life in the hands of God. Drowning was a likely prospect, as a small boat would be at the mercy of strong currents, but to make it to the other side may have been viewed as miraculous.

This early form of Christianity in south Wales was one based on movement. The eremitical ideas that came into this region promoted the seeking of solitude away from humanity. These ideas were influenced by the actions of Saint Anthony, who left behind his family and possessions to endure fasting and suffering in the desert. This test of faith and living as pure a life as possible could only be achieved away from people. As a result, shelters were set up in remote places and the holiness of the inhabitant would often attract followers. This in turn, would ensure that an association with the original occupant continued to be remembered through a church dedication or place-name. This was replicated in Wales during the fifth and sixth centuries, with remote and inhospitable places being sought to test spiritual resolve. In this way therefore, the Bristol Channel could be seen as a test of faith similar to that of Saint Anthony in the desert. It could be that the Bristol Channel was considered to have mystical properties, as it did not behave in the same way as other marine environments. The huge tidal drain may have seemed in some places as though it almost disappeared, only to flood the area again with tremendous force. The fierce currents also gave it an element of increased danger and other-worldliness. Although the southern coastline of Wales, with its river valleys made access to the sea much easier than the opposite cliffs, it also enabled the children of Brychan to journey down from the mountains to the Bristol Channel. This meant that people were more likely to embark upon sea journeys from Wales to the south and west, than to travel from the English coastline. However, accessibility alone cannot account for why some of these early ecclesiastical travellers chose to cross the Bristol Channel, as a route to the west was an alternative option. Therefore, the religious ideas of remote monasticism and tests of faith would have been a contributing factor.

Although the voyage would be a test of faith, it is unlikely that a person would just try to sail across as soon as they reached the sea. Some, who lived near the coast may already have had sea-faring experience and for those, like Brychan's children who resided inland, local knowledge would have been sought. There would have been some attempt to limit risk, even though ultimately, they were at the mercy of the elements. The weather would be a key factor in determining the success of a voyage. The Severn region is a particularly dangerous area of water with underwater rocks and sandbanks, this combined with adverse weather and strong currents has caused numerous shipwrecks

9 Griffiths, *Conquerors and Conquered*, 2–3.

to be concentrated in the area. The weather of the Bristol Channel is determined by the southwesterly gales that originate far out in the Atlantic and as a result of this dynamic climate, weather conditions can change quickly. This means that there was always the risk of being blown off-course or wrecked on rocks. Unfortunately, on its southern coast places of refuge should conditions deteriorate were limited. The unpredictability of the weather may have meant that more open water was avoided and that boats sailed near to the coast so that they had time to reach the safety of land. With the importance of being able to see the desired destination, visibility was often a deciding factor in when to travel. Misty and rainy weather is a characteristic of the region and this greatly affects visibility. Voyages during this time would have been avoided, with an inevitable delay until weather systems passed and more favourable conditions arrived.

Navigation could also be problematic in the Bristol Channel before compasses aided direction. The often-cloudy skies and occasional sea mists made locating the position of the sun difficult and sailing at night is too hazardous even today in some areas. This also meant that keeping land in sight was important and it is likely that distinctive land-markers were used in a similar way to how the Scandinavians utilized them as navigational aids centuries later. However, this was an issue with the southern coastline of the Bristol Channel. Although it can be viewed from the coastline of southern Wales, the distance, combined with a lack in variety of the topography meant that from afar, the majority of it appears to be just one big uniform land mass. But there were two main target areas that could be seen from the southeast or southwest of Wales, which a boat could aim for. To the east, the cliffs give way to lower ground which offered access inland. At the far western end, the gap between Devon and Lundy Island provided the promise of a way inland beyond, that could not be seen. Therefore, where a boat sailed from influenced which target was aimed for, as the shortest distance would be preferred.

The strong currents of the Bristol Channel also influenced which end of the coastline was chosen as the target destination. Tidal streams were a problem for maritime travel in this area in the early medieval period, as the speed that could be achieved through oar or sail power was usually not greater than the currents. Therefore, voyages had to be planned to sail with the flow of the currents, but this could be achieved, as different tides coincide with the phases of the moon. Sailing with the outgoing ebb tide towards Lundy Island meant that the island could be used as a safe haven if a boat was swept out to sea and missed the Devon coast. The subsequent following of the Devon and Cornwall coastline southwards would have been a hazardous journey, with the constant Atlantic winds threatening to wreck boats on the rocky shoreline. However, this is the route that some of the children of Brychan may have taken, as suggested by the place-names St. Endellion and St. Mabyn. The distance between the most southerly point of southeast Wales and Somerset is shorter. Sailing with the incoming flood tide would have carried a boat eastward to the lowland beaches. The tides also had an impact on when voyages could occur. If sailing from a beach, high tide was usually necessary, as boats were probably berthed beyond the tide line. However, the time of departure during the high tide was also important, not only because it influenced the direction of travel, but the destination or safe haven had to be reached before the tide turned.

The nature of the Severn region and the way it was used is likely to have affected boat design. It is probably the case that a variety of boat designs were active in the Severn region, ranging from larger, flatter cargo vessels to small, round coracles for coastal river navigation. However, for voyages involving the Bristol Channel, practicalities would have influenced design. Although there are many descriptions and depictions of boats in the hagiographies of saints active in the fifth and sixth centuries, they are the imaginings of a much later time. Therefore, they cannot be relied upon to accurately reflect the design used for religious travel in the Bristol Channel during this earlier period. However, an indication may be found in the design of craft used prior to this period. That there was a continuity in boat design for sea journeys from the earliest times to the Roman period is argued by Bowen, who cites the Bronze Age bowl from Caergwrle, Flintshire and the Iron Age Broighter gold model boat from Ireland as examples.[10] He goes on to say that this design must have continued to be used, as it is depicted on the Bantry Pillar in Ireland which has been dated to the eighth century.[11] He states that only skin-boats would have been able to deal with the conditions in open water and that they were constructed of wickerwork covered in cowhide. Although he assumes that prehistoric boats were similar to those used in western Ireland during his lifetime, he argues that the design was ideal for seafaring along the coastal areas. The size of approximately twenty-five feet long, with a width of six feet would suggest that its main function was to facilitate trade and its design meant that it was light enough to be dragged above the tide-line, without the need for moorings.[12] A description of such a boat can be found in the *Navigatio Sancti Brendani*. For his epic voyage, Saint Brendan built the lightweight boats for himself and his followers out of osier twigs and hides, with three sails and three banks of oars.[13] Although the description of Saint Brendan's voyage is not contemporary, it is possible that this type of design was used during the saint's lifetime in the sixth century.[14] The purpose of Saint Brendan's boats was to cope with open water, so it is unclear if a sail design was utilized elsewhere. But its size would provide some degree of stability to cope with the conditions of the Bristol Channel and the lightweight design meant that it could land at any type of beach, which was vital if the weather turned. Therefore, it is possible that this Irish curragh design was used in the post-Roman period. But with the design geared towards long voyages and its main function being the transport of light goods (its hide hull was not suitable for the transport of livestock or heavy items), this implies an inflexibility regarding destinations. Although this design could carry small groups of people, the very nature of trade means that they would dock at ports which

10 Bowen, *Britain and the Western Seaways*, 38.

11 Bowen, *Britain and the Western Seaways*, 39.

12 Bowen, *Britain and the Western Seaways*, 36–37.

13 *Acta Sancti Brendani*, ed. Moran, 90.

14 For a discussion of the various manuscripts associated with Saint Brendan, see Anderson, "*Navigatio Brendani*," 315. Although the earliest of these manuscripts dates from the tenth century, Anderson argues that the story of Saint Brendan's voyage was already established by the early ninth century.

provide a focus for settlement. As the objective of the early religious travellers was to find solitude away from people, these ports did not fit with this aim. It is therefore possible that smaller boats of a similar design were used for the crossings which could also be carried over land. As the trip was likely to be one-way, saints would either make the boats themselves or employ others for this task.

As the fifth century progressed, religious travel across the channel continued and remote places were still sought for spiritual purity. However, by this time not all journeys were a one-way trip to find a permanent place to dwell away from the world. Temporary off-shore hermitages were used, especially by those ecclesiastics in positions of authority, who desired some time apart from the people and responsibilities of their everyday lives. These were necessary because they were unable to completely give up everything to live a life of solitude. One of these important figures in the development of Christianity in the region was Saint Cadog, who was a grandson of Brychan. His preferred hermitage was on the island of Flat Holm. This was one of two islands that are located where the estuary of the Severn merges with the Bristol Channel, with Flat Holm being the island closest to the southeast coast of Wales. But even though the island was only a relatively short distance offshore, the boat journey to and from the island was still hazardous. These dangers are demonstrated in the *Vita Sancti Cadoci*. It relates the story of how after rowing from the island of Flat Holm to the mainland with two of his disciples, Saint Cadog, upon realising that they had forgotten his book, sent them back in the boat to get it from the island. However, by the time they made the return trip, tidal conditions had changed causing the boat to overturn and the two men drowned.[15] If such a short journey was just as hazardous as crossing the channel to find a remote retreat further afield, why did Saint Cadog choose to stay close to Wales?

Saint Cadog's island retreat was in a convenient location because it could easily be accessed from his principal monastery of Llancarfan nearby. This had become one of the main centres of learning in southern Wales and these monastic schools became very popular, attracting a large number of students. Such popularity is illustrated in the *Vita Sancti Cadoci* which tells us that, "there eagerly flowed together from various districts of the whole of Britannia very many clerics to Saint Cadog like rivers to the sea."[16] With the establishment of these monastic centres, their locations were ideally suited for sea access. Although they were some distance inland, small waterways linked these locations to the sea. For such a journey a small vessel was required either for the whole voyage or just inland from the coast. Llancarfan was ideally located to benefit from a direct crossing point from Somerset, therefore, it was well placed to accept students travelling from the south. However, from the hagiographical material, we are given a picture of students being actively recruited from throughout southern Wales. This meant that the focus for religious travel shifted away from the Bristol Channel, to the land routes of the old Roman roads, with saints moving throughout the country seeking students to study at the centres of learning.

---

15 *Lives of the Cambro-British Saints*, ed. and trans. Rees, 63–64.

16 *Lives of the Cambro-British Saints*, ed. and trans. Rees, 34.

Recruitment was not the only reason why saints travelled across southern Wales. Those saints that were associated with centres of learning were also figures of authority who travelled widely to communicate with each other. There are numerous mentions in the hagiographical material of journeys to visit members of the same kinship group, as many saints at this time were related, or to call on friends to discuss ecclesiastical matters. One of the most well-known ecclesiastical meetings of this time was the Synod of Brefi, which according to the *Vita Sancti Cadoci*, was called by Saint David to be held in west Wales whilst Saint Cadog was away, which caused friction between the two.[17]

With Saint David establishing himself as an important ecclesiastical figure of authority in west Wales, this increased religious travel along the breadth of the region, as monastic schools were not now solely in the southeast. Distribution patterns for dedications identified by Bowen in the southwest of Wales suggests that this is where saints David and Teilo started their missionary work, then they created a network of ecclesiastical settlements spreading eastwards.[18] At this point an important logistical problem may have become apparent to them. The network of Roman roads was good for establishing ecclesiastical settlements in the interior of Wales, but using them to travel long distances was time-consuming and personal risk increased through territories of other kinship groups. An alternative was to travel by boat, but this was dangerous due to the nature of the Bristol Channel. Although it was dangerous, sea travel, even with its six-hour tidal limitation, was faster than travelling by foot overland and less subject to political interventions. As a result, there was a change in the way that some religious people interacted with the Bristol Channel. The emphasis shifted from crossing it to travelling along the Welsh coastline.

Another factor which may have influenced the development of sea travel to transverse south Wales was a deterioration in the climate. The period between 400 and 600, termed the Dark Ages Cold Period, had a colder and wetter climate. The coldest period of this era follows a series of large volcanic eruptions, with the interval from 536 to about 660, known as the Late Antique Little Ice Age, being an additional environmental factor that contributed to crop failure, famine, plague and major societal changes.[19] The change in climate had an impact on the seasons, with shorter summers resulting in a more limited time for crop growth. The changes in the seasons would also have affected how long a vessel could sail for each day with the differences in daylight, which was also affected by the weather conditions. The Late Antique Little Ice Age coincided with the religious activity of Saint David, so this may have been a factor in how he chose to mitigate the dangers of sea travel in the Severn region.

With the combination of tides and available daylight, the length of the Bristol Channel could not be sailed in a day, which necessitated the need for a half-way stopover and the southern peninsula of Gower with its central position was ideal. Gower with its geo-

17 *Lives of the Cambro-British Saints*, ed. and trans. Rees, 39–40.

18 Bowen, *Settlements of the Celtic Saints*, 56–62.

19 Büntgen et al., "Cooling and Societal Change," 231.

graphical positioning, means that it has a slightly milder climate than mainland Wales.[20] With the onset of the Late Antique Little Ice Age, this would have provided a slightly more hospitable place to establish ecclesiastical settlements, with less chance of crop failure. But it was not without difficulties. A particularly dangerous part of the Bristol Channel lies off Gower's coast. To the southeast, the Mixon Shoal encompasses areas of exposed mudflats offshore from Mumbles Head, which also has strong currents. To the southwest, there are strong tidal streams around Worm's Head and the Helwick Channel is enclosed by the Helwick Sands to the south and narrows to the east into the Helwick Pass. In addition to this, the underwater shelf of Dagger Reef is also a danger.[21] The western shoreline of the peninsula is hazardous as it faces the full force of the southwesterly prevailing winds. The protruding rocky outcrops of Worm's Head to the south and Burry Holms to the north enclose the long sandy beach ensuring that there is no escape for any vessel exposed to the strong winds, currents, and wave swells of the area. To the north of the peninsula, the tide flows strongly into the mouth of the Loughor Estuary through a relatively narrow tidal channel and the large areas of sandbanks and mudflats are covered at high tide. Navigation is difficult in the area as access is limited to a few hours around high tide, with the meandering tidal channels of the low-lying saltmarsh only accessible to small boats. However, most of the dangerous waters could be avoided if travelling westwards, by sailing to the south coast of Gower, walking northwards across the peninsula, sailing from the River Loughor round Carmarthen Bay to the far west of south Wales, then the reverse trip eastwards.

That Gower was used as a trans-peninsula land routeway is supported by the fact that other land routes had already been used to avoid dangerous waters. One of these was the Camel/Fowey Corridor which transverses Cornwall, avoiding the hazardous sea off Land's End.[22] However, the main evidence that Gower was used in this way can be seen from the relationship between the positioning of ecclesiastical settlements and north/south routeways. Archaeological evidence suggests that a significant number of Gower churches had early origins with markers such as a curvilinear churchyard, inscribed stones, dedications, and place-name evidence. The positioning of the majority of Gower ecclesiastical settlements is significant in terms of their connection with travel. In Gower's peninsula, they were situated both on the bays of the south coast and bordering the estuary of the Loughor to the north, with these sites being connected by key routes running north/south. This ensured that there was not only a spiritual place to give thanks to God for the safe completion of a sea journey or prayers before setting out, but they also provided the practical function of somewhere to rest or wait for the tide. Some were also located at points along these routes, so that a traveller walking across the peninsula could rest. Saint David's personal involvement in the establishment of an ecclesiastical network in Gower is suggested through documentary and church dedication evidence. Bowen's research on the distribution of ecclesiastical settlements during

20 Oliver, "Climatology," 42.

21 Natural Resources Wales, *Carmarthen Bay*, 4–7.

22 Borlase, *Cornwall's Trans-Peninsular Route.*

the early medieval period, has been criticized for attributing church dedications to personal foundations by particular saints, as such dedications could be a result of cult activity and it cannot be determined when these associations with saints occurred. However, in Gower the positioning of churches dedicated to Saint David close to place-name evidence for centres of secular power is significant. In *Vita Sancti Davidis*, a church dedicated to Saint David in north Gower is mentioned.[23] Both this one, and another church in the peninsula dedicated to Saint David on a main north/south route, are close to locations that have evidence of secular courts. By sailing close to the coast in the direction of the tidal streams, using Gower as a land route, then continuing the sea journey on the next favourable tide, religious travellers could transverse southern Wales quicker than by just using a land route. In this way, more control over sea journeys was exerted, as risks were reduced and the Bristol Channel became part of the extensive travel network of the Severn region.

In conclusion, this body of water has many hazards that make sailing in the Severn region extremely dangerous for small boats. So why did people attempt to cross it in the fifth century? The proximity of a centre for the development of Christianity in the region explains why this body of water was used, rather than sea travel being concentrated elsewhere. But the reason why people risked their lives can be found in the religious ideas of solitude and physical tests of faith that that dominated early Christianity. Engagement by religious travellers with this water was one based on fear, as the probability of death was high. It would be down to the will of God whether a voyage would be successful. The dangers posed by weather, tides, and strong currents, influenced navigation and boat design, and as a result, some did make it across. However, with the development of centres of learning, emphasis shifted away from the water to the inland routes. In the sixth century, the desire to traverse southern Wales, combined with climatic factors meant that sea travel once again became important for religious voyages. But this time there was a change in the orientation of the direction of travel, with more of a focus on moving along the southern coast of Wales, rather than crossing the Bristol Channel. This change was more about utilizing the Bristol Channel to conduct ecclesiastical activities in a more convenient way and less about individual spiritualism. Therefore, practical solutions were sought to negate the dangers of sailing in the region, which had implications for how Christianity would develop in south Wales in the sixth century. By understanding and working with the nature of this body of water, voyages were less about a leap of faith and more about controlling the process of getting from one place to another.

---

23 *Lives of the Cambro-British Saints*, ed. and trans. Rees, 123.

Bibliography

Primary Sources

Acta Sancti Brendani: Original Latin Documents Connected with the Life of Saint Brendan, Patron of Kerry and Clonfert. Edited by Patrick Francis Moran. Dublin: Kelly, 1872.

Bede. *The Ecclesiastical History of the English People*. Edited and translated by Judith McClure and Roger Collins. Oxford: Oxford University Press, 2008.

Lives of the Cambro-British Saints, of the Fifth and Immediate Succeeding Centuries, from Ancient Welsh and Latin MSS. in the British Museum and Elsewhere, with English Translations and Explanatory Notes. Edited and translated by William J. Rees. Llandovery: printed by the editor, 1853.

Nova Legenda Anglie: As Collected by John of Tynemouth, John Capgrave, and Others, and First Printed, with New Lives by Wynkyn de Worde. Vol. 2. Edited by Carl Horstman. Oxford: Clarendon, 1901.

Secondary Sources

Anderson, John D. "The *Navigatio Brendani*: A Medieval Best Seller." *The Classical Journal* 83, no. 4 (1988): 315–22.

Baring-Gould, Sabine, and John Fisher. *The Lives of the British Saints: The Saints of Wales and Cornwall and Such Irish Saints as Have Dedications in Britain*. Vol. 1. London: Clark, 1907.

Borlase, Mark. *Cornwall's Trans-Peninsular Route: Socio-Economic and Cultural Continuity Across the Camel/Fowey Corridor*. British Archaeological Reports, British Series 653. Oxford: BAR, 2020.

Bowen, Emrys. *Britain and the Western Seaways*. Southampton: Thames and Hudson, 1972.

——. *The Settlements of the Celtic Saints in Wales*. Cardiff: University of Wales Press, 1956.

Büntgen, Ulf, Vladimir S. Myglan, Fredrik Charpentier Ljungqvist, Michael McCormick, Nicola Di Cosmo, Michael Sigl, Johann Jungclaus, et al. "Cooling and Societal Change During the Late Antique Little Ice Age from 536 to Around 660 A.D." *Nature Geoscience* 9, no. 3 (March 2016): 231–36.

Griffiths, Ralph. *Conquerors and Conquered in Medieval Wales*. Stroud: Sutton, 1994.

Nash-Williams, V. E. *The Early Christian Monuments of Wales*. Cardiff: University of Wales Press, 1950.

Natural Resources Wales. *Carmarthen Bay, Gower and Swansea Bay Local Seascape Character Assessment Final Report for City and County of Swansea*. Cardiff: Cardiff University, 2017.

North, F. J. *The Evolution of the Bristol Channel*. Cardiff: National Museum of Wales, 1955.

Oliver, J. "Climatology." In *Swansea and Its Region*. Edited by W. G. V. Balchin, 41–58. Swansea: University of Swansea, 1971.

ASTRAL FORCES AND ARTHURIAN DRAGONS IN GEOFFREY OF MONMOUTH'S *HISTORIA REGUM BRITANNIAE*

HUMMA MOUZAM

THIS CHAPTER EXPLORES the influence of Arabic and Syriac astronomy and astrology on an influential work of insular legendary history: Geoffrey of Monmouth's account of the early kings of Britain, the *Historia regum Britanniae* (ca. 1136/1138). The text's interest in astrology has been noted by Anne Lawrence-Mathers in relation to Merlin, "both boy wizard and the magus of the twelfth-century renaissance [...] an astrologer, prophet, and natural philosopher."[1] Little work, however, has been done on the cultural contexts and meanings of Geoffrey's astrological and astronomical allusions themselves, the most significant of which is the dragon. This is a figure which, I suggest, was informed by the author's engagement with twelfth-century Latin translations and re-imaginings of Arabic and Syriac works.

The Galfridian dragon is generally understood in relation to the dragon as a symbol of British national identity, as found in the "Omen of the Dragons" recorded in the ninth-century *Historia Brittonum* (attributed to Nennius, ca. 829/30), which forms the basis of Geoffrey's most significant engagement with the dragon motif in his own *Historia*.[2] The boy-prophet Merlin is summoned as a blood-sacrifice to stabilize the British King Vortigern's crumbling tower. However, Merlin prevents this bloody end by revealing a prophetic prodigy: a red dragon and a white dragon sleep beneath the falling fortress, and exemplify the past and future struggle for territory between the Britons (the red) and the Saxons (the white).[3] In the earliest "Omen" we read of *vermes* (worms), repre-

1 Lawrence-Mathers, *The True History of Merlin*, 5; Kieckhefer, *Magic in the Middle Ages*, 111.

2 See Jarman, *The Legend of Merlin*; Fulton, "Arthur and Merlin"; Jarman, "The Merlin Legend"; Padel, "Geoffrey of Monmouth."

3 "Political prophecy refers to a predominantly secular literary tradition drawing on authorities from the historical and legendary past, alongside a common stock of heroes and ciphers, to comment on near-historical and contemporary political affairs." See Flood, *Prophecy, Politics and*

Humma Mouzam is a doctoral researcher at the University of Birmingham. Her thesis, "Arabic Astronomy and Christian-Muslim Contact: Geoffrey of Monmouth's Prophetic Dragon and its Reception in Medieval Arthurian Literature," explores the far-reaching literary and cultural influences, drawn from European and Arabic sources, which informed the development of the dragon as a cultural symbol in English Arthurian literature produced between the twelfth and fifteenth centuries. The author gratefully acknowledges the support, patience, and guidance of Anne Lawrence-Mathers and Maria Carolina Escobar Vargas in the preparation of this chapter. For her wonderful and unrivalled dedication as both a supervisor and mentor, the author would also like to give a special thanks to Victoria Flood, whose advice and assistance in editing this chapter was greatly appreciated.

sentative of dragons; in Geoffrey's version, however, we encounter dragons directly, who rise up from their subterranean hiding place, and engage in combat, arguably aerial.[4] We might think here of the influence of the various dragons in the sky which appear in insular chronicles from at least the tenth-century onwards; but this is not the only possible analogue.[5] I suggest that Geoffrey's treatment of the figure of the dragon, as it appears throughout his work (as consistently aerial), may owe a debt to dragon allusions found in Arabic and Syriac astrology.

In Arabic and Syriac astronomy and astrology, the dragon (*draco*) is a feature of both constellations and eclipses: it is entwined between the Ursa Major and Ursa Minor, and responsible for causing eclipses in the sun and the moon. Although the constellation appears also in classical literature, in the writings of Ptolemy, Aratus, Virgil, and Hyginus, these presentations of the constellation possess only a very limited correspondence to Geoffrey's work.[6] The Arabic context was, as Elizabeth J. Bryan has noted, certainly known to Geoffrey's contemporaries.[7] Alongside discussion of Geoffrey's possible relationship to Walcher of Malvern's *De Dracone* (ca. 1120), one of the earliest English works to show a debt to Arabic astronomy (an influence first proposed by Bryan), I explore points of affinity with the *Liber Nemroth*, a Latin astronomical text likely of Syriac origin popular during the time of Geoffrey's writing. This is suggestive of Geoffrey's relatively broad relationship with both Arabic and Syriac influences, a reflection of the insular reception of new forms of astrological and astronomical scientific knowledge circulating during the first half of the twelfth century.

Place, 1–2. Also see Taylor, *The Political Prophecy in England*, who first coined the term. For more on the source relationship between the *Historia* and the *Historia Brittonum*, see Flood, *Prophecy, Politics and Place*, 35; Knight, *Merlin*, 23–26; Jankulak, *Geoffrey of Monmouth*, 14. For more on the *Omen* and its relationship to Welsh prophecies, see Flood, "Arthur's Return from Avalon"; Faletra, "The Conquest of the Past"; Jarman, "The Merlin Legend."

4 Geoffrey, *History of the Kings of Britain*, 144. Hereafter *HRB*.

5 See Symons, "*Wreoþenhilt ond wyrmfah*," 76.

6 Ptolemy's *Almagest*, drawing on the lost star catalogue of Hipparchus, contains the *Draco* constellation, as does the Arabic revision of his work by Abd al-Rahman al-Sufi, titled *The Book of Fixed Stars* (ca. 964). This latter work was translated into Latin in 1175 by Gerard of Cremona, four decades later than Geoffrey's *Historia*, making it an improbable analogue for Geoffrey's prophetic dragon. On the other hand, Ptolemy's *Tetrabiblos*, a text on the philosophy and practice of astrology, was indeed translated into Latin contemporary to Geoffrey's writing, by Plato of Tivoli in 1138. However, despite containing the *Draco* constellation, and although written in/ around the same year as Geoffrey's *Historia*, the Latin translation was made in Barcelona, removed from Geoffrey in Oxford, suggesting Ptolemy an unlikely influence for Geoffrey's astrological motif. The Aratean manuscripts, drawn on by Lambert of St. Omer in his *Liber Floridus* (ca. 1112–1121), as well as Virgil's *Georgics*, are more likely to have influenced the *Historia*'s final prophetic dragon (not discussed in this paper but considered at length in Chapter 2 of my doctoral thesis). For more, see Mouzam, "Arabic Astronomy and Christian-Muslim Contact."

7 Bryan, "Astronomy Translated."

Astronomy and Astrology in the Middle Ages

Throughout the Middle Ages, there was some overlap between astronomy and astrology. Both were often used interchangeably, in contrast to the modern perception of astronomy and astrology as two distinct and separate fields of study.[8] Richard Lemay describes how, while in "the mind of medieval Arab writers there is but one science of the sky with the moving bodies set in it," the subject of the heavens comprised of two individual treatments: "a purely mathematical one" (astronomy) and "a humanistic but rather conjectural one" (astrology), with the latter discipline the more "dominating interest of medieval Arabic civilisation."[9] Despite the growing medieval interest in reading the stars, some writers did possess anxieties around astrology's deterministic applications. Both Isidore and Augustine argued against those who believed that the stars (not only God's will) controlled human souls, with Augustine using the example of twins to reason that two people begotten in the same moment can possess different fates.[10] Although these authorities were enough to render the discipline of astrology questionable, the "philosophical and scientific grounding of astrology" by Arabic astrologers such as Abu Ma'shar, made the subject of astrology more respectable in the intellectual culture of the Muslim world and Christian Europe during the Middle Ages.[11] It was in the twelfth century that a true revival of Greek and Arabic astronomical and astrological knowledge occurred in the Latinate West.

Twelfth-century centres of learning, such as Chartres and the Toledo School of Learning, formed a network of notable Latinate–Arabic translators who produced scholarship on the quadrivium subjects (of which astronomy was a part). Scholars from Chartres who produced substantial astronomical materials included Hermann of Carinthia (ca. 1100), whose Latin translations of Greek knowledge and Arabic manuscripts were considered very significant in the development of astronomy in medieval Europe, and William of Conches (ca. 1090), who produced not only the first Western text which named Constantine the African (d. 1098/9) as an authority (the *Philosophia*), but later revised and expanded this treatise into his major cosmological work, the *Dragmaticon*.[12] Written in Normandy between 1144 to 1149, the writing implemented and adopted Arabic astronomical and astrological ideas from the *Liber de orbe*, a piece ascribed to medieval astronomer, astrologer, and mathematician, Māshā'allāh (ca. 740), who led the study of the stars in Abbasid Baghdad.[13] Meanwhile, active in Toledo was Gerard of Cremona (ca. 1114), whose 1175 Latinate–Arabic translation of Ptolemy's major astronomical

---

8 Lyons, *House of Wisdom*, 67; Carey, "Astrology in the Middle Ages," 889.

9 Lemay, "Astrology in Islam," 267. Also see Carey, "Astrology in the Middle Ages," 888–89.

10 Augustine, *City of God*, bk. 5.134–35; 138–39. Also see Kieckhefer, *Magic in the Middle Ages*, 127; Isidore, *Etymologies*, 99. Also see Carey, *Courting Disaster*, 28.

11 Kieckhefer, *Magic in the Middle Ages*, 130. Also see Burnett, "Adelard, Ergaphalau," 137–38.

12 Dolan, *Astronomical Transmission*, 197; Hill, *Dictionary of Theologians*, 560. For more on William of Conches, see Cadden, "Science and Rhetoric."

13 Grant, *History of Natural Philosophy*, 125; Obrist, "William of Conches, Māshā'allāh"; Samsó, "Masha'Allah."

work, the *Almagest* became "the principal channel for the recovery of the *Almagest* in the West," his presence and translation attracting other international scholars, copyists, and translators to Spain.[14]

The interest in astronomy and astrology and the transmission of Latinate–Arabic material also reached England in the twelfth century, influencing late twelfth-century English medieval translators such as Roger of Hereford, a medieval astronomer, astrologer, alchemist, and mathematician active in 1178, and Robert Grosseteste (ca. 1168), who used Graeco-Arabic astronomical knowledge to challenge traditional computistical doctrines.[15] Also widely recognized by critics are thirteenth-century English translators like Roger Bacon (ca. 1219/20), a medieval scientist, philosopher, and religious commentator, who wrote lengthily on astronomy and astrology in three key works: "the *Opus maius*, the *Communia mathematica*, and the *Communia naturalium*."[16] Geoffrey's *Historia*, however, was produced much earlier than these later translations and developments in astronomy and astrology in England, with his writing of the *Prophetiae Merlini* beginning in the 1120s, decades before England experienced a greater influx of astronomical material and a growing engagement with Arabic learning. The Latinate–Arabic astronomical ideas within his *Historia* thus stem from an earlier English interest in astronomy which occurred during the first half of the twelfth century, at a time when very few scholars in England were learned in Arabic or interested in transmitted scientific ideas from Muslim Spain. One notable figure from this earlier twelfth-century movement was Adelard of Bath (ca. 1080), a natural philosopher whose significant Latinate–Arabic translations included: Euclid's *Elements*; the *Centiloquium*, an astrological work by Abu Ma'shar and attributed to Ptolemy; Thābit ibn Qurra's *Liber Praestigiorum*, a treatise on talismanic magic; and the astronomical tables of al-Khwārizmī (ca. 750), the father of algebra and an astronomer, geographer, and mathematician from Baghdad's House of Wisdom.[17] Adelard and his works operate as part of a primary network of translators and translations actively writing on Latinate-Arabic ideas in England between 1100 and 1150, contemporary with the period of Geoffrey's work.

"Caput draconis": Geoffrey's Dragon Star and the Influence of Latinate–Arabic Astronomy

In the early 1120s, a new interest in the figure of the dragon appears in English intellectual culture, as a point of astronomical allusion. We find it, as Bryan has noted, in an astronomical treatise from the Severn Valley attributed to Walcher of Malvern, pupil of Petrus Alfonsi.[18] Described by John V. Tolan as an "intellectual emissary between two worlds,"

14 Ptolemy, *Almagest*, 3.

15 Grosseteste, *Compotus*. Also see Haskins, *Renaissance of the Twelfth Century*.

16 Hackett, "Roger Bacon on Astronomy-Astrology." Also see Hackett, "Adelard of Bath and Roger Bacon."

17 Adelard of Bath, *Conversations with his Nephew*, xi.

18 Walcher, *De Dracone*. Lyons, *House of Wisdom*, 125. For more on Lotharingia, see Welborn, "Lotharingia as a Center."

Alfonsi, a converted Jew who studied Arabic science in al-Andalus, was a notable astronomer who has been connected by historians to the English royal court, and has even been understood to have served as a physician to King Henry I.[19] Both Walcher and Alfonsi were greatly influenced by the learning of Muslim Spain, as well as by intellectual movements in Lotharingia which, in the tenth and eleventh century, served as a prominent hub for new scientific ideas that trickled into Christian Europe through contact with the Muslim-dominated Iberian Peninsula.[20] Lotharingia (particularly Liège, which, from the tenth century onwards, "became one of the most important intellectual centres of Europe") was an important site for the reading, translation, and dissemination of Arabic scientific texts, the type of work which Walcher eventually also carried out in the Severn Valley.[21] After leaving Lotharingia and arriving in England in the late eleventh century, Walcher was appointed as prior of Great Malvern Priory, Worcestershire. Walcher was greatly known for his observational use of the astrolabe, an astronomical device developed by Muslim astronomers during the Islamic Golden Age (ca. 700–ca. 1300), which he used to measure the time of both solar and lunar eclipses.[22] Based on his use of the astrolabe, Walcher then wrote a text on eclipse computation. Titled *De Dracone* (On the Dragon), the Latin astronomical treatise was written in around 1120 and draws on Arabic astronomical knowledge from Muslim Spain that Walcher's master Petrus had imparted to him. It is found in Oxford, Bodleian Library, MS Auct. F. 1. 9 alongside other arithmetical, astronomical, and calendrical works.[23] The transfer of knowledge from Petrus to Walcher leads Dorothee Metlitzki to conclude that "Walcher was the first native student of Arabic learning in England."[24] It is in this context that we first sight accounts of a dragon in the sky contemporary with Geoffrey, with a clear debt to Latinate–Arabic astronomical ideas. Philipp E. Nothaft, in his attentive study of Walcher's translations, notes that at the core of *De Dracone*, "was the insight that predicting the time of an eclipse crucially depended not only on the respective ecliptical longitude of the Sun and Moon, but also on that of the Moon's orbital nodes, known to Arabic astronomers as the head and tail of the Dragon."[25] Walcher's reference to the dragon appears as follows:

> [1.1] Among the seven planets that go around the zodiac, the Dragon roams as well, but with a contrary motion, because whereas the path of all the planets is

---

19 Walcher, *De Dracone*, 15. Also see Tolan, *Petrus Alfonsi*.

20 Walcher, *De Dracone*, 15. Also see Lyons, *House of Wisdom*, 36.

21 Welborn, "Lotharingia as a Center," 190.

22 Bryan, "Astronomy Translated," 143. For more on science in the Islamic Golden Age, see Al-Khalili, *Pathfinders*; Renima, Tiliouine and Estes, "The Islamic Golden Age"; Falagas, Zarkadoulia, and Samonis, "Arab Science." For more on the astrolabe in medieval England and Europe, see Burnett, *The Introduction of Arabic Learning*; Darby, "A Note on an Early Treatise"; *Astrolabes in Medieval Culture*; Borrelli, *Aspects of the astrolabe*; North, "The Astrolabe."

23 Walcher, *De Dracone*, 3; Lawrence-Mathers, "John of Worcester," 270.

24 Metlitzki, *The Matter of Araby*, 26.

25 Walcher, *De Dracone*, 3. For the Latin text of the *De Dracone*, see Vallicrosa, "La aportación astronómica."

> carried from Aries to Taurus, from Taurus to Gemini, and so on, only the Dragon is held to go from Aries to Pisces to Aquarius, and so on. It is, moreover, of such size that in whatever sign or degree its head is found, its tail always occupies the sign or degree opposite to it. An understanding of its circuit, however, is so essential to foreknowing an eclipse of the Sun or the Moon that without it there is no way of predicting it. For a solar eclipse never happens unless the Sun and the Moon meet with head or tail of this Dragon in one degree of a given sign, nor is there a lunar eclipse unless the Sun is in its head and the Moon in the tail opposite it-or the Sun in the tail and the Moon in its head.[26]

For Walcher the head and tail of the dragon refers to the "technical parameters" (to use Nothaft's phrase) of an eclipse, which Walcher describes in terms of the head of the dragon in the moon and the tail in the sun, or vice versa. This is caused by the movement of the *Draco* constellation, by the charting of which one might predict the time of an eclipse. Writers after Walcher were clearly fascinated by this but struggled to comprehend this borrowed concept. For example, John of Worcester (d. 1140), attempted to use "caput draconis" to describe an eclipse in his 1133 chronicle entry, as an omen preceding the death of Henry I:

> At length on the aforesaid day at midday the king went down to the sea to cross over, surrounded, as is usual with kings, by bands of knights. Suddenly a cloud appeared in the sky, which was visible throughout England, though of varying size. In some places indeed the day only appeared darkened, but in others it was so dark that men needed the guidance of candlelight to do anything. The king and his followers and many others walked about, marvelling greatly, raised their eyes to heaven, and saw the sun shining as though it were a new moon, though it did not keep the same appearance for long. One moment it was broader, the next it was narrower, now curved, now straight, now steady as usual, now moving, and seemed quivering and liquid like quicksilver. Some claim that an eclipse of the sun had taken place. If this was the case, then the sun was in the head of *Draco* and the moon in the tail or the sun was in the tail and the moon in the head of the fifth sign, Leo, in the seventeenth degree of that sign. The moon was twenty-seven days old. At the same day and hour, many stars appeared.[27]

As Charles Burnett observes, "John in using his source here confused the conditions necessary for a solar eclipse with those for a lunar eclipse."[28] He was not the only author to apply this concept to a historical account of regnal change. The term "caput draconis" appears in Geoffrey's *Historia*, applied not to an eclipse but to other astral events portending the death of a British king, including a comet. (Geoffrey presumably drew on the established relationship between comets and the deaths of rulers, a trope which goes

26 Walcher, *De Dracone*, 195.

27 John, *Chronicle*, 209–11; 210n2, which states that this 1133 entry is drawing on *De Dracone*.

28 John, *Chronicle*, 210n2.

back to the classical world, with direct application in the eleventh- and twelfth-century texts).[29] I refer to the "dragon star," a fiery symbol which appears in the sky in *Historia* Book 8, which Merlin interprets as signalling the sudden death of King Aurelius and heralding his brother Uther as his immediate successor and the next king of Britain:

> Haec dum Guintoniae gererentur, apparuit stella mirae magnitudinis et claritatis uno radio contenta. Ad radium uero erat globus igneus in similitudinem draconis extensus, et ex ore eius procedebant duo radii, quorum unus longitudinem suam ultra Gallicana climata uidebatur extendere, alter uero, uersus Hibernicum mare uergens, in septem minores radios terminabatur.
>
> (While this was happening at Winchester, there appeared a comet of great size and brightness, with a single tail. Attached to the tail was a fiery mass stretching out like a dragon, from whose mouth issued two rays, one of which seemed to extend beyond the skies of France, the other towards the Irish sea and to end in seven smaller rays.)[30]

As Bryan notes, the term "caput draconis" only appears after the episode of the dragon star, in the context of Uther's coronation—but the usage is nonetheless telling. Geoffrey writes:

> At Vther frater eius, conuocato regni clero et populo, cepit diadema insulae annuentibusque cunctis submilatus est in regem. Reminiscens autem expositionis quam Merlinus de supradicto sidere fecerat, iussit fabricari duos dracones ex auro ad similitudinem draconis quem ad radium stellae inspexerat. Qui ut mira arte fabricati fuerunt, optulit, unum in ecclesia primae sedis Guintoniae, alterum uero sibi ad ferendum in proelia retinuit. Ab illo itaque tempore uocatus fuit Vther Pendragon, quod Britannica lingua caput draconis sonamus. Iccirco hanc appellationem receperat quia Merlinus eum per draconem in regem prophetauerat.
>
> (His brother Uther summoned the clergy and people of the kingdom and took the crown, becoming king of the island with the consent of all. Remembering Merlin's interpretation of the comet, he ordered that two dragons be cast in gold, to resemble the dragon he had seen in the comet's tail. After these had been fashioned with great skill, he presented one to the cathedral in Winchester, and kept the other to take into battle. From that time he was known as Uther Pendragon, which means 'dragon's head' in British. He had received the name because Merlin had used the dragon to prophesy his succession as king.)[31]

---

29 Isidore, *Etymologies*, 105; 244. We might similarly think of the comet of 1066, mentioned by several of Geoffrey's contemporaries, including John of Worcester, as well as, of course, the Bayeux Tapestry. See John, *Chronicle*, 599–601.

30 *HRB*, 178–79.

31 *HRB*, 180–81.

Geoffrey presents "caput draconis" as a Latin calque of a Welsh or Breton phrase from which Uther takes as his title, and he does not identify its astronomical or astrological significance, but he is undeniably making use of scientific terminology. It is difficult to ascertain whether Geoffrey fully understood the science behind the astronomical term, and he omits any direct discussion of the lunar nodes (for which there was limited interest in England during the early twelfth century outside of Petrus and Walcher's work), and indeed, like John, Geoffrey may have misunderstood the precise scientific point of reference intended by Walcher—yet this is not his primary concern, for his use is more obviously literary.[32]

An Ecliptic Dragon in the *Prophetiae Merlini*

Geoffrey's astronomical analogues are not necessarily limited to those in common with Walcher. Alongside his engagement with "caput draconis" in the episode of Uther's dragon star, there is another aerial dragon in the *Historia* with a connection to the ecliptic dragon from *De Dracone*. This is found in the astrological chaos that concludes Geoffrey's *Prophetiae*. The *Prophetiae* end with apocalyptic commotion:

> Ab eis uultus auertent sydera et solitum cursum confundent. Arebunt segetes his indignantibus, et humor conuexi negabitur. Radices et rami uices mutabunt, nouitasque rei erit in miraculum. Splendor solis electro Mercurii languebit, et erit horror inspicientibus. Mutabit clipeum Stilbon Archadiae, uocabit Venerem galea Martis. Galea Martis umbram conficiet, transibit terminos furor Mercurii. Nudabit ensem Orion ferreus, uexabit nubes Phoebus aequoreus. Exibit Iupiter licitas semitas, et Venus deseret statutas lineas. Saturni sideris liuido corruet et falce recurua mortales perimet. Bissenus numerus domorum siderum deflebit hospites ita transcurrere. Obmittent Gemini complexus solitos et Vrnam in fontes prouocabunt. Pensa Librae oblique pendebunt donec Aries recurua cornua sua sopponat. Cauda Scorpionis procreabit fulgura, et Cancer cum sole litigabit. Ascendet Virgo dorsum Sagittarii et flores uirgineos obfuscabit. Currus lunae turbabit zodiacum, et in fletum prorumpent Pleiades. Officia Iani nulla redibunt, sed clausa ianua in crepidinibus Adriannae delitebit. In ictu radii exurgent aequora, et puluis ueterum renouabitur. Confligent uenti diro sufflamine et sonitum inter sidera conficient.
>
> (The planets will look away from men and alter their customary paths. Because of their wrath crops will wither and rain not fall from the sky. Roots will change place with branches, and people will marvel at the strange sight. The brightness of the sun will be outshone by Mercury's amber, to the horror of the observers. Arcadian Stilbon will change his shield, and Mars' helmet will summon Venus. Mars' helmet will cast a shadow, and Mercury's rage will know no bounds.

32 Bryan, "Astronomy Translated," 141. Bryan understands, similarly, Geoffrey's use of "caput draconis" as a "poeticised" astronomical allusion.

> Steely Orion will unsheathe his sword, and a watery sun will trouble the clouds. Jupiter will turn from his permitted course, and Venus abandon her established paths. The spite of Saturn's star will rain down and slaughter mortals with a curved scythe. The twelvefold band that is home to the stars will weep to see its travellers run amok in this way. The Twins will forgo their usual embraces and call Aquarius to the spring. The scales of Libra will hang awry until Aries supports them with his curved horns. Lightning bolts will flash from Scorpio's tail and Cancer will quarrel with the sun. Virgo will mount on Sagittarius's back and defile her virginal flowers. The moon's chariot will disrupt the zodiac and the Pleiades burst into tears. Janus will not perform his duties, but will close his door and hide in the precinct of Ariadne. In the flash of its beam, the seas will rise and the dust of the long-dead will be reborn. The winds will contend with a terrible blast and the stars will hear them howl.)[33]

Geoffrey combines apocalyptic chaos and destruction with the planetary and zodiac bodies. Though there are some studies that have stated or alluded to Geoffrey's use of astrology in this passage, most references to the topic have been brief.[34] Indeed, as Mark Williams notes of medieval apocalypticism more generally, when it comes to "assigning meaning to celestial events, apocalypticism and astrology are incompatible [...] the rise of medieval astrology is thus also, at least partially, the story of the decline of apocalypticism."[35] However, in the case of the *Prophetiae* the two are interwoven, and Geoffrey's engagement with astrology is here explicitly apocalyptic.[36]

Amidst his astrological apocalypse, Geoffrey places a (textually) hidden dragon. Although there is no explicit allusion to *Draco* anywhere within the passage, we do encounter the Pleiades, a constellation brought into conjunction with *Draco* in Syriac accounts of the astrology and astronomy of eclipses of a type with those found in medieval Arabic sources. The Pleiades are a cluster of stars commonly associated with the seven sisters of Greek mythology, but in the context of Syriac material, transmitted into western Europe in the twelfth century, are associated with eclipses.[37] We find this in the *Liber Nemroth*, also referred to as the *Liber Nimrod*, a dialogue between Nemroth

---

33 *HRB*, 158–59.

34 See Bryan, "Astronomy Translated"; Carey, *Courting Disaster*; Williams, *Fiery Shapes*.

35 Williams, *Fiery Shapes*, xxii–xxiii.

36 It is worth noting here that "The Letter of Toledo," a letter of unknown origins sent to Pope Clement III and others prophesizing the end of the world, presents a combining of astrology and prophecy very similar to that which we find in Geoffrey, an interesting precedence that appears in 1184, at the end of the twelfth century, half a decade later than the *Historia*. This demonstrates how astrology and prophecy were more clearly understood as interlinked in the later twelfth century onwards, making Geoffrey in the early twelfth century a leading writer connecting these two distinctive fields together.

37 Livesey and Rouse, "Nimrod the Astronomer." For more on the history and mythologies surrounding the Pleiades, see Andrews, *The Seven Sisters*; Bouw, "The Bible and the Pleiades"; Laoupi, "The Greek Myth of Pleiades."

the astronomer and his disciple Ioanton.[38] The treatise is divided into three units, each discussing, in turn: the universe and the sphere of the fixed stars; the solar system (in particular the planets, the sun, and the moon); and finally computistical and miscellaneous topics.[39] As Nothaft notes, the core content of the *Liber Nemroth* "very likely originated from Syria-Palestine in late antiquity, before being refashioned into a Latin treatise, most likely in the early ninth century," although it has been dated as early as the eighth and as late as the end of the eleventh century.[40] The *Liber Nemroth* enjoyed some popularity from the first half of the twelfth century onwards, quoted by the Anglo-Norman poet, Philippe de Thaon (ca. 1113), theologian Hugh of St-Victor (ca. 1141), and also the twelfth-century Chartres scholar, William of Conches.[41] This text is particularly striking, and unusual, in its two accounts of the Pleiades instigating lunar eclipses: the "tail of the Pleiades," blocks the light of the (autoluminescent) moon, dampening its glow; and the Pleiades is connected to a dragon located between the sun and the moon, which blocks the path of sunlight from reaching the moon.[42] This is the "caput draconis" by another name. It is interesting that prior to his allusion to the Pleiades, Geoffrey appears to have had the scientific terminology of the eclipse, a phenomenon "caused by a celestial shadow" in mind: "Galea Martis umbram conficiet" (Mars' helmet will cast a shadow). This is potentially another scientific allusion, made literary—here, apocalyptic.[43] Indeed, this may offer a connection which lends a unity to the whole of the *Prophetiae*: the Pleiades are a textually hidden, astronomical dragon. This suggests that Geoffrey may be reading Syriac and Arabic allusions together, and although it is unlikely that he differentiated between the origins of the two, these astronomical and astrological allusions mark his clear interest in featuring stellar dragons in his work. Certainly, Arabic, and related Syriac and classical, astrological, and astronomical precedents present a possible interpretive framework through which we might make sense out of the final passage of the *Prophetiae*, a sequence which has been previously understood in Arthurian scholarship as especially obscure.[44]

38 John, *Chronicle*, 39.

39 John, *Chronicle*, 15; Livesey and Rouse, "Nimrod the Astronomer," 204.

40 Walcher, *De Dracone*, 39; Juste, "Date of the 'Liber Nemroth'," 255.

41 Juste, "Date of the 'Liber Nemroth'," 255; Livesey and Rouse, "Nimrod the Astronomer," 237–52. Also see Draelants, "'Depingo ut ostendam'," 56. For more on Philippe de Thaon, see Philippe, "*Bestiaire*." For more on Hugh of Saint-Victor, see Coolman, *The Theology of Hugh of St. Victor*. For more on Constantine the African, see *Constantine the African*; Cambra, "The Intermediary Role of the Arabs."

42 Walcher, *De Dracone*, 40–41.

43 *HRB*, 158–59; Westfall and Sheehan, *Celestial Shadows*, 1. For an analysis of the planets at the end of the *Prophetiae*, see Boutet, *Celtic Astrology*, 205. It is interesting to add here that in 1337, Mars is associated with an eclipse: "Eclipses were inherently dangerous but this one was also linked to two dangerous planets: according to Geoffrey [of Meaux], Mars signified lies, robberies, and violence, Saturn pointed to extortion, hatred, fear and death." See Campion, *A History of Western Astrology*, 77.

44 Geoffrey, *History of the Kings of Britain*, ed. Faletra, 24-25. Also see Curley, "Animal Symbolism."

Conclusion

Geoffrey of Monmouth's *Historia* was not the only significant literary work produced in medieval England to incorporate astrological influences. Astrological allusions underlie Geoffrey Chaucer's *Knight's Tale*, which, like his *Treatise on the Astrolabe*, has been positioned by Shazia Jagot in relation to the dissemination of Arabic scientific ideas in medieval England.[45] A significantly earlier example than these, the *Historia* is an important case study into the ways in which astrological and astronomical material was translated and understood from Arabic into Latin in the first half of the twelfth century, a line of transmission often overlooked in relation to the development of the Arthurian tradition.

This chapter's discussion of the relationship between Geoffrey's dragons and medieval astronomy reveals not just the presence of astral knowledge in Geoffrey's *Historia*, but also the impact of Arabic textual transmission on literature produced in medieval Britain beyond the purely scientific. Arabic influences appear to have informed aspects of Geoffrey's literary practice, as he reimagined the ecliptic dragon as a signifier of the legendary insular past. As I argue in my work elsewhere, the astrological and astronomical qualities of the Arthurian dragon largely disappear after the twelfth century, but the point of origin is one which we cannot understand without an appreciation of Arabic influence.[46] Indeed, despite the dragon's lesser associations to the science of the stars after Geoffrey, it continues to enchant and astonish audiences both within and outside of the Arthurian world, enduring across pages and screens as perhaps the greatest of all magical creatures, with a long trans-cultural history.

---

45 For more on the influence of astronomy and astrology in Chaucer, see Jagot, "*Fin' amors*, Arabic Learning, and the Islamic World"; Jagot, "Chaucer and Ibn al-Haytham."

46 Mouzam, "The Crusading Galfridian Dragon."

Bibliography

Primary Sources

Adelard of Bath. *Adelard of Bath, Conversations with His Nephew: On the Same and the Different, Questions on Natural Science, and on Birds*. Edited and translated by Charles Burnett. Cambridge: Cambridge University Press, 1998.

Augustine, *City of God. Volume II. Books 4–7*. Translated by William M. Green. Loeb Classical Library 412. Cambridge, MA: Harvard University Press, 1963.

Constantine the African and 'Alī Ibn Al-'Abbās Al-Mağūsī: The Pantegni and Related Texts. Edited by Charles Burnett and Danielle Jacquart. Leiden: Brill, 1994.

Geoffrey of Monmouth. *The History of the Kings of Britain*. Edited and translated by Michael A. Faletra. Peterborough: Broadview, 2008.

——. *The History of the Kings of Britain*. Edited by Michael D. Reeve. Translated by Neil Wright. Woodbridge: Boydell, 2007.

Grosseteste, Robert. *Compotus*. Edited and translated by Alfred Lohr and C. Philipp E. Nothaft. Oxford: Oxford University Press, 2019.

Isidore of Seville. *The Etymologies of Isidore of Seville*. Edited and translated by Stephen A. Barney, W. J. Lewis, J. A. Beach, and Oliver Berghof. Cambridge: Cambridge University Press, 2006.

John of Worcester. *The Chronicle of John of Worcester*. Vol. 2, *The Annals from 450 to 1066*. Edited by R. R. Darlington and P. McGurk. Translated by Jennifer Bray and P. McGurk. Oxford: Clarendon, 1995.

Philippe de Thaon. "*Bestiaire*." Edited by Ian Short. *French Studies* 74 (2020): 275–339.

Ptolemy. *Ptolemy's Almagest*. Translated by G. J. Toomer. Princeton: Princeton University Press, 1998.

Walcher of Malvern. *Walcher of Malvern De Lunationibus and De Dracone: Study, Edition, Translation, and Commentary*. Edited by C. Philipp E. Nothaft. Turnhout: Brepols, 2017.

Weiss, Judith. *Wace's Roman de Brut. A History of the British: Text and Translation*. Exeter: University of Exeter Press, 2002.

Secondary Sources

Al-Khalili, Jim. *Pathfinders: The Golden Age of Arabic Science*. London: Allen Lane, 2012.

Andrews, Munya. *The Seven Sisters of the Pleaides: Stories from around the World*. Melbourne: Spinifex, 2004.

Astrolabes in Medieval Culture. Edited by Josefina Rodríguez-Arribas et al. Leiden: Brill, 2019.

Borrelli, Arianna. *Aspects of the Astrolabe: "Architectonica ratio" in Tenth- and Eleventh-Century Europe*. Stuttgart: Steiner, 2008.

Boutet, M. G. *Celtic Astrology from the Druids to the Middle Ages*. Jefferson: McFarland, 2017.

Bouw, Gerardus D. "The Bible and the Pleiades." *Biblical Astronomer* 87 (1999): 4–18.

Bryan, Elizabeth J. "Astronomy Translated: *Caput Draconis* and the Pendragon Star in Geoffrey of Monmouth, Wace, and La3amon." *Arthuriana* 26 (2016): 141–63.

Burnett, Charles. "Adelard, Ergaphalau and the Science of the Stars." In *Adelard of Bath: An English Scientist and Arabist of the Early Twelfth Century*, edited by Charles Burnett, 133–45. London: Warburg Institute, 1987.

——. *The Introduction of Arabic Learning into England*. London: British Library, 1997.

Cadden, Joan. "Science and Rhetoric in the Middle Ages: The Natural Philosophy of William of Conches." *Journal of the History of Ideas* 56 (1995): 1–24.

Cambra, Luisa María Arvide. "The Intermediary Role of the Arabs During the Middle Ages in the Transmission of Ancient Scientific Knowledge to Europe." *International Journal of Innovative Science, Engineering & Technology* 3 (2016): 422–26.

Campion, Nicholas. *A History of Western Astrology*. Vol. 2, *The Medieval and Modern Worlds*. London: Continuum, 2009.

Carey, Hilary M. "Astrology in the Middle Ages." *History Compass* 8 (2010): 888–902.

——. *Courting Disaster: Astrology at the English Court and University in the Later Middle Ages*. New York: Palgrave Macmillan, 1992.

Coolman, Boyd Taylor. *The Theology of Hugh of St. Victor: An Interpretation*. Cambridge: Cambridge University Press, 2010.

Curley, Michael J. "Animal Symbolism in the *Prophecies of Merlin*." In *Beasts and Birds of the Middle Ages: The Bestiary and its Legacy*, edited by Willene B. Clark and Meredith T. McMunn, 151–63. Philapelphia: University of Pennsylvania Press, 1989.

Darby, H. C. "A Note on an Early Treatise on the Astrolabe." *The Geographical Journal* 85 (1935): 179–81.

Dolan, Marion. *Astronomical Transmission through Illustrated Aratea Manuscripts*. Cham: Springer, 2017.

Draelants, Isabelle. "'Depingo ut ostendam, depictum ita est expositio': Diagrams as an Indispensable Complement to the Cosmological Teaching of the *Liber Nemroth de astronomia*." In *Inscribing Knowledge in the Medieval Book*, edited by Anne D. Hedeman et al., 56–92. Berlin: De Gruyter, 2019.

Falagas, Matthew E., et al. "Arab Science in the Golden Age (750–1258 C.E.) and Today." *The Faseb Journal* 20 (2006): 1581–86.

Faletra, Michael A. "The Conquest of the Past in *The History of the Kings of Britain*." *Literature Compass* 4 (2006): 121–33.

Flood, Victoria. "Arthur's Return from Avalon: Geoffrey of Monmouth and the Development of the Legend." *Arthuriana* 25 (2015): 84–110.

——. *Prophecy, Politics and Place in Medieval England: From Geoffrey of Monmouth to Thomas of Erceldoune*. Cambridge: Brewer, 2016.

Fulton, Helen. "Arthur and Merlin in Early Welsh Literature: Fantasy and Magic Naturalism." In *A Companion to Arthurian Literature*, edited by Helen Fulton, 84–101. Oxford: Wiley-Blackwell, 2012.

Grant, Edward. *A History of Natural Philosophy: From the Ancient World to the Nineteenth Century*. Cambridge: Cambridge University Press, 2007.

Hackett, Jeremiah. "Adelard of Bath and Roger Bacon: Early English Natural Philosophers and Scientists." *Endeavour* 26 (2002): 70–74.

——. "Roger Bacon on Astronomy-Astrology: The Sources of the *Scientia Experimentalis*." In *Roger Bacon and the Sciences*, edited by Jeremiah Hackett, 175–98. Leiden: Brill, 1997.

Haskins, Charles Homer. *The Renaissance of the Twelfth Century*. Cambridge, MA: Harvard University Press, 1955.

Hill, Jonathan. *Dictionary of Theologians to 1308*. Cambridge: Clark, 2010.

Jagot, Shazia. "Chaucer and Ibn al-Haytham (Alhacen): *Perspectiva*, Arabic Mathematics, and Acts of Looking." *Studies in the Age of Chaucer* 44 (2022): 27–61.

——. "*Fin' amors*, Arabic Learning, and the Islamic World in the Work of Geoffrey Chaucer." PhD diss., University of Leicester, 2013.

Jankulak, Karen. *Geoffrey of Monmouth*. Cardiff: University of Wales Press, 2010.

Jarman, A. O. H. *The Legend of Merlin*. Cardiff: University of Wales Press, 1960.

——. "The Merlin Legend and the Welsh Tradition of Prophecy." In *The Arthur of the Welsh: The Arthurian Legend in Medieval Welsh Literature*, edited by Rachel Bromwich, A. O. H. Jarman and Brynley F. Roberts, 117–45. Cardiff: University of Wales Press, 1991.

Juste, David. "On the Date of the 'Liber Nemroth'." *Journal of the Warburg and Courtauld Institutes* 67 (2004): 255–58.

Kieckhefer, Richard. *Magic in the Middle Ages*. Cambridge: Cambridge University Press, 2014.

Knight, Stephen. *Merlin: Knowledge and Power through the Ages*. Ithaca: Cornell University Press, 2009.

Laoupi, Amanda. "The Greek Myth of Pleiades in The Archaeology of Natural Disasters: Decoding, Dating and Environmental Interpretation." *Mediterranean Archaeology and Archaeometry* 6 (2006): 5–22.

Lawrence-Mathers, Anne. "John of Worcester and the Science of History." *Journal of Medieval History* 39 (2013): 255–74.

——. *The True History of Merlin the Magician*. New Haven: Yale University Press, 2012.

Lemay, Richard. "Astrology in Islam." In *Encyclopaedia of the History of Science, Technology, and Medicine in Non-Western Cultures*, edited by Helaine Selin, 267–69. Dordrecht: Springer, 2008.

Livesey, Steven J. and Richard H. Rouse. "Nimrod the Astronomer." *Traditio* 37 (1981): 203–66.

Lyons, Jonathan. *The House of Wisdom: How the Arabs Transformed Western Civilization*. London: Bloomsbury, 2009.

Metlitzki, Dorothee. *The Matter of Araby in Medieval England.* New Haven: Yale University Press, 1977.

Mouzam, Humma. "Arabic Astronomy and Christian-Muslim Contact: Geoffrey of Monmouth's Prophetic Dragon and its Reception in Medieval Arthurian Literature." PhD diss., University of Birmingham, forthcoming (2024). Especially "Chapter 4. The Post-Galfridian Crusading Dragon: Geoffrey's Middle English Reception."

North, J. D. "The Astrolabe." *Scientific American* 230 (1974): 96–107.

Obrist, Barbara. "William of Conches, Māshā'allāh, and Twelfth-Century Cosmology." *Archives d'histoire doctrinale et littéraire du Moyen Age* 76 (2009): 29–81.

Padel, O. J. "Geoffrey of Monmouth and the Development of the Merlin Legend." *Cambrian Medieval Celtic Studies* 51 (2006): 37–65.

Renima, Ahmed, et al. "The Islamic Golden Age: A Story of the Triumph of the Islamic Civilization." In *The State of Social Progress of Islamic Societies: Social, Economic, Political and Ideological Challenges*, edited by Habib Tiliouine and Richard J. Estes, 25–52. Cham: Springer, 2016.

Samsó, Julio. "Masha'Allah." In *Medieval Science, Technology, and Medicine: An Encyclopedia*, edited by Thomas Glick, Steven J. Livesey, and Faith Wallis, 331–33. New York: Routledge, 2005.

Symons, Victoria. "*Wreoþenhilt ond wyrmfah*: Confronting Serpents in *Beowulf* and Beyond." In *Representing Beasts in Early Medieval England and Scandinavia*, edited by Michael D. J. Bintley and Thomas J. T. Williams, 73–93. Woodbridge: Boydell, 2015.

Taylor, Rupert. *The Political Prophecy in England*. New York: Columbia University Press, 1911.

Tolan, John Victor. *Petrus Alfonsi and his Medieval Readers*. Gainesville: University Press of Florida, 1993.

Vallicrosa, José María Millás. "La aportación astronómica de Pedro Alfonso." *Sefarad* 3 (1943): Appendix I: 89–97.

Welborn, Mary Catherine. "Lotharingia as a Center of Arabic and Scientific Influence in the Eleventh Century." *Isis* 16 (1931): 188–99.

Westfall John and William Sheehan. *Celestial Shadows: Eclipses, Transits and Occultations*. New York: Springer, 2015.

Williams, Mark. *Fiery Shapes: Celestial Portents and Astrology in Ireland and Wales, 700–1700*. Oxford: Oxford University Press, 2010.

NATURAL AND NON-NATURAL

WEATHER, SEASONS, AND PLACE IN THE MEDICINE OF CONSTANTINE OF AFRICA

ANNE JEAVONS

THE SEASONS, WINDS, rain, and where a person lives, are now rarely considered key topics that should be covered in textbooks of medicine, yet influential medical manuals of the eleventh century regarded these as important considerations for a physician advising and treating his patients. Exploring these helps to provide an insight into an important stage in the development of medieval ideas about how the natural world worked, and how human health and disease were understood to be intimately tied up with the natural environment. It also raises the question as to why the environment was considered so important, and whether such a holistic approach proved beneficial in healthcare.

From the eleventh century, medical translations began arriving in the West from the Islamicate world, the work of a medical expert, translator, and monk, Constantine of Africa. His extensive work, a corpus of around thirty texts, was to start a medical revolution in the West. Some of the most important medical knowledge in the ancient world derived from the Hippocratic corpus of the fourth and fifth centuries BCE, and from the work of Galen in the second century CE, but most of this had been lost in the medieval West. Fortunately, they had been preserved and further developed in the Islamicate world; Constantine's translations of Arabic medical texts into Latin made them accessible, and they were widely circulated. In particular his translation of 'Alī ibn Al-'Abbās al-Maǧūsī's *Kitāb-al-Malikī* as the *Pantegni* (The Whole Art of Medicine) aimed to provide a comprehensive understanding of the human body and its treatment. Together with his widely read translation of Ḥunayn ibn Is'ḥāq al-'Ibādī's *Masā' il fī-tibb* as the *Isagoge* (Introduction to Galen's Art), this text set out the theoretical underpinnings of the new version of medicine.

One of the chief novelties of these texts was this emphasis on theory, on anatomy, physiology, and pathology, but also on understanding human beings and their health within the natural order, *medicina* now seen as part of "natural philosophy" or *physica*. There had always been both lay and clerical healers, although rarely recorded, some literate and some not, probably basing their practice on experience and treatments passed on orally. Literate doctors had some access to medical books, but these were essentially practical and remedy-based, with many lists of drugs or recipes for a condition. One

Anne Jeavons is a doctoral research student with the Graduate Centre for Medieval Studies, University of Reading, working on mental disorders and their treatment in the work of Constantine of Africa. Thanks are particularly due to Anne Lawrence-Mathers for her helpful comments on this chapter.

medical tradition from antiquity, the empiric school, had in fact avoided questions of understanding the human body and the causes of disease, as irrelevant in treatment. The new theory-based medicine, however, was extremely complex, and required a new breed of learned medical practitioners, often now called physicians. This stimulated a further proliferation of medical works and the development of more formal medical education.

It was now considered important for the educated physician to have an understanding of the seven categories of "natural" things. These were the elements (earth, water, air, and fire), the qualities (hot, cold, dry, and moist, and their various combinations), the four humours (blood, phlegm, red bile, black bile), the four principal organs (the brain, heart, liver, and the testicles). Then there were the powers (of growth, nutrition, and reproduction), the animal powers or faculties (sense, voluntary movement, imagination, reason, and memory) and the spirits (natural, vital, and spiritual) which served these functions. Then a distinction was made between these things that are "natural" and those which are "non-natural" (environmental and other factors impacting on health), and "contra natural" (disease, its causes, and symptoms).[1]

The *Pantegni* and the *Isagoge* introduced the idea of the non-naturals, and gave a great deal of detail about them. Arising from Galen's writing on the "six necessary things," these were external factors whose management is necessary to the preservation of health. Although these factors were not the "naturals," (basic components of nature or the body), they were not "unnatural" or outside nature, but they kept the naturals in their course, and could impact or change into them. The non-naturals were generally given as air, movement and rest, food and drink, sleep and waking, evacuation of the naturals, and the *accidentia anime* (the emotions). The watchword in all of these things was moderation—the patient should have moderate air, moderate exercise, baths of moderate temperature, moderate food, and neither too much sleep nor too little.[2]

The apparent importance of these external factors is exemplified in many pages on the "air," giving highly specified information regarding environmental factors, including the seasons, winds, and the qualities of different regions and terrains. Islamicate medicine had inherited Greek ideas from the Hippocratic text *Airs, Waters, Places*, and Galen's ideas that environmental air was important in the cause and prevention of disorder. The air was particularly important because it enters the body in breathing, and the *Pantegni* noted that the complexion of the body follows the complexion of the air. Physicians should therefore pay attention to the quality of air, which was potentially "a great medicine," or alternatively it could be "pestilential" associated with plagues and pandemics (Book 5, chap. 2).

According to the *Isagoge*:

> Changes of air come about in five different ways; from the seasons, from the rising and setting of the stars, from the winds, from the lands, and from the vapours that rise from them (144).

1 Constantine of Africa, "Isagoge," ed. and trans. Wallis, 140–56.

2 Constantine of Africa, "Pantegni Theorica," bk. 5, chap. 1.

It gave further detail on each of these, with the *Pantegni* devoting ten chapters to the subject. Firstly, the seasons were specified most importantly by their qualities: spring was hot and moist; summer, hot and dry; autumn, cold and dry; and winter, cold and moist. If the seasons went as expected, and people followed the dietary and health rules for the season all would be healthy, but if not, they could become ill or even *furiosi* (mad) (chap. 6). There were particular issues for each season: in winter phlegm increased, causing problems like epilepsy and apoplexy, or lung problems, whilst the summer generates bile, which changes in autumn to black bile, causing fevers, dropsy, and mania. There is a whole section devoted to the problems which arise when seasons did not go normally–if they were extreme or variable. A cold and dry spring could lead to miscarriages; an intemperate spring gave rise to fevers, apoplexy and epilepsy, mania, cough or consumption, and skin diseases (chap. 5). In unusually hot and moist conditions things decayed, generating terrible illnesses, impurities in the body grew putrid and broke out through the skin in pustules (chap. 3).

Clearly not everyone was affected equally by the seasons, and health problems were not just due to the season, or everyone would get the same illnesses. It was thought to depend partly on your complexion, the exact mixture of qualities or humours present in your body. If you were of a hot complexion, you were likely to become ill in hot seasons, but if of a cold complexion, in cold times of the year. Similarly, people's bodies had different qualities according to their stage of life and gender, and this interacted with the qualities of the season for good or ill. Summer was a healthy time for children and young people, summer and autumn best for the elderly, who were cold by nature, those in middle age were warm and dry, so did well in autumn and winter, which are cold and moist.

The air was also said to vary with the winds: the *Pantegni* explained that wind was a gas released from the earth, and its nature was determined by the place it came from. There were four parts of the world, and eight winds, two coming from each of the north, south, east, and west. The most important things to know about winds were their qualities: the northern winds were cold and dry, south winds hot and moist, whilst the east and west winds were moderate and unproblematic to health. The north wind "hardens the body, soothes the humours and cleans the spirits, heals the brain, and draws bad humours [...]" but on the other hand could cause coughs and pains in the chest. The south wind conversely "softens bodies and [...] disturbs the humours, senses, and spirit," as the brain is then filled with hot humours, leading to poor hearing, sluggishness, and even epilepsy (chap. 8).

Rain was considered a cause of problems, as "an excess of rain generates many humours in moist bodies—which quickly go off [...] The illnesses which come with much rain are long fevers, flux of the belly, infections, epilepsy, apoplexy, and quinsy [...] the brain is also filled with a great deal of humours." Dry times were healthier, although fevers could also arise if it was too dry. Heat and rain were the worst, associated with pustules and plague. In a hot summer following a wet winter and hot damp spring, women and children, by nature moist, might "expect death, due to great decay and boiling humours" (chap. 5). This seems very stark but infant and maternal mortality rates were, of course, very high at the best of times.

It was important for the physician to notice the area the patient was living in, as different regions affected the bodies, character, and culture of its inhabitants, and the kinds of illnesses they were prone to. The *Pantegni* explained that:

> It is [...] necessary for the doctor to think about the various regions when he goes into a city, that he considers the qualities and situation of a region and the nature of its water and food. From this he will be able to tell how to maintain the health of the healthy and cure the ills of the sick (chap. 10).

For example, northern cities were colder and dryer, places in the south hot and moist, the west moist and tending to be hot, and the east a little dry, and between hot and cold. There is a huge amount of detail about this, for example northern places had clear water and the healthiest air, and their inhabitants were high in the humour of bile. They had a good reddish colour, strong bodies, and were long lived, although prone to lung problems and infertility; childbirth was difficult, the women having dry bodies. In the east, the air and water were clear and soft, and the inhabitants had a moderate complexion, with a pink colour, healthy and strong bodies with few illnesses. They were "not proud or often angry [...] but humble and gentle" (chap. 9).

There is also a lot of information about altitude, terrain, and how a place was sited in relation to the position of any mountains or the sea. According to the *Isagoge*:

> There are four modalities of terrain; namely, height, depth, nearness to mountains or to the sea, and the level quality of places of terrain [...] Height produces cold and depth the contrary... If the mountains are to the south, the locality will be cold [...] If the sea is on the south the terrain will be hot and dry (145).

Those living at high altitudes enjoyed clear air from the north wind and clear water, and were likely to be large, strong, and healthy. Inhabitants of low-lying places had wet winters, but dry summers; their bodies were said to be small but broad with thick legs, with black hair, but weaker due to frequent illness. It was also apparently important for the physician to know that where there were mountains to the south, the air would be cold and dry due to the north wind, but the converse if they were to the north. If the sea was to the north the air would be cold and dry, but hot and moist if it was to the south (chap. 10). Even the nature of the ground itself was significant; stony terrain was cold and dry: thick and heavy terrain is hot and moist; clay was cold and moist (*Isagoge*, 145).

Finally changes in the air could arise due to the vapours that arose from the land, "exhalations from marshy terrain or other places where decay is going on" (*Isagoge*, 144–45). This sounds like a breeding ground for malaria, and the *Pantegni* further explained:

> If in any land there are uncultivated and uninhabited swamps, or there are ill smelling plants or trees, or underground caves, or any similar place where the natural air sits and changes, this quickly goes off. And from this the inhabitants of this place often get ill and develop fever from the fumes of this rottenness (chap. 10).

Sometimes air became so putrid as to be pestilential, this could arise if seasons "left their normal nature," where gases arose from decaying plants, ponds or ditches, from dead bodies or diseased animals. All those living in an area could then become ill with the same disease, which corrupted the humours of both men and animals. Constantine wrote that "whole populations died" and had "many terrible symptoms" such as loss of reason, pains, severe sweating, and vomiting of bile. Sometimes this pestilence fell in the middle of the period of sowing of seeds, resulting in poor crop growth and harvests; if eaten the crops also caused bad illnesses (chap. 11).

In giving this advice, Constantine was passing on Hippocrates's idea that bad air was the cause of disease, the product of contaminated water, and rotting organic matter, identifiable by a foul smell, which became known later as the miasma theory of disease. This idea persisted for centuries, people became concerned about night air and kept their windows shut, but it led to a concern with keeping cities clean, free of smells, and the importance of good sanitation. It did exclude ideas that illness could be spread by contamination from one person to another, and the miasma theory was eventually surpassed by germ theory. However, these not unhelpful Hippocratic ideas were to dominate European medieval and early modern models of medicine and public health.

The idea of pestilential air obviously had implications for preventative health, but otherwise, in all this detailed information regarding the effects of environment, seasons, and terrains, where are the treatment recommendations? This information is found, after all, in a medical text. The only advice in these chapters on the "air" is of the vaguest kind: that people should not neglect their health, should eat appropriately for the season, should purge the body of bad humours, and, by implication, should attempt to avoid bad air. Elsewhere in Constantine's writing, under particular ailments you may find dietary suggestions, but again not too much about the air. There is a little advice in the *Liber de melancholia*, that the physician should expose the melancholic patient to easterly winds and avoid the north wind, whilst those living in the north are advised to sit by flowing rivers in the summer.[3] No explanation is given for this, and nowhere is it made explicit why the physician needed to be aware of all these various environmental factors, presumably this was already understood by Constantine's readers.

On the face of it, this seems less helpful than standard seasonal advice which had been around for centuries. In the fourth century the learned Greek doctor Oribasius offered preventative recommendations, such as that in the winter people should eat more, especially when there is a north wind. In moist or cold air, they should take warm food and drink lots of wine. In the spring they should purge the body and let blood, in summer they should rest from work, and "all they do should be more cooling and moistening, than drying and warming."[4] Autumn being changeable, they should avoid the heat of midday, and not eat too much fruit.

In the eighth century, the Venerable Bede had recounted seasonal advice to prevent illness, quoting from the pseudo-Hippocratic text the *Letter to King Antigonus*, in his

3 Constantine of Africa, *Liber de Melancholia*, 143–44.

4 Oribasius, *Œuvres d'Oribase*: *Euporistes*, 415–17.

scientific work, *The Reckoning of Time*. From the winter solstice to the spring equinox, phlegm increased in a man's body so:

> At such a season, take high quality food, hot and seasoned with assafoetida, with pepper and mustard. Wash your head seldom. However, purge without ceasing. Indulge in wine and do not stint on sex.

This advice was presumably aimed at secular readers! From late March to early May blood increases, and food should be "fragrant and very pungent." Then until late June, red bile increases, people should "eat sweet foods, indulge in wine, abstain from sex, and fast very little." For the rest of the summer, as red bile decreased, black bile increased, and the diet should be sweet and cold. In the autumn phlegm increased, so one should "use all such foods as are hot and very pungent, abstain from sex, and wash very little."[5]

Bede and Oribasius both therefore gave simple directions to apply to everyone. Bede went further in giving more of a rationale for these, in terms of how the qualities of all things interacted:

> The very elements of the universe are distinguished by these divergent qualities [...]. Earth is dry and cold, water cold and wet, air wet and warm, fire warm and dry, and therefore the first is likened to autumn, the next to winter, the next to spring and the last to summer. And man himself, who is called "microcosm" by the wise, that is, "a smaller universe" has his body tempered in every respect by these same qualities; indeed, each of its constituent humours imitates the manner of the season in which it prevails. For blood which increases in the spring, is moist and warm; red bile which increases in the summer, in hot and dry; black bile which increases in the autumn is dry and cold; and phlegmatic humours, which increase in the winter, are cold and moist (100–101).

Bede just looked at the effects of the seasons on the humours, and the advice given was aimed at balancing out the qualities of the humours predominating in that season—although this was not stated directly. Similarly, Constantine's translations did not explain why they gave so much teaching about the environment, however we notice a constant theme of emphasizing the *qualities* of these environmental factors. What is new in these medical texts is that the qualities of *all* the environmental factors were taken into account, we presume in order to ascertain their effects on the body, or particular parts of the body.

Elsewhere the *Pantegni* gives the qualities and their mixtures in the human body and its various organs in detail. Most of the first book is devoted to human complexions, how they differed according to region of habitation, gender, age, and habits, how to tell the nature of the individual's general complexion, and the complexion of specific organs. The complexion of the brain for example could be determined by the shape of the head, by the hairs appearing out of it, from the eyes, and by behaviour. Someone with black or red curly hair was said to have a warm dry brain, as did someone who was quick and

---

5 Bede, *Reckoning of Time*, ed. and trans. Wallis, 87.

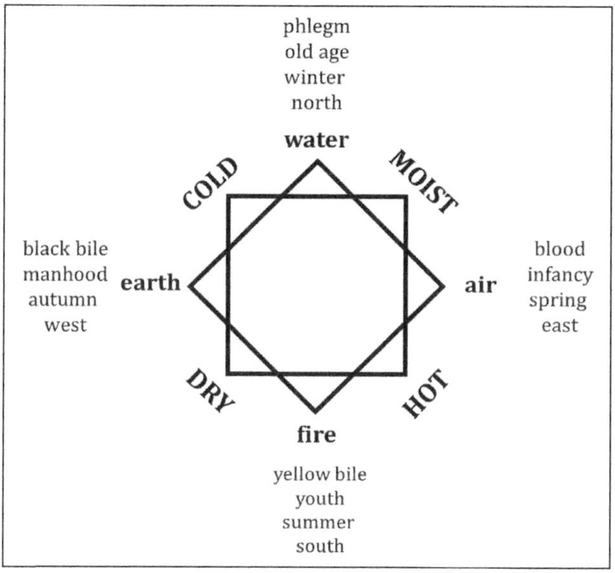

Figure 4.1: The Qualities and how they related to the Elements, Seasons, Life Stages, and Humours. Diagram by author.

alert, but boastful and unstable (Book 1, chap. 10). Whilst not in conflict with the basic ideas given by Bede, this was much more specific about the individual patient and what they might need for ideal health.

All of this provided the physician with a set of theoretical principles to enable him to work out the qualities of all the interacting factors. What was best for this particular patient with his complexion, age, and sex, according to the season, weather, and place he is living in? Then what illnesses was he vulnerable to, and what were the characteristics of the organ or organs at risk? As far as possible then, adjustments could then be made in exercise, bathing, diet or surroundings to achieve balance.

Exercise warmed the body; immoderate exercise greatly heated the body and was often drying; rest on the other hand cooled and hydrated it. Different kinds of exercise had different effects; fishing and sailing for example, acted like rest, cooling and moistening the participant (*Pantegni*, bk. 5, chap. 12). Bathing had many benefits, helping to dissolve and purge the body of excess humours. Patients could be bathed in such a way as to warm or cool, moisten or dry: for example, a long bath would cool and dry the body by dissolving the natural heat–an excessively long bath could extinguish it and even lead to death (chap. 13). Moderate sleep moderated the humours and cleared the mind, but too much sleep moistened and cooled the body; too little sleep dried out the body. Sexual intercourse was good for the health, reducing bad thoughts and anger, and cooling and drying the body. The physician should attend to the natural excretions, for example if menstruation did not occur, the liver could cool (chaps. 106–8). The easiest and most common manipulation of the qualities was however to be done using drugs and diet.

This was assisted by another of Constantine's translations, which gave further details of the precise qualities of drugs and foodstuffs. Galen had refined the basic qualities of hot, cold, wet, and dry into four levels of intensity or degrees (*gradus*), from weak (the first degree) to extreme (the fourth degree). He used these to classify drugs, and the earliest medieval access to this aspect of his work came in Constantine's translation of the *Liber gradibus* by Ibn al-Jazzar, and also included in the *Pantegni Practica*, Book 2. Elder for example was considered warm and dry in the third degree, mallows cold in the first degree and moist in the second (chap. 40). Islamicate medicine had however gone further with this and extended the system of degrees to foodstuffs, since these also had an effect on the body. The *Pantegni Theorica* lists thirty foods with their degrees of heat or cold and wet or dry, for example lentils were cold in the second degree and dry in the third, and medlar fruit cold and moist in the first degree (chaps. 33 and 83). The *Liber de gradibus* was one of the most popular and widely available of Constantine's texts, indicating that this information was particularly valued as helpful. Thanks to this new learning the physician now had not only a grasp of the qualities of seasons and environments, but also a highly specified set of remedies in drugs and foods which could be administered to restore balance and health.

This could be seen as an advance, part of a new theoretical, scholarly discipline of medicine, which offered details of anatomy, physiology, and pathology, along with rationale-based treatment–a contrast to the largely remedy based atheoretical medicine that went before. However, John Riddle complains that theory was now taking precedence over practical knowledge gained by experience, particularly of drug treatments, whilst producing little of benefit, a "retrogression in the competence of medical practice." The theory, and in particular the system of degrees, was "so complex as to be unworkable [...] physicians confronted by a patient had to make a series of judgments that no human could execute in practice."[6] A drug would have to be chosen according to its qualities and degrees, to suit the age, sex, and general temperament of the patient, their disease, the affected organ, and taking into account their place of residence, the weather, and time of year. Because of this, Riddle argues that most medical practitioners would have largely ignored this new approach in practice. There is much in this argument. By the thirteenth century things had become even more complicated, when Gerard of Cremona translated the work of al-Kindi. This gave mathematical rules to work out the degrees, and what degrees were produced by two drugs in combination. However, Roger Bacon complained that this method was "extremely difficult and almost entirely unknown among Latin physicians these days, as everyone is aware."[7] Certainly I have not seen any consideration given to degrees of drugs or food mentioned in two later medical writers I have looked at, Gilbertus Anglicus writing in the thirteenth century, or John of Gaddesden in the fourteenth.

Nevertheless, for good or ill, the new theoretical medicine had far reaching consequences. The idea of the non-naturals spawned a whole genre of medical literature in the various *Regimen sanitatis* (regimens of health) which particularly emphasized food and drink as a simpler way of regulating the non-naturals. The *Regimen Sanitatis Salernitatum* for example, probably dating from the twelfth or thirteenth century, was trans-

---

6 Riddle, "Theory and Practice in Medieval Medicine," 183, 172.

7 Bacon, "De erroribus medicorum," ed. Little and Withington, 166.

lated into nearly every European language and in use for centuries. Originally focussed on humours and complexions, later versions, at least, advised on seasons and the air in much the same terms as Constantine used:

> Yet for your lodging roomes give this direction,
> In houses where you mind to make your dwelling,
> That neere the same there be no evil sents
> Of puddle-waters or of excrements.
> Let aire be cleere and light, and free from faults,
> That come of secret passages and vaults.[8]

It gave information about the qualities of the seasons with associated recommendations about health habits and diet, the qualities of some foods were also given, for example damsons being cool and vinegar cooling and drying the body. This was all however, inevitably, general rather than individualized advice.

From the point of view of physicians' patients, learned medicine carried a certain prestige; it was a holistic, personalized medicine, although necessarily only available to the elite who could afford it. Chefs to the nobility now had to pay great attention to the qualities and temperaments of foods offered in order to preserve the health of their masters. By the fourteenth century, at the court of the duke of Burgundy, we find no less than six physicians employed, no doubt an exhibition of status; one of their tasks was to accompany the duke at dinner to advise him on the healthfulness or otherwise of the various dishes.[9] Management of the non-naturals, drug administration and medical treatment in general had become so complex that medical professionals were needed who had been highly trained in the new learning.

Theoretical medicine involved a large body of information, a science that required formal education, and led to the development of medical schools and medical faculties in universities. The required knowledge base was also ever expanding, as we shall see in Janet Walls's chapter later in this volume, it became necessary to understand the complexities of astronomy, in order to calculate the effects of planetary movements and interactions in relation to individual patients and their diseases. The planets and signs of the zodiac themselves were each ascribed qualities, Venus, for example, being cold and moist, and Virgo cold and dry, such that their influences could also be incorporated into the system described here. Formal medical education first took off in Salerno, near Constantine's base in Southern Italy, to be surpassed by prestigious centres of learning in Bologna, Montpellier, and Paris. A set of texts that every physician should know was established, the *Articella*, of which the *Isagoge* was a key component. Those wanting to train as physicians first had to study for a general degree in the arts, which included such topics as logic, philosophy, astronomy, and mathematics, before beginning their medical studies. This was in keeping with classical ideas that doctors needed to be philosophers as well as practitioners, who had an understanding of the whole natural

---

8 Taken from a seventeenth-century translation in Harington, *Regimen Sanitatis Salerni*, 29.

9 Scully, "Therapeutic Use," 66.

world and not just the human body, in order to heal and maintain health. The whole process could last eight years or more and concluded with admission to an increasingly confident and lucrative profession through various forms of qualifications and licensing. A large number of practically trained health care providers continued to serve the mass of the population, but their reputation was compromised in favour of these university-educated physicians. This may not have been to the benefit of their patients, little of this medicine being actually effective, but in the long run, attracting students with the intelligence and commitment needed to study this complex body of knowledge was probably to the good of the developing science.

Medicine was indeed now considered a science, taking its place in *physica*, natural science. Its vision was of the human being in context, as part of the natural world even stretching to the whole universe. The human body was a microcosm reflecting the macrocosm; it was made from the elements and the bodily humours were said to be their "offspring." The contribution of Constantine's translations was to provide a framework for medical knowledge, introducing the categories of things natural, non-natural, and contra-natural. The idea of the non-naturals was key; this innovation from the Galenic and Islamicate tradition affirmed the importance of the environment, the air, weather, seasons, and places, both in theory and practice. There was now a clear and comprehensive intellectual basis for viewing the patient holistically and providing individually tailored medical advice.

Bibliography

Primary Sources

Bacon, Roger. "De erroribus medicorum," In *Fratris Rogeri Bacon De retardatione accidentium senectutis*. Edited by Andrew George Little and Edward Theodore Withington. Oxford: Clarendon, 1928.

Bede. *The Reckoning of Time*. Edited and translated by Faith Wallis. Liverpool: Liverpool University Press, 1999.

Constantine of Africa. "Isagoge." In *Medieval Medicine: A Reader*. Edited and translated by Faith Wallis. Toronto: University of Toronto Press, 2010.

——. "Liber de Melancholia." In *Ishaq ibn Imran Maqala fi l-malihuliya (Abhandlung uber die Melancholie) und Constantini "Libri duo de melancholia."* Edited by Karl Garbers. Hamburg: Buske, 1977.

——. "Pantegni Theorica" and "Pantegni Practica." In *Opera omnia ysaac*. Lyon: Andreas Turinus, 1515. http://diglib.hab.de/drucke/ma-4f-35/start.htm.

Harington, Sir John. *The School of Salernum, Regimen Sanitatis Salerni*. Salerno: Ente provinciale per il Turismo, 1953.

Oribasius. *Œuvres d'Oribase*. Vol. 6, *Euporistes*. Edited by Ulco Cats Bussemaker and Charles Daremberg. Paris: Imprimerie Nationale, 1876.

Secondary Sources

Riddle, John M. "Theory and Practice in Medieval Medicine." *Viator* 5 (1974): 157–84.

Scully, Terence. "A Cook's Therapeutic Use of Garden Herbs." In *Herbs and Healing from the Medieval Garden*. Edited by Peter Dendle and Alain Touwaide, 60–71. Woodbridge: Boydell, 2008.

MATTHEW PARIS, WILLIAM OF CONCHES, AND THE USE OF DIAGRAMS TO OBSERVE THE WORLD

JUDITH COLLARD

MATTHEW PARIS, A thirteenth-century monk of St. Albans Abbey, in southern England, is now probably best known for his roles as a chronicler and as a writer of hagiography. He was a significant figure in England's cultural history, who worked also as a copyist, a collator of poetry and science, and a compiler of fortune-telling texts. Scattered throughout his manuscripts were many lively illustrations, genealogies, calendars, computistical tables, diagrams, and maps. This material occurs both in prefatory folios and integrated into the main body of manuscripts, often commentating on or complementing the written texts. These images ranged in subject matter and included observations of the natural world, as well as incorporating diagrams that were an important aspect of his work. Diagrams featured throughout his works, not only in his histories but also in less familiar works such as his editions of William of Conches's *Dragmaticon* (Cambridge, Corpus Christi College, MS 385) and the *sortes* or fortune-telling tract (Oxford, Bodleian Library, MS Ashmole 304). In this article I am particularly interested in exploring how Paris used diagrams in his exploration of the world around him.

Matthew Paris died in 1259, as recorded in his own *Chronica Maiora*.[1] He was an important figure in the writing of English history, being responsible for several chronicles that have provided us with considerable useful information about thirteenth century Europe and the Middle East. These included the *Chronica Majora*, the autograph text is now found in three manuscripts held in Corpus Christi College, Cambridge, and the British Library, the *Historia Anglorum* and the *Flores Historiarum*. The latter was initially composed for Westminster Abbey, but also provided the basis for several other monastic chronicles.[2] A copy of the *Flores Historiarum* manuscript that contains both Matthew Paris's recognisable hand and some marginal notations is found in the Chetham Library, Manchester.[3]

1 Paris, *Chronica Majora*, ed. Luard, 5:748; Vaughan, *Matthew Paris*, 7.

2 Cambridge, Corpus Christi College, MS 26, https://parker.stanford.edu/parker/catalog/rf352tc5448; Cambridge, Corpus Christi College, MS 16 I and II, https://parker.stanford.edu/parker/catalog/rb378fk5493, https://parker.stanford.edu/parker/catalog/qt808nj0703; London, British Library, MS Royal 14 C. VII, https://searcharchives.bl.uk/primo_library/libweb/action/search.do; Manchester, Chetham Library, MS 6712.

3 See also Collard, "*Flores Historiarum*," 441–66.

Judith Collard is an Honorary Research Fellow in the School of Culture and Communication at the University of Melbourne. She has previously taught at Melbourne and Monash Universities and was Programme Coordinator in Art History and Visual Culture at the University of Otago in Dunedin. She has published extensively on thirteenth-century art, particularly on Matthew Paris, as well as on twentieth-century art.

Diagrams feature in most of Matthew Paris's manuscripts. They take many forms and fulfil a multitude of different functions. They are integral to his work. Images in general form a major part of Paris's *oeuvre* and they reflect how his visual imagination was anchored in medieval intellectual thought. His diagrams provide pathways to the structuring of his manuscripts and are part of their fascinating character. This is particularly so with the presence of diagrams in his chronicles. In part they are enigmatic because the presence of these diagrams does not conform to our expectations of chronicles. However, they convey important evidence concerning thirteenth-century models of the human and natural worlds.

We have come to think of visual material, such as maps, tables and pictures as illustrations that are supplementary, as extras that are less significant than the serious business of words. This is not the case with Matthew Paris's work where the visual is integral to an understanding of what he is interested in communicating. Paris's use of this type of imagery reveals his familiarity with a range of different genres that today we often separate out into different specialities with labels such as scholasticism, science, hagiography and history. What they share is an efficient and effective means of organizing information, that sets out sometimes complex clusters of facts clearly and in often pleasing aesthetic forms. There is a real pleasure in neatly organized, carefully ruled tables with their rows of numbers, of the careful connecting together of roundels and the interweaving of explanatory texts around these rulings. Although maps and genealogies seem, at least initially, very different in types from wind diagrams or concurrent tables, it is because we are often more distracted by the outer container than the content. While family trees and maps are very familiar to us, we sometimes forget that these too are inherently diagrammatic. Mathematical tables meanwhile seem more alien in the context of a chronicle, as can liturgical calendars with their lists of holy days, although it is perhaps easier to accept the latter because of the monastic source of these manuscripts.

Recently there has been an increasing interest in the appearance of the diagram. This diagrammatic turn draws on the work of predecessors like Michael Evans, Bruce Eastwood, and John E. Murdoch, whose volume of the Album of Science focusing on antiquity and the Middle Ages presented many images drawn from early manuscripts presenting scientific ideas.[4] Faith Wallis, elaborating on the ideas of Michael Evans, helps define a diagram as a geometrical representation of a concept or abstraction. This is the case even when it may incorporate a figural image such as a wheel or a tree. It is a visual text. As she puts it diagrams are:

> Illustrations that help readers to understand a text or, in any event, deepen their appreciation of its content and implications; they incorporate textual inscriptions into the graphic schema to represent the relationship between entities or concepts; and they function as a 'visual exegesis'.[5]

4 Evans, "Geometry of the Mind," 32–55; Eastwood, *Revival of Planetary Astronomy*; Eastwood, *Ordering the Heavens*; Murdoch, *Album of Science*.

5 Wallis, "What a Medieval Diagram Shows," 1–40, esp. 3.

Bianca Kühnel has explored these ideas further, linking cosmology, time, and Christian eschatology together, arguing for example that Classical scientific schemes were reorganized in such works as Isidore of Seville's *De natura rerum* into representations of a universe created by God, thus reflecting Christian ideas about Creation.[6] Several symposia have also led to significant publications examining different types and interpretations of diagrams.[7] Each examined different aspects of medieval and early modern diagrams, acknowledging the role Jewish, Byzantine, and, particularly, Arabic scholars played in the development of diagrams. Jeffrey Hamburger's important essay "*Mindmapping*: The Diagram as Paradigm in Medieval Art–and Beyond" was published in one form in *The Visualizing of Knowledge*, while it reappeared in another form in his book *Diagramming Devotion*.[8] Barbara Obrist, Marcia Kupfer, Faith Wallis, and Adam S. Cohen have provided equally thought-provoking essays for me in this collection, each discussing different aspects of the diagram in medieval thought.[9]

As Michael Evans has pointed out, diagrammatic illustrations were generally ignored when they made up part of an illuminated manuscript.[10] In the case of Matthew Paris, although some of his diagrams such as his genealogies, have received scholarly attention, this is not the case with others. His Easter tables and his wind diagrams were not included in Nigel Morgan's otherwise majestic survey of the contents of these manuscripts. Even more tellingly, in the curious compilation of fortune-telling texts he compiled, only the two sets of portraits of philosophers and mathematicians are reproduced, while the accompanying sequences of charts are mentioned as "a series of thirteen tables and circular diagrams decorated with foliage, fruit, animals, birds and symbolic representations of cities."[11] This was later remedied by Allegra Iafrate's series of articles on this manuscript which culminated in the facsimile, *Le Moine et le Hasard*.[12] As Sophie Page has shown, diagrams played an important role in manuscript records of magic. Although she does not discuss fortune-telling, she does show how circular images appear in amulets and in ritual magic.[13] Matthew Paris's compilation, Oxford, Bodleian Library, MS Ashmole 304, is the earliest example of an illustrated *sortes* manuscript surviving.[14] To be fair, Morgan's book was a survey rather than a detailed discussion of each manuscript he included. However, there were examples of his excluding diagrams, for

6 Kühnel, *End of Time*.

7 Lutz, Jerjen, and Putzo, eds., *Diagramm und Text*; Kupfer, Cohen, and Chajes, eds., *Visualization of Knowledge*; and Hamburger, Roxburgh, and Safran, eds., *Diagram as Paradigm*.

8 Hamburger, "Mindmapping," 61–86; Hamburger, *Diagramming Devotion*, 12–32.

9 Obrist, "Idea of a Spherical Universe," 229–58; Kupfer, "Rhetoric of World Maps," 259–90; Wallis, "Visualizing Knowledge," 291–326; and Cohen, "Diagramming the Diagrammatic," 383–404.

10 Evans, "Geometry of the Mind," 32–55.

11 Morgan, *Early Gothic Manuscripts*, 140, no. 89.

12 Iafrate, *Le Moine et le Hasard*; Iafrate, "Of Stars and Men," 139–77; Iafrate, "Workshop of Fortune," 55–87; Iafrate, "'Si sequeris casum,'" 457–88.

13 Page, "Medieval Magical Figures," 432–57.

14 Iafrate, "Of Stars and Men," 142.

example, although he included the Paschal Table found in MS 26, Morgan did not include the accompanying wind diagram (fol. v verso).[15] Here Morgan was more focused on the maps and other more generally figurative imagery than such scientific images. Suzanne Lewis, in her important work on Matthew Paris's artistic activity, similarly misses out the wind diagram in her list of Paris's imagery in the *Chronica Majora* (MS 26), although she did mention it in a footnote. She did, however, include a similar diagram in her list of the images in MS 16.[16]

While the reckoning of time was of interest to historians of science, the computus table used for the calculating of the date of Easter placed opposite a St. Albans calendar in the *Historia Anglorum* has been overlooked by scholars (fols. 6v–7). The text found below it that recorded the gift of the book to St. Albans is not.[17] Neither Morgan nor Lewis provided an exhaustive list of Matthew Paris's illustrations.

The copy of William of Conches's *Dragmaticon*,[18] that Matthew Paris produced is included only in Morgan's account of John of Wallingford's miscellaneous collection of texts and images, some of which were by Paris. Here he mentions the manuscript when discussing a map of climate zones by Wallingford. "Matthew certainly knew about climate zones as is made evident by a diagram he made in his manuscript of William of Conches (Cambridge, Corpus Christi College MS 385, p. 178)."[19] It is also discussed briefly in Richard Vaughan's *Matthew Paris*.[20] Here he identified William of Conches as a well-known philosopher and teacher from Chartres. While both he and Lewis number the diagrams as twenty-three, there were twenty-seven images spread over twenty-three pages.[21] He also makes the telling point that because Matthew Paris was not a professional artist the existence of this manuscript with its diagrams "is therefore important for the light it throws on his scientific interests."[22]

Matthew Paris's chronicles are lengthy and crowded with facts, stories, commentary, and documents. These were working texts that the author seems to have continually added to and adapted and excised. Consequently, judging the ideal sequence of materials is less than clear, particularly as there are questions about whether the final placement of some images is their intended position. Suzanne Lewis, indeed, has suggested that Matthew Paris may have had a portfolio in collected drawings for later use, often reflecting his copying motifs from other manuscripts as well as trialling ideas, that were then later bound into his own or other manuscripts.[23] The appearance of short genea-

15 Morgan, *Early Gothic Manuscripts*, 137, no. 90.

16 Lewis, *Art of Matthew Paris*, 444, 496n165.

17 Lewis, *Art of Matthew Paris*, 458; Morgan, *Early Gothic Manuscripts*, 143, no. 92.

18 Cambridge, Corpus Christi College, MS 385, https://parker.stanford.edu/parker/catalog/jv228wq5037.

19 Morgan, *Early Gothic Manuscripts*, 141–42, no. 91.

20 Vaughan, *Matthew Paris*, 254–55.

21 Vaughan, *Matthew Paris*, 255, Lewis, *Art of Matthew Paris*, 441.

22 Vaughan, *Matthew Paris*, 255.

23 Lewis, *Art of Matthew Paris*, 31–32, 419–27

logical accounts of the kings of England, linked by roundels and the occasional illustration, as well as the development of distinctive galleries of kings, also reveal the flexibility of the content of these works.[24] The presence of his distinctive hand as well as his drawings appear, for example, in John of Wallingford's *Miscellany* (London, British Library, MS Cotton Julius D. VII) and the Bible now held in Corpus Christi College, Oxford (MS 2).[25] The twentieth-century removal of maps from some volumes in the British Library and the division into two volumes of the Cambridge manuscript, Cambridge, Corpus Christi College, MS 16 I and II, does signal that this moveability is still a feature of these books.

While this does suggest that Paris's manuscripts are perhaps less carefully organized than later printed books, a pattern does emerge in his chronicles at least. Integrated into these chronicles are a mix of scientific, religious, and historical material that indicate that Matthew Paris did not separate these into different categories, seeing them as interrelated. Each manuscript includes prefatory material that can include maps, genealogies and various scientific diagrams and mathematical tables. Thus, the first volume of the *Chronica Majora* (Cambridge, Corpus Christi College, MS 26) includes in its current arrangement: an itinerary from London to Jerusalem (fols. i verso–iv), a circular Paschal Table (fol. v verso), a Table of Concurrentes and a wind diagram (fol. v verso) a Calendar (fol. vi recto–verso), while at the end of the manuscript can also be found full-page illustration of a Mappa Mundi on the verso (fol. vii verso) and a genealogical diagram with extended notes (fol. viii recto–verso). The manuscript ends with a particularly grubby, torn and repaired folio (fol. ix), the verso of which is blank. The second volume of the *Chronica Maiora* (Cambridge, Corpus Christi College, MS 16) repeats a variation of this pattern. It includes in the prefatory a wind diagram (fol. ii), a drawing of an elephant and its keeper (fol. ii recto), a fragmentary itinerary (fol. ii recto), a Map of the Holy Land (fols. iii verso–iv recto), a map of Britain (fol. iv verso), and a genealogical tree from Alfred to Henry III (fols. v-v verso). These first five folios have now been detached from the rest of the volume.[26] The manuscript was rebound in 2003.[27] The third volume of the *Chronica Majora* does not follow this pattern, but it is now attached to the *Historia Anglorum*, which does include an extensive Itinerary (fols. 2–4), a Map of the Crusader Kingdom (fols. 4v–5), and a Map of Britain (fol. 5v). The *Abbreviatio Chronicorum* includes a diagram of the Heptarchy, a circular, wheel-shaped diagram depicting the seven historical kingdoms, and a Map of Britain (fol. 12v), while the *Liber Additamentorum* includes itineraries (fols. 183v–184), wind diagrams (fols. 184v–185), and another elephant drawing (fol. 169v). It also added to the collection of diagrams by including a parhelion (fol. 186), and a crude map showing Roman roads (fol. 187v).

---

24 See the discussion of these genealogies and galleries in de Laborderie, "*Genealogiae orbiculatae*," 183–202; Collard, "King John," 35–52.

25 Thomson, *Descriptive Catalogue*, 3–4.

26 Parker on the Web, https://parker.stanford.edu/parker/catalog/qt808nj0703, provides its current numbering.

27 Binski and Panayatova, *Cambridge Illuminations*, 252, no. 114.

The chronicles did not restrict the use of diagrams to the prefatory material accompanying the main body of the text. They were an integral part of the organization of these manuscripts. Paris used various types of diagrams to organize his material, to mark out the subject matter and to clarify and explicate what was discussed within the chronicle. Paris's awareness of the range of uses scientific diagrams could perform is also demonstrated in the recurrence of wind diagrams in several of his manuscripts, including the *Chronica Majora* (Cambridge, Corpus Christi College MS 26, fol. v verso, MS 16, fol. iii verso) and the *Liber Additamentorum* (London, British Library, MS Cotton Nero D. I, fol. 186). An incomplete wind rose also appeared in Cotton Nero D. 5 (fol. 184).[28] This is labelled "*Secundum magister Elyam de Derham*" and was based on a design by the Canon of Salisbury who died in 1245. A second rose on folio 184v is divided into sixteen rays. This is also followed in the *Chronica Majora* diagrams.[29] A similar wind diagram also appeared in the *Dragmaticon* (fol. 152).[30] This represented the twelve-ray rose in the centre of which is a T–O shaped map of the world. Each wind was numbered in this version. The wind diagrams in Paris's *Liber Additamentorum* were the subject of an article by E. G. R. Taylor's essay, where he suggested that it may have contained the earliest description of the sixteen-ray system. This device also added to the Latin names of the sixteen wind directions their vernacular versions, which are still in use today.[31] Barbara Obrist, in her article on such diagrams, has also pointed out that historians of science have rarely studied conceptions of the natural world such works represented, their attention being directed more to examinations of astronomy and the reckoning of time. She traces these diagrams from early medieval ideas of the world to the twelfth and early thirteenth-century depictions, which predate those drawn by Paris.[32] She did not, however, include the sixteen-ray variant found in Paris.

As much as the illustrations delight and amuse the eye, they also demonstrate how important imagery was to Matthew Paris's intellectual mindset. An examination of Paris's manuscripts that reveals a deep knowledge of the place of diagrams in the intellectual writings of the medieval period. He was also comfortable about adapting diagrams to perform his own tasks. He did not simply copy previous examples but adapted them. Surviving manuscripts in his distinctive hand also demonstrate his interest in scientific literature out of which such imagery emerged, as his ownership of William of Conches's *Dragmaticon*, that he had carefully copied and illustrated, reveals.

As Bruce Eastwood has demonstrated, diagrams in Carolingian manuscripts of astronomical and cosmological manuscripts were often adaptions of those found in the works of Pliny and Macrobius,[33] and that copyists did not always simply replicate

---

28 Taylor, "'De Ventis' of Matthew Paris," 23–26.

29 Taylor, "'De Ventis' of Matthew Paris," 23–26.

30 Vaughan, *Matthew Paris*, 255, plate xx (d).

31 Vaughan, *Matthew Paris*, 255–56.

32 Obrist, "Wind Diagrams," 33–84.

33 Eastwood, *Ordering the Heavens*, 381–84.

imagery found in their exemplars.[34] In his chapter "Carolingian Diagrams for Astronomy and Cosmology," Eastwood also briefly discussed the assumption that words and images have an oppositional relationship.[35] As he and others who work on diagrams have pointed out, diagrams often include words. He contrasts this to Gregory the Great's defence of images as the "Bible of the illiterate" and points out the teaching role they performed. Diagrams were useful as learning devices, as memory aids, and as a means of assessing a student's understanding of a text. He argues that, in astronomy at least, "the diagram could often show a higher truth than words alone." Diagrams can explain and clarify the text.[36] They operate in very different ways to traditional ideas of the pictorial, and act as intermediaries between text and image.

Steffen Bogen and Felix Thurlemann also begin their discussion on the relationship between text and images in the diagram with Gregory the Great's important justification for the role of images in religion. In their essay they argue that diagrams operate as an independent form of communication, rejecting the imposed dichotomy of word and image, and operating as a distinct medium. They draw together the role of the icon on computer programs such as Word, Isidore of Seville's *De natura rerum*, and found in the medieval *arbores consanguintatis*. They drew on theorists, such as Charles Sanders Pierce and Ferdinand de Saussure to develop a general theory of the diagram as a medium of thinking, aiding in the clarification of complexities.[37] Similarly Jeffrey Hamburger used the work of Pierce in his own study on Berthold of Nuremberg's use of diagrams in his late thirteenth-century commentary on the Carolingian writer Hrabanus Maurus.[38] Within the books of Matthew Paris, diagrams, emblems, and signs are used to communicate both ideas and complex information.

The utility and convenience of diagrams are demonstrated by Paris's diagrams of the Heptarchy, the seven kingdoms of England. This wheel diagram type, reminiscent of a rose window with spokes providing cells for each of the kingdoms, succinctly represents the complexities of Anglo-Saxon England. It does not resemble the geography of the land map, nor does it reflect the fluidity of these kingdoms through conquest, marriage, and the death of dynasties are found traced in brief king lists. What the Heptarchy diagrams do ably is delineate the division of the country into individual monarchies that were ultimately became unified under the kings of Wessex, best personified by Alfred, at least for Matthew Paris.[39] He divided this image into seven separate compartments, each representing one kingdom. These kingdoms are Northumbria, East Anglia, Essex, Kent, Sussex, Mercia, and Wessex. If not invented by Paris, his use of it was the earliest surviving examples of its appearance. That his chronicle is the earliest in which this format appears

34 Eastwood, *Ordering the Heavens*, 391.

35 Eastwood, *Ordering the Heavens*, 420–25.

36 Eastwood, *Ordering the Heavens*, 424.

37 Bogen and Thürlemann, "Jenseits der Opposition von Text und Bild," 12–15.

38 Hamburger, *Diagramming Devotion*, 13, 24–25, 27–28.

39 Collard, "Art and Science," 18.

is generally accepted.[40] The Diagram of the Heptarchy appeared with a genealogy of the kings of England in the *Chronica Maiora* (MS 26, fol. iv verso) as well as in John of Wallingford's *Miscellany* (fol. 49v). The *Chronica* Heptarchy rose contains at its centre a bust of Alfred describing him as the "proto-monarch," the first ruler of all England.[41] The format of the genealogical diagrams themselves seems to have evolved from those produced for Peter of Poitiers's *Compendium Historiae in Genealogia*, that began to appear in the late twelfth century.[42] A fine illustrated example of this text was produced probably in St. Albans sometime between 1245 and 1254 and is roughly contemporary with the creation of Matthew Paris's genealogy.[43] The shape of the Heptarchy diagrams was one way of describing the makeup of England in diagrammatic form, another form of mapping.

Another representation of Britain in Matthew Paris's historical texts was included in the *Liber Additamentorum* (fol. 187v). It is a sketch outline showing the four main Roman Roads labelled here the "Scema Britannie." These roads are Icknield Street, the Fosse Way, Ermine Street and Watling Street. In this version the sketch map is positioned with west at the top. As Vaughan points out, the roads are shown intersecting, incorrectly, at Dunstable.[44] Once again this is quite a crude depiction and demonstrates his interest in jotting down information that broadened his understanding of the world.

The copy Paris produced of William of Conches's *Dragmaticon Philosophiae* (Cambridge, Corpus Christi College, MS 385) also revealed his familiarity with such diagrammatic schemes used to explain the natural world as well as other texts such as Peter of Poitiers's *Compendium Historiae in Genealogia Christi*.[45] The *Dragmaticon Philosophiae* was an illustrated edition of William's work dating originally to the late 1140s and was addressed to his patron Geoffrey Plantagenet, Duke of Normandy and Count of Anjou, the father of Henry II of England.[46] Italo Ronca, who has edited and translated the work, dates it to between 1147 and 1149.[47] William was familiar with the work of the Arabic astronomer Māshā'allāh ibn Atharī (762–ca.815).[48] As Obrist has pointed out, William adopted several arguments made by Māshā'allāh, including proving that the world was round and the explanation he gives for the apparent irregularity of Saturn's move-

---

40 Monroe, "Roll-Manuscript," 206–7; Monroe, "13th and Early 14th Century Illustrated," 1:265; Collard, "Gender and Genealogy," 20.

41 See Collard, "Gender and Genealogy," 42

42 See, for example, Worm, "Visualizing the Order of History," 243–63.

43 Eton, College Library, MS 96; Monroe, "Roll-Manuscript," 106–7; Morgan, *Early Gothic Manuscripts*, 140–41.

44 Vaughan, *Matthew Paris*, 244.

45 Collard, "Gender and Genealogy," 11–35. For an account of Peter of Poitiers's genealogies, see Monroe, "Roll-Manuscript," 92–107.

46 A very useful account of William of Conches's career and influences, as well as the scholarship around him can be found in Ramirez-Weaver, "'So that You Can Understand This Better,'" 319–48, esp. 319–22.

47 William of Conches, *Dialogue on Natural Philosophy*, trans. Ronca and Curr, xvii.

48 Obrist, "William of Conches," 30.

ments, as well as including three of his diagrams.[49] His use of this Arabic source is further detailed in her article "The Idea of a Spherical Universe and Its Visualisation in the Earlier Middle Ages."[50]

Paris's version is unusual because we know that it was produced by him, probably for his own use given his general interest in science. It is much annotated by Paris and others. It is one of four manuscripts that he copied out himself in his distinctive hand.[51] It is very rare that we can identify so precisely a medieval scribe who was also a significant author in his own right. His edition was one of many copies of this dialogue that had initially been written as an aid to Count Geoffrey's sons.[52] As Ramirez-Weaver has pointed out, there have been at least eighty-one copies made of the *Dragmaticon* and in each "these complex recombinations of text, image, and illustrative potential reveal the individual identities of their makers through selective but creative artistic renderings of the nevertheless hegemonic designs."[53] The work of Matthew Paris is no exception to this. His individual response is revealed in the care taken with each image, his individual touches in the treatment of the planets shown, in the flaming red of the Sun and the black Earth, and in the depictions of the towered structures that represent individual cities in these diagrams. The manuscript that he based his copy on is unknown, and the diagrams may have varied from the prototype that was used. What is clear is that it did contain most, if not all, of the diagrams that William of Conches planned. The instructions included in the text demonstrated that William was aware of the need to instruct and explain the work's content.

> So that you can understand this better I shall sketch a figure in which I shall draw a line for the flat earth and the two ends of it two cities, and above it I shall draw in the curve of the sun and above each of the two cities the [rising and setting] sun, in this way.[54]

This image was found on page 173 of Matthew Paris's manuscript. His characteristically colourful touch is reflected in his representation of a pair of fortified cities, linked by two red and blue lines that trace the movement of the sun through the sky. The sun itself is represented by two flaming red balls set low over the towns.[55]

---

49 Obrist, "William of Conches," 31.

50 Obrist, "Idea of a Spherical Universe," 239–49; Obrist, "Guillaume de Conches," 123–96.

51 These are Bernard Silvestris, *Liber Experimentarius and Other Fortune-Telling Texts* (Oxford, Bodleian Library, MS Ashmole 304); Henry of Avranches, *Poetry* (Cambridge, University Library, MS Dd.9.78); and Robert Grosseteste, *Tract on the Virginity of the Blessed Virgin Mary* (London, British Library, Royal MS 4 D VII, fols. 246v–249). The collection of Henry of Avranches's poetry was given by Matthew Paris to his monastery. See Vaughan, *Matthew Paris*, 18n5.

52 Vaughan, *Matthew Paris*, 255.

53 Ramirez-Weaver, "'So that You Can Understand This Better,'" 324.

54 William of Conches, *Dragmaticon*, bk. 6, 2.3, 121 and fig. 25.

55 Cambridge, Corpus Christi College, MS 385, https://parker.stanford.edu/parker/catalog/jv228wq5037.

The *Dragmaticon* was a useful encyclopaedic account of the nature of the world. It was divided into six books, all of which included diagrams. The only section without any was the final one that concentrated on humanity and included discussions on sperm, intercourse, conception, the natural virtues, the brain, sleep, the senses, and the soul amongst other matters. Matthew Paris carefully copied these illustrations into his version of the text.

The work had been planned with diagrams from the beginning. This is apparent within the text itself where William explained their presence several times to the reader, including this comment on an astronomical figure:

> But since what one sees with one's eyes is better retained [by the mind], a diagram of each syzygy should be provided.[56]

Matthew Paris incorporated most of these into his copy. They appear on twenty-three pages, which sometimes contain more than one diagram. For example, on page 130 of Cambridge, Corpus Christi College, MS 385 there are two. That on the left shows the Earth, the Sun, and the epicycles of Venus and Mercury, that on the right depicts the order of the planets according to Plato. These are, from the top: Saturn, Jupiter, Mars, Venus, Mercury, the Sun, Moon, and Earth.[57] In Matthew Paris's manuscript the first image is in the centre of the page, again in descending order: Venus, Mercury, Sun, Venus, Mercury. Each planet is drawn as a brown circle, its name given in red. The Earth shown at the bottom of the diagram, coloured black, except where "*Terra*" is written in red. Around the small circle of the Earth is a green rim. The epicycles are drawn in red. There are three, the two outer circles are also given a green hue. These are also labelled, describing the orbits of each planet, including the sun. This is written in blue. The second diagram is simpler in design, a sequence of descending red circles, each planet named in blue lettering, with a green inner border alternating with a very faint red or orange one.

The *Dragmaticon* extends from page 89 to page 212 in this collection, which also included several works not by William of Conches, Matthew Paris nor, indeed, from St. Albans. It was the second section. The first contained the *Tractatus monachi peccatoris,* on the sins of monks, the third consists of several Middle English sermons and tracts by Richard of Saint-Victor, Beniamin minor and others, compiled in the fourteenth century, whilst the fourth part was the apocryphal gospel, the *Euangelium Nicodemi*, and some exempla and stories.[58]

Matthew Paris, in his edition, replicated twenty-seven of the twenty-eight illustrations found in more complete editions.[59] In this he was not exceptional. As Vaughan pointed out, there were many copies of this work and Paris differed from these only

56 William of Conches, *Dragmaticon*, bk. 2, 5.2, 30, fig. 2.

57 William of Conches, *Dragmaticon*, 64–65. The image is available online: https://parker.stanford.edu/parker/catalog/jv228wq5037.

58 James, *Descriptive Catalogue*, 2:232–35.

59 William of Conches, *Dragmaticon*, for examples of these diagrams.

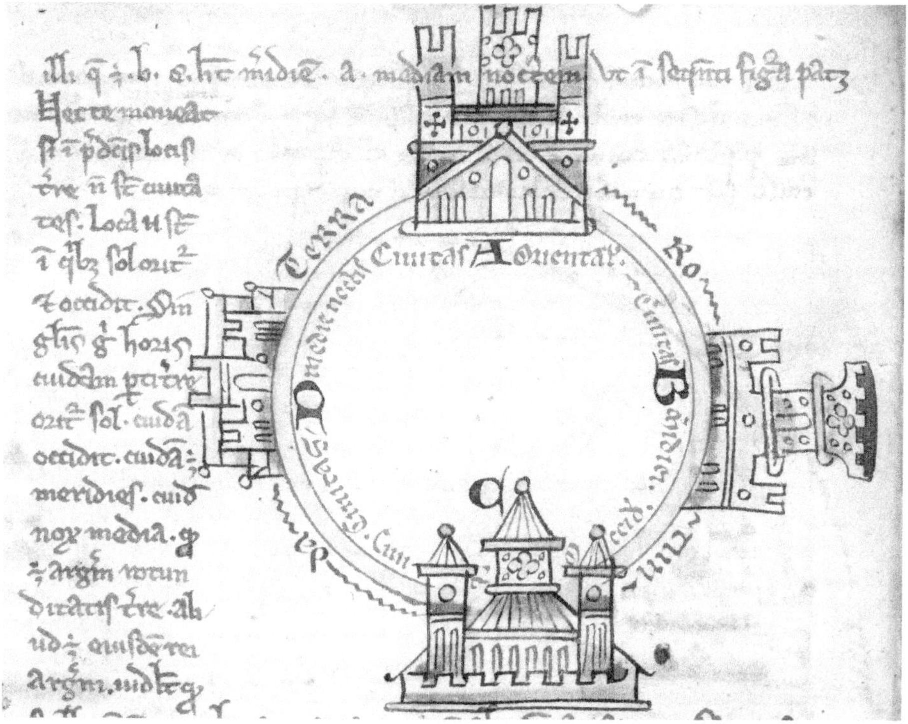

Figure 5.1: "Proof for the roundness of the Earth." William of Conches, *Dragmaticon Philosophiae*. Cambridge, Corpus Christi College, MS 385, p. 174. Image used courtesy of the Parker Library, Corpus Christi College, Cambridge.

in the artistry shown in his diagrams.[60] Paris generally followed the imagery closely, although there were exceptions. On page 174, on the following page to that already discussed, instead of representing the diagram showing another proof for the roundness of the earth with a circle containing four additional discrete circles within its circumference, Paris draws a circular diagram with four cities at each of the cardinal points (Fig. 5.1). They were done in his distinctive hand, reminiscent of his treatment of the various cities that populate his itineraries. They are symmetrical, each with a central tower, three being crenelated, and one with three small spires.

Two diagrams in Paris's edition were very similar to those found in John of Wallingford's *Miscellany* (London, British Library, MS Cotton Julius D. VII, fol. 46). These are the diagrams that William intended to represent the earth's climate zones. They are found on pages 123 and 175, although Paris reorientated them by placing north rather than east at the top. In the explanatory text accompanying the second of these, William labelled these as the Frozen Zone in the North, Our Temperate Zone, the Torrid Zone, the Other Temperate Zone, and the Frozen Zone in the South. He represented all the zones

60 Vaughan, *Matthew Paris*, 255.

in these diagrams, as did Paris here, and further elaborates the nature of these zones in two extensive texts.[61] Paris followed the diagram closely on page 123, but on page 175 he varied it by adding into the second temperate zone a small depiction of Africa and Europe separated by the Mediterranean, reflecting a T–O shaped map form imposed onto this drawing. In the section on the waters and the tides of the ocean he represented on page 166 the tides of the ocean and on 167 the oceanic currents and their collateral winds. The former is shown in a circular form, which Matthew Paris annotated in red in his characteristic hand, around the outer edge water is shown, with two additional zones of water occupying the top half of the image. A third zone, not coloured with green waves, depicts two more seas, one of which is clearly marked the Mediterranean. The second image is simpler, showing the Earth once again surrounded by water, although this time divided into sixteen compartments, and dissected by the Great Ocean. These outer compartments alternate between coloured waves and text, referring to the winds. Once again William explained the diagram:

> But because we shall save labour by providing a visible figure, I shall make a sketch similar to the previous one, not in the middle [of the earth] as with the first figure, but on both sides of it. So we may understand the cardinal winds from that figure and the collateral ones from this. But because we cannot show more than two collateral winds in one figure, the others may be understood by analogy with these.[62]

Throughout the manuscript Matthew Paris put his own mark on these images, as with the explanation of the concept of syzygy. This was originally an astronomical term that William of Conches defined for the duke in the following way:

> "The conjunction, through a mean, of bodies that differ in qualities: as earth and fire are joined by two means; earth and air, or water and fire, for one. Furthermore, the syzygy of two extremes through two means is solid, because the contrariety of those extremes involves three qualities, just as solid bodies are three-dimensional, or because they are conjoined to resemble solid [that is, cubic] numbers."[63]

Given the density of the description, the diagram did give the reader some direction in how to interpret this information. In this case, Paris provided only one diagram, rather than the two suggested by the text. This took the form of a circle with a quatrefoil overlay. It represented the four elements: fire, air, water and earth. Within each was also a description of the qualities of each element, thus water is described as cold and moist, earth as cold and dry, air as moist and hot, and fire as dry and hot.

The fifteenth-century Bohemian example studied by Ramirez-Weaver (Madrid, Biblioteca Nacional de España, MS Res. 28, fol. 29r) similarly only represented one of the

61 William of Conches, *Dragmaticon*, bk. 3, 7:6–13, 54; bk. 6, 3:2–8, 124.

62 William of Conches, *Dragmaticon*, bk. 5, 9:11, 112.

63 William of Conches, *Dragmaticon*, bk. 2, 2, 30.

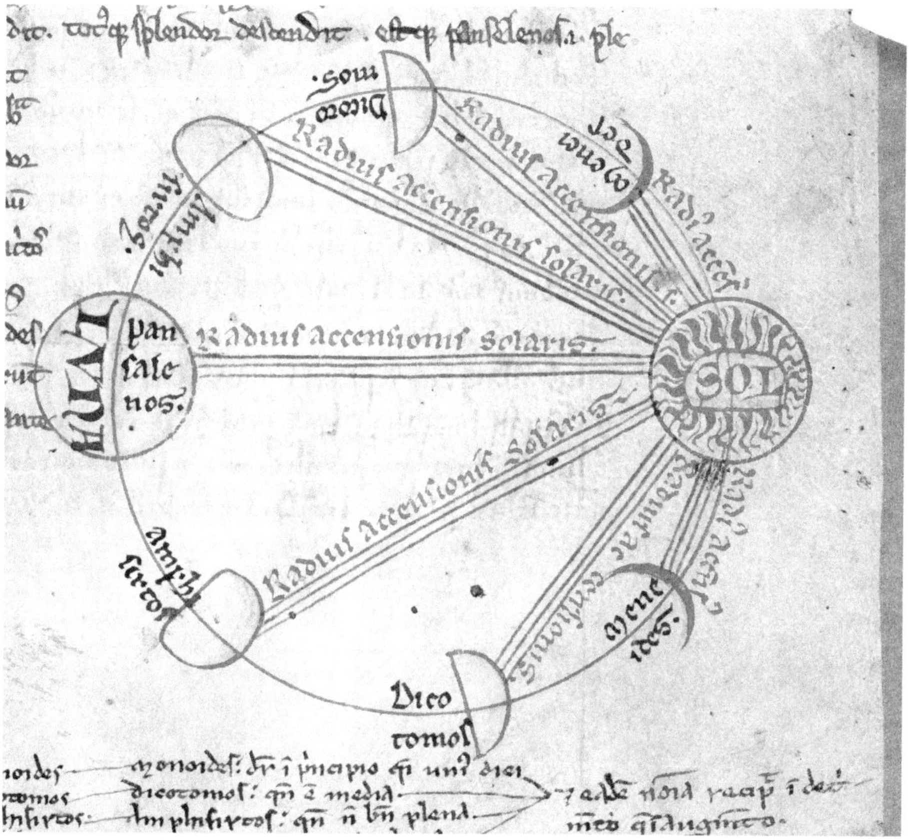

Figure 5.2: "The Phases of the Moon." William of Conches, *Dragmaticon Philosophiae*. Cambridge, Corpus Christi College, MS 385, p. 147.
Image used courtesy of the Parker Library, Corpus Christi College, Cambridge.

two syzygies described in the original text.[64] As Ramirez-Weaver points out, the seventh-century writer Isidore of Seville provided the precedence for this type of round diagram in his *De natura rerum*. This type of diagram is derived from traditions of classical medical handbooks and cosmological treatises which were common in antiquity. Isidore adapted and Christianized the understanding of the universe as divine, something that William of Conches then reused, borrowing the earlier Isidorean model.[65] The use of such circular diagrams is prominent throughout William's and, indeed, Isidore's work.

One particularly fine example was found on page 147 in Matthew Paris's copy (Fig. 5.2). This presents the phases of the moon. In the version provided by Ronca and Curr, it is shown schematically, with a series of circles representing the eight phases

64 Ramirez-Weaver, "William of Conches," 8–10.

65 Ramirez-Weaver, "William of Conches," 12.

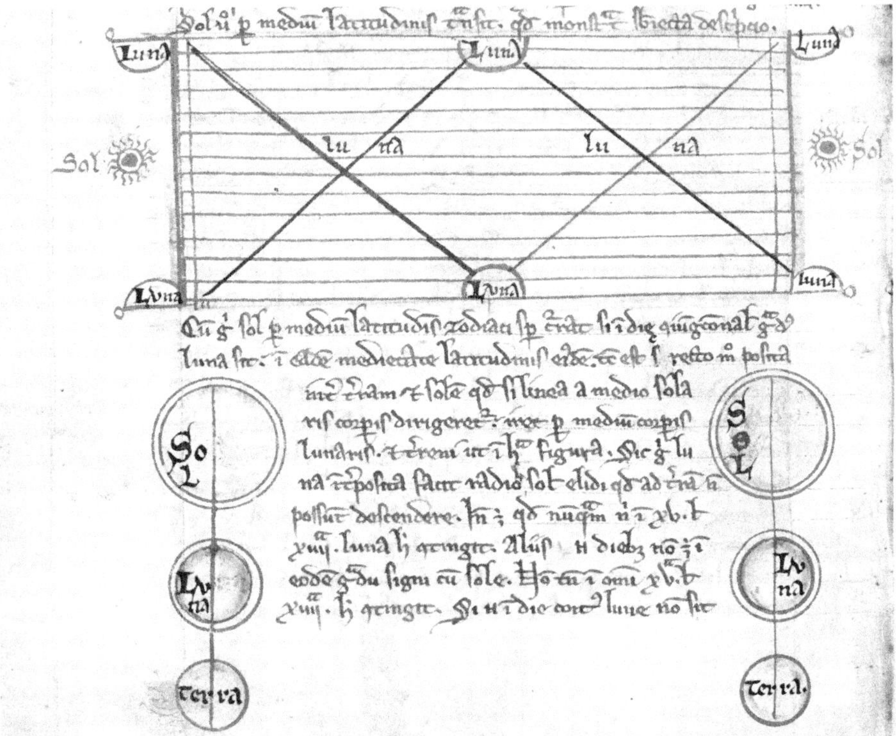

Figure 5.3: "The paths of the Sun and the Moon through the Zodiac; The Moon in Middle Latitude; The Moon not in Middle Latitude." William of Conches, *Dragmaticon Philosophiae*. Cambridge, Corpus Christi College, MS 385, p. 142. Image used courtesy of the Parker Library, Corpus Christi College, Cambridge.

of the moon, including the new moon, the full moon, half-moons, crescent and gibbous moons, as coloured circles that show how these different phases are manifested. All are linked together in a circle at the centre of which is the Earth. To the right is a slightly larger circle from which project rays. This is the Sun. The resulting diagram is simple and elegant. The moon is described as lacking its own heat and brightness, being illuminated by the sun.[66] In contrast, that by Matthew Paris is more dynamic. It is also more contained, consisting of a more integrated image. The Sun, named "SOL," is drawn as a red ball containing red flames. From it extends seven sets of blue lines that connect to each of the phases of the moon, drawn as crescents, half and three-quartered circles, with the full moon, called "LUNA" in blue lettering, is placed directly opposite the Sun. Connecting all, and intersecting each of the phases, is a red circle. There is a real energy in the way a red text runs down each set of blue lines, explaining that they represent a ray of solar ignition. Curiously, there is no new moon shown.

---

66 William of Conches, *Dragmaticon*, bk. 4, 7–11, 86–87.

While most of the images are circular, or incorporate the circle as the dominant feature, there is one exception, although half-moons and the sun are included (Fig. 5.3). The sun is shown twice. It is shown as circles, coloured in red; around each extend red rays. This diagram represents the paths of the sun and the moon through the Zodiac. Only the sun and the moon are labelled. It takes the form of a rectangle, across run fourteen horizontal red lines, while at either end run two more lines, creating a border to the form. Dissecting this are eight brown lines producing two X shapes. It is possible that this was unfinished, as the example given in Ronca and Curr's edition is more complicated, giving not only the moon's movements but also that of the sun, which runs along the central axis in a wave formation. Below this graph-like diagram, in Matthew Paris's work, are two additional diagrams that represent the Moon between the Sun and the Earth, both in and out of middle latitude. Here the text is crucial for the interpretation of these images, all three of which concern the eclipse of the sun. They also demonstrate that the Sun is larger than the Earth. This latter concern is also explored on page 144, where this is dramatically shown in three diagrams that depict the shadows that would be created if the Sun was equal in size, smaller or larger. The Earth is always shown at the top of each image, and above it extends the shadow, which is coloured black. This is cylindrical, top-like or cone-like, depending on the sizes of each figure. Once again both text and image work together to explain the proposition being presented.

The use of diagrams as an effective tool for explaining complicated ideas was well established by the thirteenth century, as this discussion has shown. Macrobius, for example, in the fourth century, had intended that diagrams be included in his *Commentary on the Dream of Scipio*, writing: "Since our eyes often open the way to the understanding of a problem, it would be well to draw a diagram."[67] This type of explanatory image was found in encyclopaedias and other scholarly texts including Lambert of St.-Omer's *Liber Floridus* or Isidore of Seville's *Entymologies*.[68] The variety and beauty of these diagrams, and the wealth of surviving manuscripts are now receiving increasing attention.[69]

Matthew Paris used diagrammatic imagery as an important part of his work and showed his awareness of its ability to communicate quickly and without excessive explanation. His fascination with the potential of diagrams was expressed not just in his depictions of the heptarchy and of genealogies, but also in more specific images such as wind diagrams. His copy of William of Conches's *Dragmaticon* reveals this commitment and his passion. The possession of this manuscript amongst his *oeuvre* also shows his interest in furthering his understanding of the wider world. William's own use of these diagrams demonstrates his interest in conveying scientific information and ideas to his readers simply and unambiguously, overcoming the difficulty of conveying this material in written form. Matthew Paris shared this interest in exploring and conveying ideas and information in visual form. The frequent appearance of maps, wind diagrams and other

67 Macrobius, *Commentary on the Dream of Scipio*, trans. Stahl, 175.

68 De Coene, de Reu, and de Maeyer, *Liber Floridus*, 75–88.

69 See for example Kühnel, *End of Time*; Kühnel, "Carolingian Diagrams, Images of the Invisible," 359–89; Obrist, "Wind Diagrams," 33–84; Ramirez-Weaver, "William of Conches," 1–41.

images reveal his active engagement with such forms and appreciation of their potential to enrich his work. His love of diagrams is not only seen in their proliferation throughout all his manuscripts but also in the care with which he drew them. It also reveals this was more than a passing fancy. Matthew Paris's decorative but robust treatment of diagrams move them beyond the strictly functional into a major feature of the manuscripts.

Bibliography

Manuscripts

Cambridge, Corpus Christi College, MS 16.
Cambridge, Corpus Christi College, MS 26.
Cambridge, Corpus Christi College, MS 385.
Cambridge, University Library, MS Dd.9.78.
Eton, College Library, MS 96.
London, British Library, MS Cotton Julius D. VII.
London, British Library, MS Cotton Nero D.I.
London, British Library, Royal MS 4 D VII.
London, British Library, MS Royal 14 C. VII.
Manchester, Chetham Library, MS 6712.
Oxford, Corpus Christi College, MS 2.
Oxford, Bodleian Library, MS Ashmole 304.

Primary Sources

Macrobius. *Commentary on the Dream of Scipio*. Translated by William Harris Stahl. New York: Columbia University Press, 1952.

Matthew Paris. *Chronica Majora*. Edited by H. R. Luard. 7 vols. London: Rolls Series, 1872–84.

William of Conches. *A Dialogue on Natural Philosophy (Dragmaticon Philosophiae)*. Translated by Italo Ronca and Matthew Curr. Notre Dame: University of Notre Dame Press, 1997.

Secondary Sources

Binski, Paul, and Stella Panayatova. *The Cambridge Illuminations: Ten Centuries of Book Production in the Medieval West*. London: Harvey Miller, 2005.

Bogen, Steffan, and Felix Thürlemann. "Jenseits der Opposition von Text und Bild: Überlegungen zu einer Theorie des Diagramms und des Diagrammatischen." In *Die Bildwelt der Diagramme Joachims von Fiore: Zur Medialität religiös-politischer Programme in Mittelalter*. Edited by Alexander Patschovsky, 1–22. Ostfildern: Thorbecke, 2003.

Cohen, Adam S. "Diagramming the Diagrammatic: Twelfth-Century Europe," In *The Visualization of Knowledge in Medieval and Early Modern Europe*. Edited by Marcia Kupfer, Adam S. Cohen, and J. H. Chajes, 383–404. Turnhout: Brepols, 2020.

Collard, Judith. "Art and Science in the Manuscripts of Matthew Paris." *Medieval Chronicle* 9 (2014): 79–116.

——. "*Flores Historiarum* Manuscripts: The Illumination of a Late Thirteenth-Century Chronicle Series." *Zeitschrift für Kunstgeschichte*, 71, no. 4 (2008): 441–66.

——. "Gender and Genealogy: English Illuminated Royal Genealogical Rolls from the Thirteenth Century." *Parergon* n.s.17 (2000): 11–34.

——. "King John and the Symbol of the Falling Crown in the Chronicles of Matthew Paris." *Studies in Medieval and Renaissance History* 3rd ser., vol. 6 (2009): 35–52.

De Coene, Karen, Martine de Reu and Philippe de Maeyer. Liber Floridus *1121: The World in a Book.* Tielt: Lannoo 2011.

Eastwood, Bruce. *Ordering the Heavens: Roman Astronomy and Cosmology in the Carolingian Renaissance.* Leiden: Brill, 2007.

——. *The Revival of Planetary Astronomy in Carolingian and Post-Carolingian Europe.* Aldershot: Ashgate, 2002.

Evans, Michael. "Geometry of the Mind." *Architectural Association Quarterly*, 12, no. 4 (1980): 32–55.

Hamburger, Jeffrey F. *Diagramming Devotion: Berthold of Nuremberg's Transformation of Hrabanus Maurus's Poems in Praise of the Cross.* Chicago: University of Chicago Press, 2020.

Hamburger, Jeffrey F. "Mindmapping: The Diagram as Paradigm in Medieval Art—and Beyond." In *The Visualization of Knowledge in Medieval and Early Modern Europe.* Edited by Marcia Kupfer, Adam S. Cohen, and J. H. Chajes, 61–86. Turnhout: Brepols, 2020.

Hamburger, Jeffrey F., David J. Roxburgh and Linda Safran, eds. *The Diagram as Paradigm: Cross-Cultural Approaches.* Washington: Dumbarton Oaks Research Library and Collection, 2022.

Iafrate, Allegra. *Le Moine et le Hasard: Introduction au facsimile du MS Ashmole 304.* Paris: Garnier, 2015.

——. "'Si sequeris casum, casus frangit tibi nasum': La raccolta delle sorti del MS Ashmole 304." *Aevum* 85 (2011): fasc. 2, pp. 457–88.

——. "Of Stars and Men: Matthew Paris and the Illustrations of MS Ashmole 304." *Journal of the Warburg and Courtauld Institut*e 76 (2013): 139–77.

——. "The Workshop of Fortune: St Albans and the Sortes Manuscripts." *Scriptorium* 66 (2012): 55–87.

James, M. R. *A Descriptive Catalogue of The Manuscripts in the Library of Corpus Christi College Cambridge.* 2 vols. Cambridge: Cambridge University Press, 1912.

Kühnel, Bianca. "Carolingian Diagrams, Images of the Invisible." In *Seeing the Invisible in Late Antiquity and the Early Middle Ages: Papers from "Verbal and Pictorial Imaging: Representing and Accessing Experience of the Invisible, 400–1000" (Utrecht, 11–13 December 2003).* Edited by Giselle de Nie, Karl F. Morrison, and Marco Mostert, 359–89. Turnhout: Brepols, 2005.

——. *The End of Time in the Order of Things: Science and Eschatology in Early Medieval Art.* Regensburg: Schnell and Steiner, 2003.

Kupfer, Marcia. "The Rhetoric of World Maps in Late Antiquity and the Middle Ages." In *The Visualization of Knowledge in Medieval and Early Modern Europe.* Edited by Marcia Kupfer, Adam S. Cohen, and J. H. Chajes, 61–86. Turnhout: Brepols, 2020.

Kupfer, Marcia, Adam S. Cohen, and J. H. Chajes, eds. *The Visualization of Knowledge in Medieval and Early Modern Europe.* Turnhout: Brepols, 2020.

Laborderie, O. de "*Genealogiae orbiculatae*: Matthew Paris and the Invention of Visual Abstracts of English History." In *Thirteenth Century England, XIV: Proceedings of the Aberystwyth and Lampeter Conference, 2011.* Edited by Janet Burton, Phillipp Schofield, and Bjorn Weiler, 183–202. Woodbridge: Boydell and Brewer, 2013.

Lewis, Suzanne. *The Art of Matthew Paris in the* "Chronica majora." Berkeley, University of California Press, 1987.

Lutz, Eckhard Conrad, Vera Jerjen, and Christine Putzo, eds. *Diagramm und Text: Diagrammatische Strukturen und die Dynamisierung von Wissen und Erfahrung*. Wiesbaden: Reichert, 2014.

Monroe, W. H. "A Roll-Manuscript of Peter of Poitiers' *Compendium*." *Bulletin of the Cleveland Museum of Art* 65 (1978): 92–107.

Monroe, W. H. "13th and Early 14th Century Illustrated Genealogical Manuscripts in Roll and Codex: Peter of Poitiers' *Compendium*, Universal Histories and Chronicles of the Kings of England." 3 vols. PhD diss., University of London, Courtauld Institute of Art, 1989.

Morgan, Nigel. *Early Gothic Manuscripts 1190–1250*. London: Harvey Miller, 1982.

Murdoch, John E. *Album of Science: Antiquity and the Middle Ages*. New York: Scribner, 1984.

Obrist, Barbara. "Guillaume de Conches: Cosmologie, physique du ciel et astronomie; Textes et images." In *Guillaume de Conches: Philosophie et science au XIIe siècle*. Edited by Barbara Obrist and Irene Caiazzo, 123–96. Florence: SISMEL, 2011.

——. "The Idea of a Spherical Universe and its Visualisation in the Earlier Middle Ages (Seventh to Twelfth Century)." In *The Visualization of Knowledge in Medieval and Early Modern Europe*. Edited by Marcia Kupfer, Adam S. Cohen, and J. H. Chajes, 229–58. Turnhout: Brepols, 2020.

——. "William of Conches, Māshā'allāh and Twelfth-Century Cosmology." *Archives d'histoire Doctrinale et Littéraire du Moyen Age* 76 (2009): 29–87.

——. "Wind Diagrams and Medieval Cosmology." *Speculum*, 72, no. 1 (1997): 33–84.

Page, Sophie. "Medieval Magical Figures: Between Image and Text." In *The Routledge History of Medieval Magic*. Edited by Sophie Page and Catherine Rider, 432–57. London: Routledge, 2019.

Ramirez-Weaver, Eric M. "'So that You Can Understand This Better:' Art, Science, and Cosmology for Courtiers in William of Conches' *Dragmaticon Philosophiae*." In *Diagramm und Text: Diagrammatische Strukturen und die Dynamisierung von Wissen und Erfahrung*. Edited by Eckhard Conrad Lutz, Vera Jerjen, and Christine Putzo, 319–48. Wiesbaden: Reichert, 2014.

Ramirez-Weaver, Eric M. "William of Conches, Philosophical Continuous Narration and the Limited Worlds of Medieval Diagrams." *Studies in Iconography* 30 (2009): 1–41.

Taylor, Eva G. R. "The 'De Ventis' of Matthew Paris." *Imago Mundi* 2 (1937): 23–26.

Thomson, Rodney M. *A Descriptive Catalogue of the Medieval Manuscripts of Corpus Christi College, Oxford*. Cambridge: Brewer, 2011

Vaughan, Robert. *Matthew Paris*. Cambridge: Cambridge University Press, 1953.

Wallis, Faith. "Visualizing Knowledge in Medieval Calendar Science: A Twelfth-Century Family of 'Graphic Glosses' on Bede's *De Temporum ratione*." In *The Visualization of Knowledge in Medieval and Early Modern Europe*. Edited by Marcia Kupfer, Adam S. Cohen, and J. H. Chajes, 291–326. Turnhout: Brepols, 2020.

——. "What a Medieval Diagram Shows: A Case Study of 'Computus.'" *Studies in Iconography* 36 (2015): 1–40.

Worm, Andrea. "Visualizing the Order of History: Hugh of Saint Victor's *Chronicon* and Peter of Poitiers' *Compendium Historiæ*." In *Romanesque and the Past: Retrospection in the Art and Architecture of Romanesque Europe*. Edited by John McNeill and Richard Plant, 243–63. Leeds: Maney, 2013.

ASTROLOGY: SCIENCE OR DIVINATION?

THE EXAMPLE OF ASTRO-METEOROLOGY

ANNE LAWRENCE-MATHERS

MODERN UNDERSTANDING OF the nature and uses of medieval astrology is still often affected by the assumption that it was primarily focused on the casting of birth horoscopes and the making of predictions concerning the futures of individuals. This view is partially supported by the fact that medieval condemnations of astrologers and their works tend only to mention these "judicial" or "genethliacal" types of astrology. However, such condemnations were never intended to describe all of medieval astrology, and there were several forms which were accepted not simply as unproblematic but actually as socially useful. One of these was weather forecasting by astrological techniques, which came to be known as "astro-meteorology," and this chapter will focus on that as an important example of valued astrology. The question of the power of celestial bodies over earthly phenomena such as winds, rain, and storms is also one of special relevance to this volume. It raises important issues concerning both the perceived boundaries of the natural and permissible sources of knowledge. This problem, of the difficulty of precise distinction between activities which harnessed "occult" natural powers and those which involved demonic contacts, was also an ongoing concern for medieval theologians.

Lack of clarity on the term astrology itself, as well as on types of astrological practice and their levels of spiritual danger, is already found in key patristic sources on the topic. This ambiguity continued throughout the medieval period, which can make exact translations of texts into modern English problematic. St. Augustine, whose hostility to "astrology" is frequently cited, confessed to having been deeply interested in it when younger. In his very influential *On Christian Doctrine* he defined casters of birth-charts (*genethliaci*) as followers of a specific form of superstition. He acknowledged that these practitioners, called *mathematici* in Latin, were only one type of astrologer, and that they worked hard to establish the accurate positions of the planets and stars at the time of someone's birth. Their error, which was a serious one, was in making predictions which denied free will and made human beings "the slaves of Mars or Venus or all the stars." It was this, not the practical difficulties which made such horoscopes faulty, which made these practitioners so dangerous. Their beliefs and predictions are placed "in the same class as if they were leagues and covenants with devils."[1]

---

1 Augustine, *On Christian Doctrine*, bk. 2, chaps. 20–22. See *De doctrina Christiana*, ed. and trans. Green.

Anne Lawrence-Mathers is Professor of Medieval History at the University of Reading and a Fellow of the Royal Historical Society and the Society of Antiquaries. Her other publications include: (with Carolina Escobar-Vargas) *Magic and Medieval Society* (2014); *The True History of Merlin the Magician* (2012); *Medieval Meteorology* (2019).

However, even Augustine, in this same text, is clear that the movements of the stars conform to fixed patterns, set by God, which order times and seasons. Moreover, as he points out, knowledge of the course of the moon is widespread and is central to the calculation of Easter each year. Knowledge of the movements of other heavenly bodies, although much scarcer, "involves no superstition" and is impressive in some ways for granting the possibility of making "sure calculations" concerning the positions of celestial bodies in the past and the future as well as the present.[2] The danger lies in the seductive possibility of gaining "information as to our own acts and fates" which is pernicious madness.[3] It is important that the concept of "astronomy" is not invoked here as a distinct category, and neither are all forms of astrology classed together. A very similar stance is expressed in the discussion of the luminaries as "signs" in Augustine's commentary *On the Literal Meaning of Genesis*. Chapter 14.29 of this work dismisses the superstitious observation of such signs as "sheerest folly." But reading the celestial bodies as signs which: "forecast the weather" through the changing seasons; can help travellers; and enable the calculation of calendars and the precise measurement of time, is both good and useful.[4] From this evidence it can be argued that Augustine accepted that it was appropriate and useful for humans to create and apply knowledge concerning the cycles of celestial bodies and their relationship to changes in the natural world below on Earth. However, he did not attempt to produce an overview as to the exact natures and powers of the planets, or just how their influences worked.

Also important, though less often discussed by historians, are the views of St. Jerome, especially in his commentary on the biblical story of Daniel. Chapter 2, verse 2 of that book includes a list of the various practitioners of divination and magical arts in the service of King Nebuchadnezzar. This leads Jerome into brief discussions of the problems of translating from Hebrew and Greek into Latin in these cases. Once again, key terms in analysing astrology are *genethliaci* and *mathematici*, which apply to those who cast birth horoscopes.[5] These are less sinister than those whose divinations involve sacrificed animals, blood and dead bodies, but are viewed negatively. More ambiguous are the *magi*. Jerome records that the term has come to be used for malevolent enchanters, but does not entirely accept this since the word was originally applied to the Chaldean philosophers who studied the stars. Moreover, it was this study which led the experts to Bethlehem when they followed the star. Having pointed out this discrepancy, Jerome refrains from passing further judgement.[6]

---

2 For the ecclesiastical "science" of computus, and the complex calculations underlying the Church calendar, see Nothaft, *Scandalous Error*.

3 Augustine, *On Christian Doctrine*, bk. 2, chap. 29.

4 Augustine, *Literal Meaning of Genesis*, trans. Hill, 208. See also Nothaft, *Scandalous Error*, chaps. 1 and 2.

5 Jerome, *Commentary on Daniel*, trans. Archer, 24.

6 Jerome, *Commentary on Daniel*, trans. Archer, 25. Medieval interpretations of the astrological expertise of the magi are helpfully discussed in Collins, "Scholastics, Stars, and Magi."

A much fuller attempt to make sense of terms for experts in types of astrology, and their relationship to practitioners of other forms of superstitious and magical prediction, is provided by Isidore of Seville, in Books 3.24–71 and 8.9 of his *Etymologies*. This remained a key reference work from the seventh to the twelfth century. Unfortunately, Isidore's handling of the issue, together with its varied presentation in manuscripts, created further ambiguity. The key section of text is in Book 8 and headed *De magis*, which in some ways echoes Jerome's comment on the widening meaning of that term. However, "magi" are only explicitly discussed in the first part, with attention switching to practitioners of divination thereafter.[7] This has led leading historians of magic to conclude that, for Isidore, magic and divination were one and the same. Perhaps most influential has been Lynn Thorndike's view that "from the first Isidore identifies magic and divination" in this section.[8]

That conclusion has perhaps been over-emphasized, since elsewhere Isidore uses "magi" less pejoratively. Thorndike himself points out that Isidore states, in his discussion of the mathematical subjects of the *quadrivium*, that astrology is only superstitious in parts, with other parts being acceptable as study of the natural world.[9] This refers to Book 3.27, on the difference between astronomy and astrology, where Isidore accepts that astrological study of the movements of the planets and their positions at chosen times is licit. Astrology becomes superstitious, and the terrain of *mathematici*, when attempts are made to practise augury by the stars or to link zodiac signs to parts of the human soul, or to make predictions about chosen individuals.[10] Yet in the section *De magis* the familiar terms *genethliaci*, *mathematici*, and *horoscopi* are listed together with *astrologi* and *magi* as a subgroup of diviners. Such confusion is perhaps best explained by the fact that the tools required for the types of precise calculations needed to draw up detailed astronomical charts had ceased to be available in the Latin West and did not return until the twelfth century. Simpler substitutes were available, as discussed below, but did not conform to the late-classical descriptions. Ambiguity of learned terminology was thus a puzzle for those engaged in textual commentary but not an immediate issue for those dealing with living people and their errors.

That was certainly the case, for instance, for Bede, writing about a century later than Isidore and with reference to his works. In his textbook on the calculation of the Christian calendar, *De temporum ratione* (The Reckoning of Time), he expounds on the calculation of the positions of the sun and moon on the ecliptic and thus in relation to the zodiac. These rather basic matters are treated as presenting some difficulties for students, and there is no sense that they will be able to work out the longitudes of other planets. Even in his more wide-ranging work on natural philosophy, *De natura rerum* (On the Nature of Things), he is only able to add general information on the spheres of

7 Klingshirn, "Isidore of Seville's Taxonomy."

8 Thorndike, *A History of Magic*, 1:629.

9 Klingshirn, "Isidore of Seville's Taxonomy."

10 Isidore of Seville, *Etymologies*, trans. Barney et al., 181–83 and 99.

the planets and the time taken by each to complete a circuit around the earth.[11] The first serious change in this situation was presented in the late tenth century by the arrival of the collection of texts now known as the *Alchandrean corpus* or *Liber Alchandrei*.

This was a collection of short, primarily astrological or divinatory treatises which, like other books offering new and strange knowledge, linked much of its contents to Alexander the Great and his supposed tutor, Aristotle. Several of its treatises claimed to make it possible to offer astrological predictions—although no technical, astronomical knowledge of planetary positions was required.[12] These texts were clearly based on or translated from treatises in Arabic, and incorporated names and terms transliterated from both Arabic and Hebrew. Some Greek terminology is also apparent. The compilation, in its Latin form, was almost certainly made in Catalonia and in a Christian context. Surviving manuscripts give it varying titles, sometimes using the name *Mathematica Alhandrei summa astrologi*, which clearly transgresses the condemnations of the Church Fathers.

The texts assume that the user will be giving advice to someone seeking answers to questions concerning the outcomes of illness, marriage, or business and legal affairs. This is the traditional function of the *mathematici* and is clearly problematic. Even more so is the provision of methods of identifying key elements of a birth horoscope. The basic method is of clear Arabic origin since it uses lunar mansions, something which had not previously appeared in any Latin text. Happily for the client who did not know their date and time of birth, all that was needed was their name together with that of their mother (or sometimes the day in a lunar month most closely related to the question). These were to be written down in accordance with the instructions given, and the numerical values attributed to their component letters (in a table provided) were to be added together. The total was divided by twenty-eight and the remainder could then be applied to the numbered list of lunar mansions. Ideally the indicated mansion would be placed within the 30° of the ecliptic occupied by a zodiac sign, and the relevant sign would thus be the client's "ruling sign." A similar, though simpler, procedure was expounded for the identification of the planet ruling a client's birth horoscope.

However, the same process could be used, together with a diagram known as the *Sphere of Apuleius*, or *Sphere of Life and Death*, to deduce whether a sick person would or would not recover.[13] Augustine had not condemned medical applications of astrology; and it is also possible that priests would value guidance as to whether to give extreme unction to a sick person. Similarly, there was no ban on study of the courses and positions of the planets—Augustine had simply emphasized the practical difficulties involved in making calculations with any degree of accuracy. Therefore, the instructions concerning the movements of the planets, found in some manuscripts together with the

---

11 Bede, *The Reckoning of Time*, trans. Wallis, 54–63; *On the Nature of Things*, trans. Kendall and Wallis, 80–87.

12 For texts included in the collection see Juste, *Les Alchandreana primitifs*. Juste provides editions of the texts, based on a corpus of seventy-one manuscripts, together with a full commentary.

13 See chapter by Joanne Edge in this volume.

core Alchandrean texts, were not problematic in themselves; and nor was their claim to be derived from the work of Ptolemy of Alexandria. Such information is found, for instance, in the volume which is now London, British Library, Harley MS 2506, together with texts and images taken from prestigious works of classical astronomy.[14] This manuscript was possibly produced in the abbey of Fleury ca. 1000, but the Alchandrean texts continued to be used in the twelfth century and enjoyed a revival in popularity during the Renaissance. An example of a twelfth-century copy of selected texts is found in London, Wellcome Collection, MS 21.[15] This in fact appears to be a part of a larger volume, but now contains two versions of the *Sphere* together with a treatise on the powers of the planets and an anonymous text on physiognomy.

A much greater advance in Latin knowledge of the science of the stars began to gather speed in the twelfth century, originating in newly-Christian-dominated regions of Iberia and carried from there by enthusiastic scholars. An impressive part of this was an impressive and fascinating Islamicate astronomical device, the astrolabe.[16] Even this very important piece of new technology did not make it possible on its own to draw up the kind of horoscope needed for full natal or judicial astrology. What it did offer was nevertheless revolutionary and provided incontrovertible evidence of the superiority of Islamicate astronomical science. For a start, an astrolabe came equipped with interchangeable plates, calibrated to represent the heavens as observed from specific locations. The appropriate plate was used together with the overlaying "star-net" or *rete*, whose pointers made it possible to locate and identify major stars.[17] The accompanying instructions advised not only on how to construct an astrolabe but also on how to use it for such practical applications as telling the time, measuring distances, and measuring heights or depths.[18] An astrolabe could also be used to measure the exact location (to fractions of a degree) of readily identifiable planets such as the sun and the moon. The instructions explain that the same procedure could also be used to establish the position of any other visible planet.[19]

---

14 A digitized version of this manuscript is available on the British Library website at: www.bl.uk/manuscripts/FullDisplay.aspx?ref=Harley_MS_2506 (currently unavailable, May 10, 2024).

15 This manuscript has been digitized and can be viewed online at: https://wellcomecollection.org/works/ufns95hv (accessed May 10, 2024).

16 See Burnett, "King Ptolemy"; and McCluskey, *Astronomies and Cultures*, 179–80

17 For a helpful commentary on the parts of an astrolabe see the website of the Whipple Museum of the History of Science in Cambridge: www.whipplemuseum.cam.ac.uk/explore-whipple-collections/astronomy/medieval-astrolabe/parts-astrolabe.

18 A helpful, brief account of the development, construction, and uses of Islamicate astrolabes by Emily Winterburn is at: https://muslimheritage.com/using-an-astrolabe/ (accessed May 10, 2024). For discussion of the study of the astrolabe in medieval England see Falk, *The Light Ages*. The same author's website offers very helpful blog posts and videos on medieval astronomy and technology: www.sebfalk.com/blog.

19 An extremely useful edition and translation of the most important thirteenth-century Latin compilation on the astrolabe has been published online by Ron Thomson at: https://shareok.org/handle/11244/14221.2 (accessed May 10, 2024).

The tool which made it possible both to identify visible planets and to calculate the positions of planets not currently visible, was a set of planetary tables. These covered all seven planets, as well as the nodes of the moon (the points at which the observed path of the moon crossed the ecliptic). The latter move through the zodiac and were often treated as if they were planets. The tables were based on the work of Claudius Ptolemy, drawn up ca. 150 CE, as part of his great astronomical work, the *Mathematical Compilation* or *Almagest.* Ptolemy's tables were updated and revised by Islamicate astronomers and mathematicians, drawing upon Hindu and Persian sources as well as the work of many prominent Arabic astronomers. This meant that the tables first translated into Latin, especially those produced for use in al-Andalus, were based on much more recent observations, and on latitudes closer to locations such as Paris or London. However, they still presented many challenges to new users, and it is a tribute to their perceived value that so many scholars worked so hard to overcome these difficulties.[20] Not the least of the problems was that the differing models and assumptions underlying varying early versions of the tables could produce results at odds with one another.[21]

A particular problem was that an early Latin translation, popularized especially in England, was of the *Zīj* of al-Khwārizmī (d. ca. 850), as updated for Cordoba in the late tenth century by Maslama al-Majrīṭī (d. ca. 1007). These were the tables used by Adelard of Bath, who brought his Latin version to England.[22] The original tables had used the Persian year (of 365 days) and the era of Yazdegird III, but Maslama revised them for the Arabic lunar calendar and the Hijra era. Some tables were also recalculated for the meridian of Cordoba, although the introductory instructions in the Latin version continued to use the mysterious city of Arim as "the central place of the earth" and to explain that "the corrections for the planets and [the reckoning] of time are made with reference" to it.[23] Less likely to cause confusion were the more up to date *Toledan Tables*. These were put together in about 1080 and for the meridian of Toledo, as the name suggests. The leading astronomer on the project was al-Zarqālī, known in Latin as Azarquiel (d. ca. 1100), usually named as the author of the tables in the Latin versions. These tables drew on the earlier works, as well as providing new figures for some planets, including the sun.[24] A scholar equipped with tables like these, and with the mathematical ability to adapt them for a specific location and date, could draw up horoscopes for individual clients, for communities, or for the benefit of those ruling medieval states and kingdoms. Inevitably this would mean that it was much more

---

20 For full presentation and discussion see *Computational Astronomy*, ed. Chabas.

21 A helpful outline is given by Chabás and Goldstein, "Computing Planetary Positions."

22 See Burnett, ed., *Adelard of Bath*.

23 For the tables see *The Astronomical Tables of al-Khwarizmi*, ed. Neugebauer. For brief details of al-Majriti see Vernet and Samsó, "The Development of Arabic Science in Andalusia." See also Mercier, "Astronomical Tables in the Twelfth Century."

24 More than two hundred copies of the Latin versions of the Tables of Toledo are cited in *The Toledan Tables*, ed. Pedersen. This supersedes the work of Toomer, "A Survey of the Toledan Tables"; but Toomer's discussion of the variations in the tables included in the hundred manuscripts he used remains helpful.

possible for precisely the type of astrological enquiry which the Church Fathers had condemned to be undertaken, alongside enquiries concerning "natural" phenomena such as weather. That being the case, it is hardly surprising that the great scholastic theologians of the thirteenth century showed a revived concern with the examination, definition and judgement of the varying types of astrology which were once again possible. Once again, their debates reveal much about what was perceived as "natural" in the case of astrology.

Many such judgements were apparently passed on the basis of theory, without the theologian engaging directly in astrological practice. However, there were some exceptions to this rule, with one such being the scholarly bishop of Lincoln, Robert Grosseteste (ca. 1170–1253). In his early treatise *On the Liberal Arts* (ca. 1200) Grosseteste already referred with confidence to technical terminology from the "modern" study of the stars. Indeed, he here asserted that astronomical/astrological knowledge was fundamental not only to proper understanding of natural philosophy but also to successful work in areas such as farming, medical healing, and the transmutation of metals. He even states that "lower nature does not act except when celestial power moves it"[25] and goes on to explain that the moon plays a crucial role in mediating and transmitting the influences of the other planets as they pass through its sphere on the way down to Earth. The first part of this may sound surprising but is in fact in line with the views of both St. Augustine and Thomas Aquinas. In Part One of his *Summa theologica* (completed by 1269) Aquinas deals with the powers of the stars over earthly things (in Question 115) and quotes Augustine to confirm that: "Bodies of a grosser and inferior nature are ruled in a certain fashion by those of a more subtle and powerful nature."[26] Planetary influences are thus placed safely within the natural workings of the created universe.

In the same passage Grosseteste also shows understanding of technical matters, such as whether a planet is at mid-heaven, and whether it is in "aspect" with other planets (in other words whether its position in the zodiac is separated from those of other planets by a significant number of degrees). It will be clear that judgement on such questions required knowledge of specific planetary positions. Grosseteste says that a positive aspect between the waxing moon and a fortunate planet, such as Jupiter, could have very beneficial results for crops planted at that time; but an aspect with the cold, destructive force of Saturn would damage the plants, as would an aspect with the burning heat of Mars.[27] Moreover, even in his condemnation of judicial astrology, Grosseteste does not hesitate to show his technical expertise. He asserts that the claims of judicial astrologers depend upon their ability to calculate not only planetary positions and aspects but also celestial houses, ascendancies, and much more, to a level which is in fact impossible.

25 Grosseteste, *De artibus liberalibus*, chap. 11. See *The Scientific Works of Robert Grosseteste*, vol. 1, *Knowing and Speaking*, ed. Gaspar, 88–89.

26 Thomas Aquinas, *Summa theologica*, 1a q.115. The relevant passages are available at: www.newadvent.org/summa/1115.htm (accessed May 10, 2024).

27 *De artibus liberalibus*, 88–91

This criticism was made in Grosseteste's *Hexaemeron*, or commentary on the creation, which is one of his later works; however, even here, he notes the positive comments of the Fathers concerning the planets as signs of coming weather.[28]

Grosseteste's criticisms could not have been made without knowledge of astrological textbooks, such as the widely-known *Introductorium in astronomiam* of Abu Maʿshar (written before 900 and twice translated into Latin before 1150). The use of "astronomy" in the most frequent Latin title for this work is significant for demonstrating continuing looseness in terminology, despite the increased attention being given to superstitious applications.[29] A leading figure in this critical attention was Aquinas, whose views on the powers of higher bodies were mentioned above. After a long exposition of the categories of effects and events of which the stars cannot be the cause, and which they also cannot predict, he then specifies: "On the other hand if one were to apply the observation of the stars in order to foreknow those future things that are caused by heavenly bodies, for instance, drought or rain and so forth, it will be neither an unlawful nor a superstitious divination."[30]

Grosseteste's details concerning practical problems suggest more personal study of the science of the stars than that of Aquinas. It is significant that his example is taken not from judicial astrology but from what Isidore called "natural" astrology—which was coming to be known as "mundane" or world astrology. He outlines the problems of drawing up a chart for the "revolution of the year" (in other words, the moment of the Sun's entry into the sign of Aries, closely related to the timing of the vernal equinox), something which was central to making predictions concerning the forces acting upon weather, agriculture, and human health in the relevant year. As the discussion above shows this was not viewed as divination or superstition; however, Grosseteste asserts, astronomers could not "exactly identify this revolution of the year for a given location." Islamicate astronomers had in fact found ways to deal with the problem; but personal experience informs Grosseteste's reference to "those who have laboured hard with astronomical calculations and tables." Thus, while such applications of astrology were not superstitious, practitioners were guilty of fraudulent claims.

These distinctions were very clear in theory. However, in intellectual centres such as universities there was an ever-growing body of work involving applications of the science of the stars, such that it was very difficult in practice to keep track of it all. This made it necessary to commission the critical survey and catalogue of works in the field,

---

28 Grosseteste, *Hexaemeron*, eds. Dales and Gieben, especially Part Five, chaps. 7, 8 and 9. For translation of relevant passages see *Robert Grosseteste: On the Six Days of Creation*, trans. Martin, 164–68.

29 For discussion of the reception and importance of Abu Maʿshar's work see Lemay, *Abu Maʿshar and Latin Aristotelianism*. It is worth noting that Adelard of Bath had translated a shorter version, giving only the "practical instructions" in this work rather earlier, in the 1120s. See Abu Maʿshar, *The Abbreviation of the Introduction to Astrology*, ed. and trans. Burnett et al.

30 Thomas Aquinas, *Summa theologica*, 2a2ae q.95, art. 5: www.newadvent.org/summa/3095.htm#article5 (accessed May 10, 2024).

known as the *Speculum astronomiae* and attributed to Albertus Magnus.[31] This work lists and discusses an impressive range of titles, drawing on older booklists in the process. Overall, it provides a survey of the state of knowledge concerning all branches of the science of the stars by the 1260s, together with clear statements that many necromantic works were being concealed under that heading.

Helpfully, Chapter One confirms that the Latin term *astronomia* covered two different areas of study. The first, which dealt with the structure of the cosmos and the regular movements of the heavenly bodies, corresponded to the modern definition of astronomy and was defined as "a great wisdom." Both planetary tables and astrolabes are included here. More complex is the "science of the judgements of the stars" which is subdivided into valuable and detestable parts. The former is defined as knowledge of the ways in which changes in the heavenly bodies bring about changes in material things on Earth. It is acknowledged that this was acquired from other languages, but that does not detract from its importance. Chapters Four and Five of the *Speculum astronomiae* provide a short textbook on the basics of this valuable science, including the zodiac signs, houses, planets, and technical terminology. Works by Ptolemy of Alexandria, Albumasar (Abu Maʿshar), and numerous others are commended. This leads into a summary of how to interpret the "revolutions" of the planets, all of it dependent on being able to make the sorts of calculations discussed by Grosseteste. The problem of establishing the exact time of the Sun's entry into Aries, and its correlation with the equinox, is sidestepped. What is discussed instead is the astrological "new year," defined as the planetary positions at the new or full Moon immediately preceding the Aries entry.[32]

As noted above, this was crucial for forewarning of impending events in relation to things such as floods, storms, droughts, earthquakes, disasters, crops, and animal herds. All these would affect food supply, food prices, and human health, and were thus of great economic and political significance. As Chapter Seven of the *Speculum astronomiae* states: "this information shows what God, who is glorious and sublime, will bring about in a given year, through the applications of the stars, on the rich men of some climes and on the whole of their populations, concerning the price of grain, whether there is war or peace, earthquake and floods, falling stars and terrible prodigies, and other such things." On a more detailed level, a survey is also provided as to how the movements of the planets affect the atmosphere surrounding the Earth and thus bring about changes in the weather. This is the core of what came to be known as astro-meteorology, and shows that it was always closely related to the making of judgements concerning the impacts of weather as well as forecasts of the weather itself. Detailed knowledge of the techniques involved is shown here, together with an impressive list of works on the subject, demonstrating the level of importance attributed to this field of knowledge. Terminology taken from Latin translations of Arabic texts is used, including both the lunar mansions and the concept of "gates of the moon" which determined whether and when rain would fall.

---

31 For discussion of the authorship and importance of this work see Giralt's chapter above. For full discussion and translation see *The* Speculum astronomiae *and Its Enigma*, trans. Zambelli.

32 *The* Speculum astronomiae *and Its Enigma*, trans. Zambelli, 208–31.

A reading list of five key works is provided, starting with the relevant parts of Ptolemy's *Quadripartitus* (Work in Four Parts) and proceeding through both direct translations of Arabic texts and what were claimed as new compositions by Latin authors.

Subsequent parts of the *Speculum astronomiae* turn to the much more problematic branches of the science of the stars, and deal not only with genethliacal and judicial astrology but also with texts instructing on the making and uses of images and talismans. These sought to draw on the powers not only of stars and planets but also of "spirits" associated with them. The proliferation of such necromantic and divinatory texts, and their adoption of misleadingly reassuring titles, were significant parts of what led to the survey and report underlying the *Speculum*.

How then were astro-meteorological forecasts—or prognostications, to use the medieval term—made? The basics were set out in Ptolemy's *Quadripartitum*. This established the various natures and powers of the planets, their inter-relationships with one another and with the climatic zones of the Earth, and then the role of such technicalities as Houses and Exaltations. These latter are important because of their perceived effect on the inter-relationships, and the degrees of power, of the planets. For instance, if two planets with differing powers are placed opposite one another in the zodiac then their effects might simply cancel one another out. However, if one planet is placed in a sign or house which enhances its power—or, obviously, which weakens it—then the outcome will be significantly affected. If a planet was "retrograde" that should also be taken into consideration, as should whether it was moving closer to another, slower-moving planet.

The idea of the "New Moon of the year," and its significance for choosing the date for which to draw up a detailed chart or horoscope in order to make a prediction, is explained in Book Two.[33] Chapter 11 of this book lists the general weather conditions associated with each sign of the zodiac, and the subdivisions of each sign, while Chapter 12 is titled "The Investigation of the Weather in Detail." Longer-term forecasts are to be made by taking the date of a new Moon and drawing up a chart for a specific location (using Ptolemy's planetary tables). Monthly, weekly and even daily forecasts can be produced by bringing increasingly technical details into the interpretation of the chart, including the risings and setting of powerful stars and their positions in relation to the Sun.

The wide-ranging, updated textbooks on the science of the stars, written in the ninth and tenth centuries by Islamicate scholars, included techniques based on Ptolemy's work—but also added new concepts and procedures. These drew on developments in both astronomical observation and mathematics, which made it possible to update Ptolemy's planetary tables and to produce a new response to the problem of the precession of the equinoxes. However, the philosopher who achieved the earliest recognition in the Latin world specifically for his expertise in weather forecasting was al-Kindi. This great,

33 Unfortunately, there is no modern, critical edition and translation of a twelfth-century, Latin version of this work. Most are based on the Greek original or a later, abridged paraphrase known as the "Proclus Paraphrase." The thirteenth-century version of William of Moerbeke, based on a Greek text, is now: *Ptolemy's Tetrabiblos in the Translation of William of Moerbeke*, eds. Vuillemin-Diem and Steel.

ninth-century expert on both natural philosophy and the science of the stars wrote a long work *On the Revolutions of the Years of the World* which was translated first into Hebrew and then (in 1278) into Latin. However, extracts and short treatises ("Letters") on the causes and forecasting of meteorological phenomena were sought out earlier and translated into Latin under the title *De mutatione temporum* (On Weather Changes).[34] This survives in thirty manuscript copies, which is a high total for such a technical work. Part of its attraction was probably that it did not deal with weather forecasting in isolation, but set it within an overview of the forces which cause atmospheric and meteorological changes, and those which cause heat, cold, dryness, and wetness. The fundamental driving force is stated to be the physical movements of the planets, since these generate energy and, especially, heat. This basic heating process is magnified by the power of the Sun, and modified by the changing position and force of the Sun in relation to the Earth. Actual weather, and its fluctuations in any given locality, are modulated by the interactions between the Sun and other planets, and between pairs and groups of those other planets, as they also move and interact. Someone equipped with the tools and basics provided by Ptolemy should now be able to produce a forecast for any chosen date and place, without any need to call upon spirits or intelligences.

However, al-Kindi goes further than this and identifies specific planetary positions and groupings as especially significant. Practical help for the making of prognostications is given by tables, setting out planetary combinations and assigning values for the level of heat each will generate. Again, pride of place is given to the Sun. As in Ptolemy, the Moon is identified as playing the next important role in determining the weather, due to its power over the elements of both earth and water. Twelve key points in the Moon's circuit of the Earth are identified, and at each the relationship between the Moon and the Sun must be examined in detail. The significance of this is that it will make possible a forecast of coming winds, since cooler air will contract and hotter air will then expand into those zones, both causing winds of varying strengths and determining their directions. For a full weather forecast the positions of all the planets must be established, so that their groupings can be identified. The final stage is the calculation of the relative strengths of these groupings. For this, the astrometeorologist must also chart the aspects between each planet and each grouping, and apply expert judgement to interpret their overall outcomes. This will include attention to the effect on each planet of the qualities of the zodiac sign in which it is placed at the time in question.

That may sound time-consuming but in fact a full forecast needed to take still further factors into account. Of these, perhaps most important was whether a planet was moving around the zodiac in the "normal" direction or was moving in reverse (retrograde). However, the lunar mansions—which have already been mentioned—should also be considered, since these sections of the zodiac could also affect the qualities and strength of planets occupying them. Like the zodiac signs, the lunar mansions were based on stellar groupings. In this case, twenty-eight major stars or star-groups were

---

34 See Bos and Burnett, *Scientific Weather Forecasting*; and Burnett, "Weather Forecasting in the Arabic World."

fundamental; and their identifications and evaluations were accepted as having been made by Indian astrologers. Each mansion had a name and a set of qualities; and, at least for purposes of weather-forecasting, they were increasingly significant.[35] What was particularly useful was that they established four key times each month when the Moon's position would be especially influential in relation to the weather. This removed the need for frequent forecasts, since the forecast for each key time would hold until the next. However, some activities were so time-sensitive that daily forecasts were still required. Since the time needed for this was considerable, and the supply of astro-meteorologists able to make such forecasts was limited, it follows that these were available only to the rich and powerful.

That fact, together with concerns about the practical difficulties of full-blown astrometeorology, may underlie the ongoing production of new treatises offering "improved" ways of making forecasts. Several of these, issued under the names of highly-regarded experts in the science of the stars, set out the favoured method and tips of the expert in question. One such was Guido Bonatti, who enjoyed a very successful career in Italy, working for Guido da Montefeltro (1223–1298), ruler of Urbino, amongst others. Bonatti wrote an encyclopaedic survey of astrology, which is notable for its practical approach and its lasting popularity.[36] This had six main parts, one of which was entirely devoted to the subject of astrometeorology. An edited version of Bonatti's work, with expensive illustrations, was presented to King Henry VII of England and is now in the British Library as MS Arundel 66.[37] The section on weather forecasting is here headed "On Deluges and Airs" (*De ymbribus et aeris*) and begins on folio 243v.[38] Bonatti provides both information on the wet and dry mansions of the Moon and a table of all the mansions, as well as guidance on when Saturn is likely to be powerful enough to prevent rain. This practicality is taken further in the reduction of technical details and the provision of brief guides on likely outcomes when the Moon is in specified aspects with each of the other planets. Whether the king would have made personal use of these materials is unknown; but scholars or physicians in attendance on his court would have been able to do so, and without causing anxiety about illicit divination.

However, one thirteenth-century treatise took a more radical approach. This is an anonymous text, widely believed in the medieval period to be the work of Grosseteste, entitled *De impressionibus aeris* (On Atmospheric Impressions).[39] It sets out a highly

---

35 For discussion see Burnett, "Weather Forecasting, Lunar Mansions and a Disputed Attribution."

36 The text was edited by Johannes Angelus and printed in Augsburg, 1491, by Erhard Ratdolt; also in Venice by Penzio, 1506; and in Basel, 1550, by Jakob Kundig. The Ratdolt edition is accessible from the website of the Bayerische Staatsbibliothek: https://bildsuche.digitale-sammlungen.de/index.html?c=viewer&bandnummer=bsb00025600; for the Basel version see http://hardenberg.jalb.de/display_page.php?elementId=5363 (both accessed May 10, 2024).

37 On this manuscript see Fronska, "The Royal Image and Diplomacy."

38 The manuscript has been digitized and can be seen here: www.bl.uk/manuscripts/FullDisplay.aspx?ref=Arundel_MS_66 (currently not available).

39 For the text see *Die philosophischen Werke des Robert Grosseteste*, ed. Baur. Extracts are given in English translation in Dales, *The Scientific Achievement of the Middle Ages*, 65–67.

simplified method for making an astro-meteorological weather forecast and then argues that such work is a duty for good Christians since it will enable provisions to be made against coming disasters and famines. This reads like a textbook for those who have no wish to become fully trained astrologers but do accept the need to be able to make prognostications of the weather. It survives in seventeen manuscripts, so was clearly less popular than Bonatti's work, but is interesting for its demonstration of the social and practical value attributed to astrometeorology. The procedure involves the drawing of a circular diagram, comprising eight concentric circles, divided into thirty-degree segments. Each planet is then entered into the correct sign for the chosen day, using tables not provided, and the power of each in the relevant sign can be found in the text. The technical issue of aspects is much easier to handle, since the circular diagram makes them directly visible. This method effectively reduces the judgement of the interactions between planets to a matter of simple arithmetic, and makes it possible to produce a weather forecast very quickly. No interest is shown in theory, and an even more pedagogical note is struck by the "worked example" of a forecast for April 15, 1249, with an illustrative diagram. It is also noted that the forecast was correct. This leads into the forecast that July 1249 would be unusually hot and dry and that provision must be made against this, and also against the famine likely to result from the long stay of Saturn in the sign of Capricorn, which would begin in 1255 and last for five years. Both estate managers and those with a duty to provide charity for the starving would be interested in such guidance.

This analysis has strongly suggested that by the end of the thirteenth century the distinction between "mundane" astrology and judicial or genethliacal astrology was both clear and long-established. The value placed upon the benefits provided by the first is demonstrated by a compelling quantity of evidence. What had been a new science of the stars had gained a place in natural philosophical studies as well as in medicine; but its value was not purely academic, as the careers of famous figures like Guido Bonatti and Michael Scot demonstrate. Of course, the very fact that Bonatti and Scot were credited with providing secret advice to their patrons, Guido da Montefeltro and the Emperor Frederick II, meant that they were suspected of indulging in the forbidden forms of astrology as well as the "natural" ones. However, there was no condemnation of all types of astrology. Indeed, knowledge of the regular movements of the celestial bodies, with at least basic understanding of how these related to such things as seasonal patterns of weather, daylight and tides, became more widely available.

At the level of university study this was provided by textbooks such as *De sphaera mundi* (On the Sphere) by John of Sacrobosco (written ca. 1230). Moreover, something almost akin to a space race was under way by the fourteenth century, in the form of the appearance of publicly-displayed astronomical clocks. Basic clock-making had been a recognized trade, at least in Cologne, since the late twelfth century, and trade was good enough for that city to have a street of clockmakers by 1220. In 1232 the Emperor Frederick II received from the Sultan of Damascus a much more advanced, astronomical clock. This had "images" of the Sun and Moon which moved mechanically around models of their courses and thus "infallibly" indicated the hours of both day and night. Its value was estimated at the impressive figure of more than 20,000 marks, but the chronicler sounds still more impressed by its scientific accuracy.[40] The clock designed by Richard of Wallingford for his abbey of St. Albans is impressively described in his treatise *Tractatus Horologii Astronomici* (On the Astronomical Clock, 1327) was one of the earliest recorded. This clock does not survive but at least parts of others which were completed before the end of the fourteenth century remain in Wells, Rouen, and Bad Doberan.[41] Equally impressive was the development of *equatoria* which provided schematic, working models of celestial orbits and positions. These were made up of discs bearing graduated scales, which simulated the movements of the planets.[42]

Nevertheless, the science of the stars remained a challenging field of study, as the appearance of new "teaching aids" in the fourteenth century demonstrates. A leading figure in this pursuit was John of Saxony, who was trained in Paris in the 1320s. By 1327 he had composed a new set of "canons" or instructions for using the Alfonsine Tables, which was rapidly followed by a textbook designed to introduce Latin readers to the basic concepts and procedures of mundane astrology.[43] In a later work he moved on to produce a detailed guide to the Tables, even providing worked examples for Paris in 1355. He also drew up an *Almanach scilicet temporale* (effectively a set of lists of ready-calculated planetary positions) for 1336 to 1380, for the meridian of Paris. This innovation heralded the production of more such ready-calculated tables, often combined with medical and health advice, for wealthy patrons.

The increasing integration of astrology into medical theory and practice, like its use for weather prediction, did not end hostility on the part of theologians towards judicial and genethliacal astrology. Accordingly, experts went out of their way to support mundane astrology. John of Eschenden, writing in Oxford in the 1340s, wrote a *Summa iudicialis de accidentibus mundi* (Summa on Mundane Astrology)[44] which rebutted criticisms. He and his work achieved a very positive reputation after the disaster of the Black Death, since he successfully claimed to have predicted that catastrophe as early as 1345, on the basis of eclipses and planetary conjunctions. Evidence that Eschenden's skills were valued is provided by commissions for him to draw up astro-meteorological forecasts.[45] One of these covering the years 1368 to 1374, opens with five charts for major planetary conjunctions in 1365. These conjunctions laid down the prevailing conditions

---

40 Part 7 (*continuatio IV*) of *Chronica regia Coloniensis*, ed. Waitz, 263 (www.dmgh.de/mgh_ss_rer_germ_18/index.htm#page/263/mode/1up, accessed May 10, 2024).

41 See Falk, *The Light Ages*; on Richard of Wallingford's achievements see North, *God's Clockmaker*.

42 For an overview see North, "The Quadrivium." For discussion of the equatorium see Falk, *The Light Ages*, chap. 7; and "Vernacular Craft and Science."

43 Translations of extracts from John's "Rules" or canons, with extracts from his "edition" of the Tables, are provided in *A Source Book in Medieval Science*, ed. Edward Grant (Cambridge, MA: Harvard University Press, 1974), 465–88.

44 John's name appears in different forms. Thorndike, who has given the fullest account of John's works in *A History of Magic*, 3:325–46, uses Eschenden. John North prefers the form Ashenden; see for instance "Astrology and the Fortunes of Churches," in his *Stars, Mind and Fate: Essays in Ancient and Mediaeval Cosmology* (London: Hambledon, 1989).

45 These are found in Oxford, Bodleian Library, MSS Ashmole 192 and 393.

for the forecast, while two in 1369 would further affect the years from 1370. On these bases Eschenden forecasts a prolonged period of disturbed weather, with floods likely up to 1370 and droughts in the last three years.

Such forecasts were clearly immensely valuable if correct but always open to error. This may well be the driving force behind a clear trend in the fourteenth and fifteenth centuries towards improving their accuracy. Interest in checking forecasts against actual weather is demonstrated in surviving manuscripts from Oxford, Wurzburg, and (probably) Basel. The earliest example is found in Bodleian Library, MS Digby 176, where weather is recorded from January 1337 to January 1344 in *Consideraciones temperiei pro 7 annis Christi* ("Notes on Weather for 7 Years").[46] Their author, William Merle, has been identified as rector of Driby, Lincolnshire, but had repeated licences to live and study in Oxford. His notes on weather relate both to Oxford and Lincolnshire and accompany both work on natural "signs" of coming weather and study of astrometeorology. The records from Wurzburg and Basel are slightly different in approach, since they are embedded into textbooks on mundane astrology and on astro-meteorology in particular. Both seem to record past weather as evidence that astro-meteorological techniques would have been able to predict it.[47] A curious fact is that no instructions for making astro-meteorological predictions are found in treatises and collections concerning agriculture and estate management. These contain only simple guides to the positions and interactions of the Sun and Moon, together with short prognostic texts, at most. The implication of this is that full forecasts continued to be the preserve of the highly trained expert.

That conclusion is further supported by the instant popularity of the annual forecasts of weather, economic conditions, and largescale disasters (including war) when they began to be part of the duties of university-based professors of astronomy and astrology in the fifteenth century. Competition for such experts, and their predictions, is shown by the frequency with which they moved from one centre to another and the speed with which their prognostications were rushed into print. Charles V had sponsored a chair in Paris in 1379, and this was quickly followed by others. John of Gmunden, who died in 1442, was the first professor of astronomy at Vienna, and he was succeeded by Georg Peurbach, who was also employed by Ladislaus V of Hungary and the Emperor Frederick III. Experts were in place at the universities of Bologna, Padua, Louvain, Krakow, Ingolstadt, Leipzig, Wittenberg, and Salamanca (to name only those with surviving records) during the fifteenth century.

46 For facsimiles of the weather records, with accompanying translation, see William Merle, *Merle's MS.*, ed. Symons. Brief details on Merle's career, with notes on his meteorological terminology, are given in the *Dictionary of Medieval Latin from British Sources* at: www.dmlbs.ox.ac.uk/web/william-merle-consideraciones-temperiei.html (accessed May 10, 2024).

47 The Wurzburg record is now Nuremberg, Stadtbibliothek, MS Cent V 64, part 1. It is discussed in Thorndike, *A History of Magic*, 3:143–46. The Basel manuscript is Basel, Universitätsbibliothek, MS F. III. 8. A digital facsimile is available at: www.e-codices.unifr.ch/en/list/one/ubb/F-III-0008 (accessed May 10, 2024). For discussion see Thorndike: "A Weather Record for 1399–1406" and "A Daily Weather Record from the Years 1399 to 1401." The later article is followed by a "Climatological Analysis" by Frederick, Landsberg and Lenke.

The career of Joannes Vesalius illustrates the demand for these predictions and forecasts. This Vesalius studied at Cologne and Pavia before coming to the new University of Louvain/Leuven in 1429. By 1455 he was one of the most important physicians in Brussels and was also being consulted and paid by Duke Philip the Good of Burgundy. Already in 1430 the council of Louvain commissioned from him an almanac (or set of planetary calculations) and accompanying prognostication for 1431. This was presumably successful, since others are recorded for 1439 and 1440, and he was commissioned to produce later almanacs for the duke. When Jan van Westfalen, Leuven's first printer, arrived in the 1470s he began almost immediately to publish annual prognostications of this type, thus making them more widely available. The production of such forecasts was speeded up by the growing availability of ready-calculated *Calendars* or *Almanacs* showing full sets of planetary positions, and eclipses, for periods of several years. Most celebrated of all such works was that of Johann Müller, better known as Regiomontanus, whose work was printed by Ratdolt, the publisher of many astronomical and astrological works. Indeed, Ratdolt's first publication in Venice was Regiomontanus' *Calendar*, issued in 1476, and followed in 1481 by the *Ephemerides*.[48] Both were reissued many times, and in rival editions. Publications of printed prognostications, with accompanying tables of varying complexity, spread across Europe alongside printing workshops themselves. Demand was such that they were a main source of income for printers, and became the basis of a lucrative monopoly for the Crown and the Company of Stationers in seventeenth-century England, despite ongoing literary satires.

Strikingly, support for astro-meteorology survived both the new discoveries of astronomers in the sixteenth and seventeenth centuries and the rising persecution of witches and practitioners of magic. Astro-meteorology was practised and strongly supported by Tycho Brahe (1546–1601) and Johannes Kepler (1571–1630) amongst others.[49] Moreover, sales of almanacs remained respectable until the end of the eighteenth century.[50] Astro-meteorology both gave rise to and was finally subsumed into the increasing trend of keeping weather diaries and delivering reports to the learned societies which sprang up across Europe. This was very different from the fate of horoscopic astrology and emphasises the complex yet fundamental differences between different branches of the medieval "science of the stars."

48 A digital copy of Ratdolt's version of Regiomontanus' *Ephemerides* 1484–1506 is hosted online by the Europeana website. The work belongs to the University of Vienna. A rival edition, also produced in Venice, but in 1498, can be viewed via the Gallica website at: https://gallica.bnf.fr/view3if/ga/ark:/12148/bpt6k596433 (accessed May 10, 2024).

49 On Brahe see Adam Mosley, "Tycho Brahe and Weather Prediction," (Cambridge: Department of History and Philosophy of Science, University of Cambridge, 1999), at: www.sites.hps.cam.ac.uk/starry/tychoweather.html (accessed May 10, 2024). For Kepler's *Ephemerides* see vol. 11, pt. 1 of *Johannes Kepler Gesammelte Werke*.

50 See Kassell, "Almanacs and Prognostications"; and Capp, "The Potter Almanacs." The classic work on the subject remains Capp's *English Almanacs*. The most recent survey is that of Kusukawa, "Incunables and Sixteenth-Century Books."

Bibliography

Manuscripts

Basel, Universitätsbibliothek, MS F III 8.
London, British Library, MS Arundel 66.
London, British Library, MS Harley 2506.
London, Wellcome Collection, MS 21.

Primary Sources

Abu Maˁshar. *The Abbreviation of the Introduction to Astrology: Together with the Medieval Latin Translation of Adelard of Bath*. Edited and translated by Charles Burnett, Keiji Yamamoto, and Michio Yano. Leiden: Brill, 1994.

Al-Khwarizmi. *The Astronomical Tables of al-Khwarizmi*. Edited by Otto E. Neugebauer. Historisk-filosofiske Skrifter, Det Kongelige Danske Videnskabernes Selskab. 4, no. 2. Copenhagen: Munksgaard, 1962.

Les Alchandreana primitifs. Edited by David Juste. Leiden: Brill, 2007.

Augustine. *De doctrina Christiana*. Edited and translated by R. P. H. Green. Oxford: Clarendon, 1995.

——. *The Literal Meaning of Genesis*. Translated by Edmund Hill, in *The Works of St Augustine: A Translation for the 21st Century*. Part 1, Vol. 13, *On Genesis*. New York: New City, 2002.

Bede. *The Reckoning of Time*. Edited and translated by Faith Wallis. Liverpool: Liverpool University Press, 1999.

——. *On the Nature of Things*. Translated by Calvin B. Kendall and Faith Wallis. Liverpool: Liverpool University Press, 2010.

Bonatti, Guido. *Liber astronomiae*. Edited by Johannes Angelus. Augsburg: Erhard Ratdolt, 1491.

Brahe, Tycho. *De Nova stella, 1573*. Copenhagen: Regia Societas Scientiarum Danica, 1901.

Chronica regia Coloniensis. Edited by Georg Waitz. MGH SS rer. Germ. 18. Hannover: Hahn, 1880.

Computational Astronomy in the Middle Ages: Sets of Astronomical Tables in Latin. Edited by José Chabás. Estudios sobre la Ciencia 27. Madrid: Consejo Superior de Investigaciones Cientificas, 2019.

Isidore of Seville. *The Etymologies of Isidore of Seville*. Edited and translated by Stephen A. Barney, W. J. Lewis, J. A. Beach, and Oliver Berghof. Cambridge: Cambridge University Press, 2006.

Jerome. *Commentary on Daniel*. Translated by Gleason Archer. Grand Rapids: Baker, 1958.

Kepler, Johannes. *Ephemerides novae motuum coelestium*. Edited by Volker Bialas. Vol. 11 part 1 of *Johannes Kepler Gesammelte Werke*. Munich: Beck, 1983.

Mashaˀallah (Pseudo-). *On the Astrolabe*. Edited and translated by Ron Thomson. Toronto, 2020 (https://shareok.org/handle/11244/14221.2).

Merle, William. *Merle's MS. Consideraciones temperiei pro 7 annis. Per Magistrum Willelmum Merle, socium domus de Merton: The earliest known journal of the weather: kept by the Rev. William Merle, Rector of Driby, Lincolnshire 1337–1344*. Edited by George J. Symons. London: Stanford, 1891.

Regiomontanus, *Ephemerides 1484–1506*. Venice: Ratdolt, 1506. Available at: https://www.europeana.eu/portal/en/record/9200209/o_225215.html.

Robert Grosseteste. *De artibus liberalibus*. In *The Scientific Works of Robert Grosseteste*. Edited and translated by Giles E. M. Gasper et al. Vol. 1, *Knowing and Speaking*. Oxford: Oxford University Press, 2020.

——. *Hexaemeron*. Edited by Richard C. Dales and Servus Gieben. Oxford: Oxford University Press for British Academy, 1982. Translated by C. Martin, *Robert Grosseteste: On the Six Days of Creation*. Oxford: Oxford University Press for British Academy, 1996.

—— (attrib.). *De impressionibus aeris*. In *Die philosophischen Werke des Robert Grosseteste, Bischofs von Lincoln*. Edited by Ludwig Baur. Münster: Aschendorff, 1912.

The Speculum astronomiae *and Its Enigma: Astrology, Theology, and Science in Albertus Magnus and His Contemporaries*. Translated by Paola Zambelli. Dordrecht: Kluwer, 1992.

Thomas Aquinas, *The Summa Theologica of St. Thomas Aquinas*. 2nd (rev.) ed. London: Burns, Oates, and Washbourne, 1920.

——. *Summa theologiae*. Translated by Fathers of the English Dominican Province. New York: Benziger, 1947–48. The Aquinas Institute. https://aquinas.cc/la/en/~ST.I. Also at www.newadvent.org/summa.

The Toledan Tables: A Review of the Manuscripts and the Textual Versions. Edited by Fritz S. Pedersen. 4 vols. Historisk-filosofiske Skrifter 24, Det Kongelige Danske Videnskabernes Selskab. Copenhagen: Reitzel, 2002.

William of Moerbeke. *Ptolemy's Tetrabiblos in the Translation of William of Moerbeke*. Edited by Gudrun Vuillemin-Diem and Carlos Steel. Leuven: Leuven University Press, 2015.

Secondary Sources

Bos, Gerrit and Charles Burnett. *Scientific Weather Forecasting in the Middle Ages*. London: Kegan Paul, 1999.

Burnett, Charles. "King Ptolemy and Alchandreus the Philosopher: The Earliest Texts on the Astrolabe and Arabic Astrology at Fleury, Micy and Chartres." *Annals of Science* 55 (1998): 329–68.

——. "Weather Forecasting in the Arabic World." In *Magic and Divination in Early Islam*. Edited by Emilie Savage-Smith, 201–10. Aldershot: Ashgate, 2004.

——. "Weather Forecasting, Lunar Mansions and a Disputed Attribution; the *Tractatus pluviarum et aeris mutationis* and *Epitome totius astrologiae* of 'Johannes Hispalensis'." In *Islamic Thought in the Middle Ages (Studies in Text Transmission and Translation in Honour of Hans Daiber)*. Edited by Anna Akasov and Wim Raven, 219–66. Leiden: Brill, 2008.

——, ed. *Adelard of Bath: An English Scientist and Arabist of the Early Twelfth Century*. Edited by Charles Burnett. Warburg Institute Surveys and Texts 14. London: The Warburg Institute, 1987

Capp, Bernard. *English Almanacs, 1500–1800: Astrology and the Popular Press*. Ithaca: Cornell University Press, 1979.

——. "The Potter Almanacs." *Electronic British Library Journal* 2004, article 4 (11 pp.).

Chabás, José and B. R. Goldstein. "Computing Planetary Positions: User-Friendliness and the Alfonsine Tradition." *Journal for the History of Astronomy*, 44 (2013): 257–76.

Collins, David J. "Scholastics, Stars, and Magi: Albert the Great on Matthew 2." In *The Sacred and the Sinister: Studies in Medieval Religion and Magic*. Edited by David J. Collins, 255–76. University Park: Pennsylvania State University Press, 2019.

Dales, Richard C. *The Scientific Achievement of the Middle Ages*. Philadelphia: University of Pennsylvania Press, 1973.

Falk, Seb. *The Light Ages: A Medieval Journey of Discovery*. London: Allen Lane and Norton, 2020.

——. "Vernacular Craft and Science in the *Equatorie of the Planetis*." *Medium Ævum* 88 (2019): 329–60.

Frederick, Ralph H., Helmut E. Landsberg, and Walter Lenke. "Climatological Analysis of the Basel Weather Manuscript." *Isis* 57 (1966): 99–101.

Fronska, Joanna. "The Royal Image and Diplomacy; Henry VII's *Book of Astrology* (British Library, Arundel MS 66)." *Electronic British Library Journal* 2014, article 7 (28 pp.).

Kassell, Lauren. "Almanacs and Prognostications." In *The Oxford History of Popular Print Culture*. Vol. 1, *Cheap Print in Britain and Ireland to 1660*. Edited by Joad Raymond), 432–45. Oxford: Oxford University Press, 2011.

Klingshirn, William E. "Isidore of Seville's Taxonomy of Magicians and Diviners." *Traditio* 58 (2003): 59–90.

Kusukawa, Sachiko. "Incunables and Sixteenth-Century Books." In *Thornton and Tully's Scientific Books, Libraries and Collectors*. Edited by Andrew Hunter, 115–63. 4th ed. London: Routledge, 2016.

Lemay, Richard J. *Abu Maʿshar and Latin Aristotelianism in the Twelfth Century: The Recovery of Aristotle's Natural Philosophy Through Arabic Astrology*. Beirut: American University of Beirut, 1962.

McCluskey, Stephen C. *Astronomies and Cultures in Early Medieval Europe*. Cambridge: Cambridge University Press, 1998.

Mercier, Raymond. "Astronomical Tables in the Twelfth Century." In *Adelard of Bath: An English Scientist and Arabist of the Early Twelfth Century*, edited by Charles Burnett, 87–118. Warburg Institute Surveys and Texts 14. London: The Warburg Institute, 1987.

North, John. "The Quadrivium." *A History of the University in Europe*. Edited by W. Ruëgg. Vol. 1, *Universities in the Middle Ages*, edited by Hilde de Ridder-Symoens, 337–58. Cambridge: Cambridge University Press, 1992.

——. *Stars, Minds and Fate: Essays in Ancient and Medieval Cosmology*. London: Hambledon, 1989.

——. *God's Clockmaker, Richard of Wallingford and the Invention of Time*. London: Hambledon, 2005.

Thorndike, Lynn. *A History of Magic and Experimental Science*. 2 vols. New York: Columbia University Press, 1923.

——. "A Weather Record for 1399–1406 AD." *Isis* 32 (1940): 304–23.

——. 'A Daily Weather Record from the Years 1399 to 1401." *Isis* 57 (1966): 90–99.

Toomer, G. J. "A Survey of the Toledan Tables." *Osiris* 15 (1968): 5–174.

Vernet, Juan, and Julio Samsó. "The Development of Arabic Science in Andalusia." In *Encyclopedia of the History of Arabic Science*, ed. Roshdi Rashed, 1:243–75. 3 vols. London: Routledge, 1996.

MAGIC AND SCIENCE IN THE MIDDLE AGES

THE BUILDING OF THE BOUNDARIES BETWEEN NATURAL MAGIC AND NECROMANCY, ca. 1230–ca. 1310

SEBASTIÀ GIRALT

LEARNED MAGIC ARRIVED in Western Europe along with the other bodies of knowledge from the Greco-Arabic tradition thanks to the Latin translations that were completed primarily on the Iberian Peninsula during the twelfth and thirteenth centuries. In contrast to sorcery and other practices hitherto disdained by the intellectual elites as rural superstitions, learned magic enjoyed considerable power of attraction and prestige due not only to its world view and complex techniques but also to the authority conferred by its ancient, often mythical origins. When the new natural sciences and occult arts spread throughout Western Europe, university scholars were faced with the need to filter them to integrate them into high culture if they were considered licit, or if not, strongly refute them by means of faith and reason.

Thus, it was primarily during the thirteenth century that theologians and natural philosophers began to distinguish between two types of learned magic. One, which we can call natural magic, is compatible with religion and included in the sciences, insofar as it seeks to know and exploit those mechanisms of nature that are hidden, because they elude rational knowledge. The other type, usually called necromancy, and currently referred to as ritual, ceremonial, or addressative magic, is seen as incompatible with religion, as it is aimed at the domination of spirits, which the scholastics always consider to be demons, with the objective of using their power. Therefore, the natural or supernatural causality attributed to one or the other is the basis for differentiating between natural magic and necromancy. Causality is the factor that distinguishes both types of magic from rational knowledge, since the causes attributed to them, whether natural or supernatural, are occult.

This chapter seeks to review the opinions of scholastic thinkers during the key period from the thirteenth century to the beginning of the fourteenth century, in order to define exactly what can be considered natural magic, as opposed to necromancy, and to discern which bodies of knowledge and practices concerning the occult were perceived by the intellectual elites as licit and which were considered dangerous or forbidden.

Sebastià Giralt is a senior lecturer of Classics (Latin) at the Universitat Autònoma de Barcelona. His research has primarily focused on Latin and Romance texts regarding medieval medicine, magic, and astrology, especially related to the Crown of Aragon and Arnau de Vilanova.

Occult Properties and Natural Magic

In the intellectual circles of late medieval Latin Europe, it was common to postulate the existence of hidden properties in nature, with diverse nomenclature, which establish a relationship between all the elements of the universe and are the cause of portentous effects in our world. This is what Nicolas Weill-Parot referred to as the "natural occult."[1] Hereinafter, we will use the name "natural magic" to refer to the use and study of these properties in writings on the natural world and medicine, although during the Middle Ages, this nomenclature was used only by William of Auvergne and only became widespread during the Renaissance. In contrast, late medieval authors tended to restrict the term "magic" to illicit practices. Most of them attributed the origin of occult properties to the stars. Such properties served to justify such diverse phenomena as the attractive force of magnets, certain virtues attributed to stones, animals or herbs, the electric discharges of the ray, premonitions, or the evil eye, with the common denominator being that they existed outside the rational framework of natural scholastic philosophy.

The only medieval scholar to use the term natural magic (*magica naturalis*) to refer to the science (*scientia*), that is the study of the wonders "that nature works with the virtues infused by God," was William of Auvergne in his works *De legibus* (1228–1230) and *De universo* (1236–1240). William, theologian and bishop of Paris, considered natural magic to be the eleventh part of natural science and equivalent to what philosophers called, very improperly, "necromancy according to physics" (*nigromantia secundum physicam*).[2] Of course, this should not be confused with "necromancy" in the more usual sense of demonic magic but in the general sense of "magic."[3] According to William, it was not possible to comprehend the numerous and amazing "occult virtues," although their effects are found in the books of researchers and in those on secrets and admirable virtues of animals.[4] According to him, such occult virtues function on the basis of sympathetic and antipathetic relations between them by their *aspectus* and *habitudo* within the framework of a cosmic connection (*colligantia*).[5] This doctrine with its neoplatonic roots would be set aside by later theorists on occult properties.[6]

The more general conception of occult properties was developed in the medical field, based on Galen, the treatise *De physicis ligaturis* attributed to Costa ben Luca,[7] and Avicenna. Avicenna developed the most influential formulation of these properties within the framework of his pharmacological theory set forth in the *Canon*, which was translated by Gerardo da Cremona in the twelfth century, and in *De viribus cordis* which

---

1 Weill-Parot, *Points aveugles de la nature*, 25–136; Draelants, "Notion of 'Properties.'"

2 *De legibus*, 24, William of Auvergne, *Opera*, 1:69; *De universo*, 1.1.43, William of Auvergne, *Opera*, 1:648.

3 Sannino, "*Nigromantia secundum physicam.*"

4 *De universo*, 2.3.22 and 2.1.32, William of Auvergne, *Opera*, 1:1060 and 1:883.

5 *De universo*, 1.1.46 and 2.2.75, William of Auvergne, *Opera*, 1:657 and 1:930.

6 Weill-Parot, *Points aveugles de la nature*, 103–5.

7 Wilcox and Riddle, "Qusta ibn Luqa's Physical Ligatures."

was translated by Arnau de Vilanova in the last third of the thirteenth century. In the *Canon*, Avicenna explains these properties by the perfection of matter coming from the *forma specifica* or, according to the Galenic expression, *a tota substantia*, beyond the primary qualities and the complexion.[8] In the Latin version of *De viribus cordis*, it is called *proprietas*, and its cause is attributed to "a superior influence," which would be "a divine emanation" according to another passage.[9] Weill-Parot has convincingly argued that the *proprietas* is infused by the "giver of forms," one of the intelligences emanating from the first intellect, which proceeds from God.[10] However, Latin authors interpret this as being due to the influence of the stars.

The theologian Albertus Magnus appeared open to natural magic in his works on nature, in which he claimed to have collected information on animal, vegetable, and mineral substances with amazing virtues coming, not from their components or composition, but brought about in the species as a whole by the faculties of heaven or the soul, understood through experience (*experimentum*) and used by the magicians. If one is well-acquainted with the *virtus celestis*, as he called it, one can employ natural means to achieve everything that can be achieved by means of the magical sciences.[11] Albertus made a sharp distinction between licit and illicit magic in his theological writings, but in his natural works he is even interested in necromancy. In my view, he followed the tendency, as he himself acknowledged, to respect the authorities in each of the fields of knowledge he dealt with—religious authorities for theological works, philosophical authorities for the natural sciences and medical authorities for medicine.[12]

Roger Bacon restricted the term "magic" to illicit practices, but at the same time, he referred to amazing natural effects as "secret workings of nature and technology" (*secreta opera nature et artis*). In the set of treatises in which this English Franciscan developed his theory of *scientia experimentalis* between 1266 and 1278, these "secret workings" fall within the scope of what he defines as *scientia experimentalis*; this is one of the specific natural sciences which has its basis in experience, and which the philosopher should employ to discern true science and technology from the fallacies of the magicians.[13] Bacon's criteria for distinguishing between false knowledge and true knowledge were based not only on their moral legitimacy or theological arguments, but also on their utility for philosophy, as the practices and knowledge acquired by illegitimate means are either unreliable or ineffective. More specifically, the criteria he took into account in order to delimit the illicit are as follows: first, astrological determinism; second, invocation by means of conjuring and sacrifices to demons, who act primarily out of spite and may give true or false information; third, the contamination of astral

---

8 Avicenna, *Canon*, fol. 28v.

9 Avicenna, *De viribus cordis*, 125–34.

10 Weill-Parot, *Points aveugles de la nature*, 51–53.

11 Albertus Magnus, *De vegetabilibus*, 474–75; Albertus Magnus, *De mineralibus*, 2.2.10 and 2.3.6; and Albertus Magnus, *Opera omnia*, 5:40 and 55.

12 *Super II Sententiarum*, 13.C.2, Albertus Magnus, *Opera omnia*, 27:247.

13 Bacon, *Opus maius*, 1:392 and 394–96; *Communia naturalium*, 2, Bacon, *Opera*, 2:5 and 9.

observations with circles, figures, meaningless characters, foolish formulas and irrational supplications; fourth, the recourse to fraudulent means, with accomplices, mechanical tricks, and sleight of hand.[14]

Likewise, Thomas Aquinas recognized the existence of natural occult properties and considered their use legitimate. However, his concern was primarily directed towards discerning between occult operations of natural causation and those of supernatural origin, whether diabolical or miraculous. In particular, he devoted an epistle entitled *De operationibus occultis nature ad quendam militem ultramontanum* (ca. 1270), to the causality of what he called the "hidden workings of nature."[15] Aquinas distinguished between workings generated by the form imprinted by the stars (*forma specifica*) and those caused directly by a superior agent (supernatural), because the latter are not found in all individuals of a species, while the former are, insofar as they have their origins in an intrinsic principle of that species. The corollary of his reasoning is that natural occult workings cannot be introduced into an object by means of technology (*ars*).

In the *questio* 5.41 to Aristotle's *Metaphysica*, written during the 1270s, the Averroist philosopher Siger of Brabant advocated for what he understands as "magic," or that which we herein term "natural magic," to be classified as science.[16] Siger framed his own discourse on magic in tacit opposition to those of Aquinas and Avicenna.[17] Faith prevented him from denying the existence of demons and their intervention in the world. However, these questions were not the object of science, which is concerned with universal truths. Therefore, the works of intelligent entities, whether good or evil, were not the subject of science. Thus, Siger considered magic, that which we herein refer to as "natural magic," to be "technology and science" (*ars et scientia*), as opposed to necromancy.

Some of the most illuminating passages defining occult properties are found in two works by physician Arnau de Vilanova: *Speculum medicine* (ca. 1308), and *De parte operativa*, unfinished at his death in 1311.[18] In pharmacological compounds, the primary and secondary qualities, which develop from the primary qualities, can be predicted by means of reason. That said, in addition to these complexional qualities, everything that is created *per naturam* or *per artem*, whether mineral, vegetable, animal or artificial, acquires properties originating from the influence of the stars. Their knowledge and use are truly difficult, because they are accessible only through experience and not by means of reason as are the common qualities. For this reason, Arnau sometimes called them *vires occulte* or *virtus occulta*, although he usually referred to them simply as *proprietas*.[19]

---

14 *Tractatus brevis*, Bacon, *Opera*, 5:1–24; Bacon, *Opus maius*, 1:240–42.

15 Aquinas, *Letter of Saint Thomas Aquinas*.

16 Siger of Brabant, *Quaestiones in metaphysicam*, 279–85.

17 Maurer, "Between Reason and Faith."

18 Arnau de Vilanova, *Speculum medicine*, 142–43 and 254–56.

19 Giralt, "*Proprietas*"; McVaugh, "Development of Medieval Pharmaceutical Theory," 17–20, 115–22, and 249–52.

When speaking of these properties, the distinction made by Arnau and other authors between specific and individual faculties is fundamental. Indeed, the occult properties are called *forma specifica* when they cover the entire species and, therefore, occur in each and every individual of the species, although to varying degrees. But in other cases, the *propietas* is exclusively individual, produced by a fortuitous concurrence of factors, such as the position of the stars at the given moment in which the individual is conceived, born, or in an object of human creation such as astrological figures or images, when its manufacture is completed.

Similar to that of Arnau is the conception of occult properties developed by his contemporary Pietro d'Abano, also a physician, in *Conciliator differentiarum philosophorum et medicorum* (1310). According to him, the differences in the magnitude of the *forma specifica* between individuals of the same species are due to the divergences between their complexions and materials, in addition to the complexions and materials of the external agents that have introduced it into them, i.e., the stars.[20]

Power of the Soul, *Fascinatio*, and Prodigious Faculties

Magical and astrological literature conveys the idea that magicians and astrologers possess extraordinary faculties, either through the power of their souls or due to the astrological conditions that influenced their birth. This question was the subject of great controversy among the scholastics.

The fundamental starting point for the late medieval debate on the power of the soul is Avicenna's *De anima*, 4.2. The latter, after exposing the power of the soul over one's own body, which was accepted by the Latin scholars without reservation, moves on to the subject of its external influence, which is more controversial, because it advocates action at a distance, which was not acceptable in Aristotelian physics, i.e., a soul can naturally influence foreign bodies through *fascinatio*, but in addition, if it is noble, constant and powerful, it can subdue matter to heal or destroy, cause rainfall and fertility or drought and death.[21] Unlike Avicenna, some of the scholastics related it to an astrological influence.[22]

Avicenna's influence can already be found in William of Auvergne, who hesitatingly took up the possibility that the souls of certain animals, such as the basilisk, and of certain persons can work wonders outside their bodies, which are the object of natural magic.[23] It is also from Avicenna, as well as from al-Ghazāli, that Albertus declared having derived the definition of *fascinatio* that he gives in his early commentary on the *Sentences*, 2.7.7.[24] Albertus, however, had reservations, for the reason that neither *fascinatio* nor magical art can harm those whose faith in God is steadfast. Several years later,

20 Federici Vescovini, *Medioevo magico*, 192–204.

21 Avicenna, *Liber de anima*, 65–66.

22 On *fascinatio*, see Delaurenti, "La fascination et l'action à distance."

23 *De universo*, 1.1.43, William of Auvergne, *Opera*, 1:648.

24 Albertus Magnus, *Opera omnia*, 27:153.

however, he no longer expressed such reticence when he related *fascinatio* to the exaltation of man as the only link between God and the world which, coming from the Hermetic *Asclepius*, he took up in *De animalibus* and other writings; men of auspicious birth accomplish wonders, devise incantations, and make prophecies thanks to the power to transmute the bodies that the stars imbue in their souls.[25]

The theory of *fascinatio* appears in some of Bacon's works which were also based on Avicenna. According to the Franciscan, this phenomenon is explained by a contagious faculty received by the bodily complexion of a person born under an inauspicious constellation. With the corrupt vapours and spirits produced by his unfortunate complexion and transmitted primarily through the porosity of his eyes, he contaminates those around him. And if the wickedness of the soul, the burning desire, the conviction of his power, a firm intention and the selection of astral conditions are added in, there can be no doubt that nature obeys his thoughts. The wise men, in contrast, rely on the benevolence of the soul and an auspicious complexion.[26]

Equally inspired by Avicenna, Pietro d'Abano stated that the noblest souls are endowed with exceptional natural faculties that have their origins in the position of the stars at their birth. This gives them the ability to overcome earthly bonds, exercise *fascinatio*, and dominate and transform earthly matter, including healing the sick. This is one of two causes, along with the strength of the patient's imagination which is induced by trust in the physician; here, we see the influence of *De physicis ligaturis* by which the *precantatio*, a formula with therapeutic value, can produce results. For Pietro, *fascinatio* takes place when the soul of the magician, agitated by a violent feeling, alters his body and his eyes, through which he then alters the air, and this in turn alters the body of the one to whom the incantation is directed.[27]

The proliferation of Avicenna's theories of origin around *fascinatio* and the power of the soul met with strong opposition, which was expressed, for example, in their condemnation in 1277 by Étienne Tempier, bishop of Paris, who attacked, among other things, the ideas that one soul can have power over another or that astrological conditioning affects the inclinations of the soul.[28] Likewise, based on Aristotle, according to whom all natural movement works by means of contact, Aquinas explicitly replied to Avicenna in *Summa theologica*, 1a q.117, art. 3 (1270–1272), denying that the human soul has the capacity to affect an external body without an intermediary bodily agent. He recognized only that, through the effect of a particularly powerful imagination, the soul can alter the humours of its own body, particularly in the eyes, through which it affects the surrounding air within a certain radius; common examples include the gaze of a menstruating woman or the venomous gaze of sorceresses. In the latter case, the intervention of the devil cannot be ruled out.

---

25 Sturlese, "Intelletto acquisito e divino."

26 Bacon, *Opus maius*, 1:142–43 and 398–99; *Opus tertium*, Bacon, *Opera*, 1:98.

27 *Differentiae* 64 and 135, Pietro, *Conciliator*, fols. 94v and 191v–192v; Paschetto, *Pietro d'Abano*, 135–37 and 235–42; Delaurenti, *La puissance des mot*, 347–64.

28 *Chartularium*, 549, no. 112 and 555, no. 207.

As for the assertion that, of all men, magicians are graced by the stars, at the moment of their birth, with the power to perform magical operations, in *Summa contra gentiles*, 3.105 (ca. 1260) Aquinas responded that neither celestial bodies nor human words can ever have the power of influencing the intellect.

Siger of Brabant also rejected the explanation developed by Avicenna for *fascinatio*. His argument was not far removed from Aquinas's naturalistic justification, as Siger sought an explanation that would agree with Aristotle and Averroes, i.e., that a soul can only affect a foreign body indirectly, by means of its own body.[29]

The position of Arnau de Vilanova lies somewhere between the two; he accepted the effects of *fascinatio* and the extraordinary faculties of certain individuals without attributing them to the power of the soul or to action at a distance. According to Arnau, people can possess occult properties which are also imbued by the position of the stars at the moment of their birth, and which interact with the faculties coming from the favourable or unfavourable situation in the heavens at the moment the procedure is performed. Therefore, it is thanks to such properties rather than to their operations or instruments that, on certain occasions, some magicians, sorcerers and *fascinatores* perform their operations with great effectiveness, while at other times, or if performed by other people, the failure is absolute. The medium of transmission is the air, which they corrupt or affect with the vapours they emit.

Magical Figures, Words, and Characters

Late medieval theologians and natural philosophers agreed both in rejecting the practices included in magical books that are explicitly addressed to spiritual beings, such as sacrifices, propitiations, fumigations or adorations. Another series of technical resources, among which characters, figures, words and images stand out, require a deeper reflection to discover whether they are of a diabolical character or whether their effects can have a natural origin. In this section, we focus on characters (symbols, letters and other markings), figures (both geometrically based and figurative representations) and the word, meaning an oral formula or incantation (*carmen, incantatio*).[30]

Following Augustine, who considered all magical practices, including characters, formulas, and rituals, as signs of a pact with demons (*De doctrina christiana*, 2.20.30; *De civitate Dei*, 21.6), most detractors of necromancy consider the use of words, formulas, characters, and figures to be a clear line of demarcation between natural magic and necromancy. William of Auvergne argued that, like images, characters, and figures have no effect unless they function as signs by which demons can recognize their worshippers. Therefore, they constitute an obvious indication of the necromancers' pact with the devil. Likewise, William denied that words and formulas have magical power in and

29 Siger, *Quaestiones in metaphysicam*, 287.

30 On the power of the word, see Delaurenti, *La puissance des mots*.

of themselves. They only take effect through the work of the demons whom magicians venerate.[31]

Thomas Aquinas came to the same conclusion as William of Auvergne in affirming that the natural matter of human words are the sounds emitted, and their form is the meaning expressed by the ideas of the mind; therefore, they do not have the capacity to alter a natural body by means of a natural faculty but only by means of a spiritual substance. Likewise, for Aquinas (*Summa contra gentiles*, 3.105–7), characters and figures are signs, because they have no active or passive value in terms of preparing matter to receive a natural effect. Therefore, if they are signs, they must be addressed to intelligent beings, the only beings who can be honoured with the sacrifices and prostrations that are usually addressed to them. Who are these beings? The evil nature of the practitioners of these arts and the means they use, as well as the material and immoral character of their objectives, prove that the targets must be demons. However, even when the purposes are not evil, such as the acquisition of knowledge in the *Ars notoria*, the use of figures and unknown words, and not instituted by God, shows that it is based in an agreement with the devils, which cannot enlighten the intellect (*Summa theologica*, 2a2ae q.95, art. 8).[32] Although he does not state it so clearly, the thoughts of Albertus Magnus on characters and words must not have been very different from those of Aquinas, if several of the allusions scattered throughout his work are taken into account.[33]

For his part, Arnau de Vilanova responded in *De reprobacione nigromantice ficcionis* (1276–1288) to the belief that spirits are naturally subdued by figures, arguing that it is impossible for these, or any other accident, to dominate a substance. The power to coerce demons can be provided to figures neither by their matter nor by their artificer nor by the stars. The words contained in incantations, as the accidents that they also are, are subject to the same limitations and also cannot obtain such coercive capacity from the air, the vocal organs or the soul.[34]

Pietro d'Abano dedicated the *differentia* 156 of the *Conciliator* to the efficacy of enchantment (*precantatio*) which, according to him, derives from an internal cause, the soul, and an external cause, the stars. He who utters it must be a wise man—a doctor or an astrologer—with a good reputation to arouse confidence and must have a strong and well-disposed soul.[35]

The scholastic who went the furthest in accepting the power of signs and words was Bacon. He distinguished between characters and formulas based on astrological conditions and those that are fraudulent. As for the former, he elaborated his theory on the properties of characters, letters, images, formulas and incantations on the basis of the

---

31 *De legibus*, 27, William of Auvergne, *Opera*, 1:89–90; Sannino, "*Nigromantia secundum physicam*."

32 The angelic magic of the *Art notoria* is generally condemned or silenced in the sources here studied. See Véronèse, "L'Ars notoria au Moyen Âge," 112–15, 249–50, 637–47.

33 *Super II Sententiarum*, 7.50.12, Albertus Magnus, *Opera omnia*, 27:163–64; Albertus Magnus, *De vegetabilibus*, 6.1.34 and 7:458.

34 Arnau de Vilanova, *Epistola de reprobacione*, 226–27.

35 Delaurenti, "Pietro d'Abano et les incantations."

ineffable power that the astrologer can imprint on words by selecting the most suitable time thanks to the combined *species* of the rational soul and heaven, which can dominate not only natural beings but even minds, taking into account that the free will cannot be oppugned. Indeed, images, formulas, and characters receive powers from the constellation under which they have been crafted. But workings and words contain still other special faculties, because they also receive power from the soul, if it is rational and righteous. The body also plays a role in the process as an instrument of the soul, because its complexion influences them, as well as the very physical reality of the word, i.e., the form it gives to the air when it is uttered. Therefore, four types of *species*—coming respectively from the stars, the soul, the body and the word—must be considered in order to distinguish between the workings of *scientia experimentalis* and those of *magic*.[36] Baconian theory was developed primarily under the dual influence of al-Kindī's *De radiis*, not referenced, and Avicenna's *De anima*.[37]

The Magic of Images

Images and talismans provide a particularly privileged point of observation for perceiving the diversity of sensibilities and opinions expressed by medieval scholars dealing with the occult arts.[38] These can take the form of statuettes, rings, gems, medals, or engravings (seals) and were among the principal instruments used in magic. The most well-known treatises in this field were *De imaginibus* attributed to Tābit ibn Qurra, which describes talismans for warding off harmful animals or obtaining fortune, wealth, power, and love. But the two twelfth-century versions of this work that circulated were received very differently—the one entitled *De imaginibus*, by Juan de Sevilla, was praised as an example of the art of images by the *Speculum astronomie* and by Bacon. In contrast, the version written by Adelard of Bath, entitled *Liber prestigiorum*, was rejected by the *Speculum*. What was the reason for such a different reception? To understand this, we must first examine the classification of magical images set forth in the *Speculum*, a treatise in defence of astrology, written around 1260, later falsely attributed to Albertus Magnus.[39]

In dealing with that which it terms the "science of images" the *Speculum astronomie* distinguished between three types—the images of the first two usurp the name of astronomy, but are in fact necromantic and should be avoided because of the danger to faith, while those of the third are astronomical.[40] The first category is abominable and

36 *Opus tertium*, Bacon, *Opera*, 1:96–99; Bacon, *Opus maius*, 1:395–97.

37 Fanger, "Things Done Wisely by a Wise Enchanter."

38 The reference study on astrological images between the thirteenth and fifteenth centuries is Weill-Parot, *Les "images astrologiques"au Moyen Âge* (see esp. 40–62, 27–153, 215–302, 316–39, 456–531).

39 Paravicini Bagliani, *Le Speculum astronomiae une énigme?*; *Speculum astronomiae*, ed. Zambelli, 1–41 and 121–25.

40 *The* Speculum astronomiae *and Its Enigma*, trans. Zambelli, 240–50 and 270.

consists of the worst kind of idolatry, as it involves fumigations and invocations. The second type is somewhat less unacceptable but nonetheless detestable—it consists of images with inscribed characters that must be exorcised by certain names.

The third type is more clearly distinct—it consists of a single image, without fumigations, invocations, exorcisms, or inscribed characters, but only engraved at the astrologically propitious moment, after the example of *De imaginibus*. The effects of this type of image come from the *virtus celestis* of the constellations according to whose template they have been crafted. However, the treatise ends up considering it admissible to record some single words or utter a phrase, as long as they have a clear and direct meaning.

Weill-Parot concludes that the argumentative strategy of the *Speculum astronomie* uses the classification of images in order to include the notion of the astrological image (*imago astronomica*) as a third way. His intention was to remove the suspicion of necromancy from a certain type of image by attributing its effects to a natural astrological causality while condemning the other two types. In its origin, the *imago astronomica* was a "phantom notion," because in practice, there were no texts on images devoid of any ritual apparatus or without any inscription or formula not intended for supernatural beings.[41]

The *Speculum astronomie*, therefore, included Adelard's translation among those necromantic books that were to be rejected, while that of Juan de Sevilla appeared as an example of a very useful astronomical book. The reason is clear: Adelard translated an Arabic version of Tabit's book to which fumigations, prayers and explicit invocations of spirits had been added. The dissemination of the two translations was very different; while sixty-one manuscript copies of the Juan de Sevilla are known, only four of the Adelard translation have survived.[42] In fact, in general, many more copies of the treatises on images not condemned by the *Speculum astronomie* are preserved than of those considered illicit. Thus, this treatise had a decisive influence on the dissemination of books on images. On the other hand, the total or partial scholastic condemnation of texts on images did not prevent copyists from considering them as belonging to the natural realm, and so they were usually included in compilations of natural knowledge, astrology and medicine, but almost never in manuscripts of necromantic texts.[43]

The separation between at least two types of images responded to a trend that could already be observed in some previous works. A clear precedent is a text that begins *Ut testatur Ergaphalau*, found in a manuscript from the twelfth century, and that, according to its editor, Charles Burnett, could even have been written before the end of the tenth century. In the division of the sciences that it offers, it distinguishes between a *scientia imaginaria pura*, in which the images are based not on incantations or exorcisms, but only on astrological observation, and a *scientia imaginaria exorcismalis* intended for the spirits, that does include the support of incantations and exorcisms.[44]

41 Weill-Parot, *Les "images astrologiques"au Moyen Âge*, 27–153 and 215–19.

42 Bohak and Burnett, *Thabit ibn Qurra*, 48–50, 68–73, 201.

43 Klaassen, *Transformations of Magic*, 23–24 and 39–40.

44 Burnett, "Adelard, Ergaphalau and the Science of the Stars."

The categories of images established by William of Auvergne and the first Albertus Magnus also point in the same direction, even if they were not yet as well defined as in the *Speculum* and rejected them all. Indeed, in the *De legibus*, 23,[45] he went to great lengths to demonstrate that magical images, both those made solely with attention to astrological conditions and those which also demand sacrifices, prayers, characters, or figures, are a form of idolatry. In *De universo* 1.1.46, William presented a *questio* on whether terrestrial images obey not only the images of the firmament or constellations but also their representations, arguing with numerous reasons of various orders against the different types of magical images.[46]

In the commentary on the *Sentences* (1246–1249), Albertus Magnus also disapproved of any use of images, because this represented a risk of falling into idolatry and was oriented to evil ends.[47] Nevertheless, in later works, Albertus expressed different and, at least on first sight, contradictory opinions; in the *De celo et mundo* 2.3.5 (written in 1250), he stressed the difficulty of knowing whether the stars have an effect not only on natural beings but also on artificial ones such as images.[48] In *De fato*, 4, he justified the power of images on the basis of astrology[49]. In the *Summa theologica* (after 1270), he only alluded to astrological images to condemn them as an illusion caused by demons.[50] But the work to which he devoted most space was *De mineralibus* (1251–1254), in which he first speaks of the powers conferred on certain stones by the *forma specifica* of astral origin (2.1.4); later, in 2.3.1, he refers to traces of figures produced in certain stones by celestial influence, which as a starting point for his defence of the use of artificial images.[51] The solution of Albertus to the dichotomy between *natura* and *ars* was to position the image in a causal chain in which the craftsman manufactures the talisman by subjecting his technology (*ars*) to the natural causality coming from the stars by selecting the astrologically convenient moment according to the theory of the *electiones*. In my opinion, the diverse treatment of the issue in the writings of Albertus can be explained by the orientation and use of different authorities depending on the work, as we have seen before.

With a stance similar to that of al-Kindī, Bacon accepted certain images, at the same level as some characters and formulas, without specifying what type in particular, but emphasized that they meet the appropriate astrological conditions, and also cited Tābit ibn Qurra as the highest authority. He described these images, characters, and formulas as "philosophical," perhaps with the intention of differentiating between them and the *imago astrologica* as coined by the *Speculum astronomie* from which Bacon differed,

45 William of Auvergne, *Opera*, 1:65–67.

46 William of Auvergne, *Opera*, 1:658–66.

47 *Super II Sententiarum*, 7.50.9 and 11–12, Albertus Magnus, *Opera omnia*, 27:157–58 and 162–64.

48 Albertus Magnus, *De caelo et mundo*, 150a.

49 Aquinas, *Opuscula omnia*, 5:412–13. *De fato*, previously attributed to Thomas Aquinas, is now thought to be Albertus Magnus's work.

50 Albertus Magnus, *Opera omnia*, 2:327.

51 Albertus Magnus, *Opera omnia*, 5:28 and 48.

because he accepted images with inscriptions, which in principle are rejected in that book, and left it up to the wise man to discern, by means of "experimental science," those which are valid and those which are not.[52] The basis for the differing attitudes of the two is that the Franciscan recognized the power of words, as we have seen above. His position, which was eccentric in his time, goes so far as to argue that the *ars* is capable of going beyond the simple imitation of nature to the point of perfecting it.

Aquinas's attack on this practice was apparently based on the justification given in the *De radiis* of magical and astrological images.[53] Indeed, he was of the opinion that, while it is acceptable to make use of natural occult workings which emanate from their substantial form, the effects of objects created by technical means are caused by something else.[54] The basis of this reasoning was his conception of the *forma specifica*, since, as we have already seen, according to Aquinas, it was the only type of natural occult properties admissible, as he rejected the individual properties. Therefore, as artificial forms such as images or sculptures are accidents not inherent to the entire species, they cannot give an individual the capacity to receive from a celestial body the natural faculty which would allow them to produce effects transcending the virtues of the elements forming the material composition of that celestial body. In any case, these effects must come from an extrinsic agent, from malign spirits.

The proof of demonic intervention is that it is necessary to inscribe characters and figures on the talisman, which would be completely unnecessary for a natural operation. While some convey express invocations to demons that imply an explicit pact with them, others represent tacit pacts with malign spirits, as shown by the engraved drawings and inscriptions. Thus, Aquinas rejected not only the necromantic images but also the astrological images defended by the *Speculum astronomie*.

Up to now, we have considered only a purely theoretical debate; however, around 1300, the practices of physicians such as Arnau de Vilanova and Pietro d'Abano included the use of astrological seals. In the case of Arnau, his interest is attested to both in his works, in which he justifies the therapeutic effects of this method as the result of occult properties, and by evidence based on its use in his professional practice.[55]

Pietro, for his part, used the notion of "astrological image," under the influence of the *Speculum astronomie*, but also combined the two classes of rejected images established by this treatise into a single category of illicit images. In the *Conciliator* and other works, Pietro spoke of the virtues and methods for making forty-eight astrological images that, according to *electiones* and *interrogationes*, can mitigate, modify or increase astral influences. He attributed a therapeutic function to them, as they have the power to attract

52 Bacon, *Opus maius*, 1:394–98; Bacon, *Part of the Opus tertium*, 53.

53 *The* Speculum astronomiae *and Its Enigma*, trans. Zambelli, 38–39.

54 The attitude of Aquinas towards images is set forth primarily in the *De operationibus occultis nature*, following the line of reasoning outlined above, but here it is supplemented by passages from the *Summa contra gentiles*, 3, 104–5, and *Summa theologica*, 2a2ae q.96, art. 2, 2.

55 Giralt, "Astrological Works Attributed to Arnau de Vilanova."

beneficial celestial rays to patients and to protect them from harmful rays.[56] However, the references of Pietro to the images generally appeared to be inserted within theoretical expositions, and only two witnesses are found regarding a possible therapeutic application of the seals of Leo and the Serpentarium to counteract kidney disease and poisons, respectively.[57]

The Frontiers of the Forbidden

While sacrifices and rituals were unanimously rejected by all scholastic authors, the question of whether other magical resources such as formulas, characters or images generally serve to invoke demons or whether some of them may have properties of natural origin, was a subject of debate. Everyone also agreed that, in reality, human beings do not have any natural or supernatural mechanism, except for the power provided by God to certain saintly people, to subdue demons. It is the demons themselves who teach such practices to necromancers in order to make them think they can bring them under their control and force them to do their bidding. Demons pretend to obey and are even capable of working certain wonders, but in reality, their false submission is nothing more than a deception, permitted by God, to drag sinners who practise necromancy to the perdition of their souls.[58]

Throughout this study, we have seen how the establishment of the boundaries between the newly permitted and forbidden knowledge became the subject of a profound debate in natural philosophy and theology during the thirteenth and early fourteenth centuries. Philosophy provided the theories on the mechanisms by which the natural universe is governed and, therefore, served to determine which were natural and which were supernatural, which were divine and which were diabolical, while theology established the permissibility or otherwise of the use of these mechanisms according to the doctrine of the Church. Faced with the ever vigilant and distrustful attitude of the more orthodox ecclesiastical sectors, the scholars of natural philosophy were interested in clearly delimiting this frontier in order to free the newly imported knowledge of pagans and infidels from suspicion.

Therefore, one must ask what specific interests or uses were served by the legitimization of natural magic. From the outset, it seems evident that physicians such as Arnau de Vilanova and Pietro d'Abano were driven by an immediate, professional stimulus—to take advantage of the powers of a series of substances and instruments and incorporate them into their therapeutic arsenal. The motivations of the developers of natural philosophy, the mendicant orders, are less clear. For the Dominican tradition, in which William of Auvergne, Albertus Magnus, and Thomas Aquinas were the most distinguished, the

---

56 Federici Vescovini, "Pietro d'Abano e l'astrologia-astronomia," 9–28.

57 Pietro, *Conciliator*, fol. 17v (*differentia* 10); Pietro, "El *De venenis*," 79; Weill-Parot, *Les "images astrologiques"au Moyen Âge*, 500–31.

58 Three works focus on such a conception of necromancy as a deception: Aquinas, *Quaestiones disputatae*, 6, 10; Arnau de Vilanova, *Epistola de reprobacione*; Bacon, *Opera*, 1:523–51. Arnau's epistle seems to be inspired by Aquinas's question.

natural wonders, so admirable for their lack of rational explanation and so beneficial for humanity, would represent a magnificent proof in favour of the goodness of Creation and against the Cathar dualism that it fought against. On the other hand, for a Franciscan like Roger Bacon, the occult properties would link perfectly with his study of the *virtutes* of the elements of the natural world and with his marked neoplatonic bias.[59]

From this study we can conclude that, when it came to discriminating between that which is permitted and that which is not, within the scholastic viewpoints in favour of accepting Greco-Arabic natural knowledge and harmonizing them with faith, there was a consensus on some fundamental points. First, compared with necromancy or magic judged illicit according to Christian doctrine because it is based on the invocation of spirits, in reality demons, there is another perfectly legitimate magic—although most avoid calling it so, based on amazing natural properties, imbued by the stars and called occult, because they are not comprehensible to human reason but only through experience. As these have a natural cause, it is both licit and beneficial for mankind to employ them. Second, necromancy represents a deception, whether performed by its practitioners in front of others, or inflicted on those who believe in it by the demons they invoke. Third, characters, figures, and words used in a given working are what serve as a guideline for distinguishing between demonic magic and natural magic.

It is in this last aspect, as well as in two more that are closely linked to it—the use of images and the power of the soul—that the principal divergences within scholasticism arose. Scholars such as Albertus Magnus (in his natural works), the unknown author of the *Speculum astronomie*, Roger Bacon, Siger of Brabant, Arnau de Vilanova, and Pietro d'Abano had more open viewpoints in comparison to William of Auvergne and Thomas Aquinas. The latter condemned all practices based not only on characters and words but also on images, and asserted that their effects cannot be due to astral influence alone but imply the direct intervention of demons. In doing so, they denied the possibility that human beings can channel occult properties by technical means (*ars*), a limitation that considerably restricts the margins of natural magic as much as it widens those of diabolical magic. Two sensitivities were thus formed—one more concerned with the dangers that could arise from knowledge of the occult arts on the part of the more "theological" tendency embodied by William, Aquinas, and the religious works of Albertus, and the other more "naturalistic" and interested in the benefits that the new knowledge and its applications could bring to humanity. These, then, represent two attitudes towards knowledge—one more inhibited by the fear of falling into *curiositas* or an excessive desire for knowledge, and the other more daring and driven by a fascination and an optimistic yearning towards the theoretical (*scientia*) and technological (*ars*) knowledge provided by the new translations.

More specifically, we can see that, starting from the two poles mentioned above, the positions held by the scholastics were varied when it came to defining the criteria for distinguishing between that which is licit from that which is dangerous or prohibited, and that which is possible by natural means and that which is not (see Table below).

---

59 French and Cunningham, *Before Science*, 7–268.

Table of Opinions of Scholars on Magic and Science						
	Forma specifica or occult properties common to the entire species	Technical mastery of occult properties (images)	Power of the soul	Extraordinary powers from the stars	Power of the word	Characters
Albert (theological works)	×					
Thomas Aquinas	×					
William of Auvergne	×		perhaps			
Siger of Brabant		×				
Speculum astronomie		×				
Arnau de Vilanova	×	×		×		
Albert (natural works)	×	×	×			
Pietro d'Abano	×	×	×	×	×	
Roger Bacon	×	×	×	×	×	some

We can attempt to classify the range of different opinions by taking five variants as a touchstone: first, the technical mastery of occult properties; second, the power of the soul, understood as action at a distance; third, the extraordinary faculties imbued in certain persons by the stars; fourth, the power of the word; and fifth the use of characters. The resulting positions can be graduated as follows: (1) Albertus in his theological works and Aquinas, who rejected the five possibilities as susceptible to the intervention of demons; (2) William, who did not consider the power of the soul impossible; (3) Siger and the *Speculum astronomie*, who defended the channelling of natural magic through technique—Siger in general, and the *Speculum* with a focus on the *astronomical imago*[60]; (4) Albertus, in his natural works, who accepted the power of the soul; (5) Arnau, who admitted the existence of extraordinary personal powers; (6) Pietro, who recognized the power of the word; (7) Bacon, for whom certain characters could have natural effects.

60 One technical application of natural magic that William of Auvergne considered possible was the acceleration of the spontaneous generation of certain animals such as worms, frogs or lice (*De legibus*, 24.1.70, William of Auvergne, *Opera*, 1:69), but it is a resource to which he referred only briefly, and has scarcely been contemplated by anyone other than this author.

Lastly, we may wonder whether the debate over the limits of necromancy and the licit occult had consequences for the practice of magic or whether it was ever settled in any way. As shown by the bishop of Paris's condemnation in 1277, the persecution of necromancy certainly gained strength beginning in the second half of the thirteenth century, in accordance with the concerns generated by the diffusion of the new magical texts, and would intensify during the subsequent centuries. In the long run, the criteria of Aquinas, which were more restrictive, rationally founded, and clearer than the indefinite and oscillating criteria of Bacon and Albertus, respectively, as well as his formulation of the pact with the devil, contributed to the theoretical cementing of the witch-hunt. However, throughout the following centuries, the repression of necromancy was fundamentally directed against books and magical workings explicitly aimed at supernatural beings, which were considered illicit by all scholastic thinkers. At the same time, it generally left a wide margin of tolerance for works and practices that could fall into the categories of natural magic and astrology. However, this did not mean that they did not continue to be questioned frequently by the more orthodox. The debate therefore continued.

Bibliography

Primary Sources

Albertus Magnus. *De animalibus*. Edited by Hermann Stadler. 2 vols. Münster: Aschendorff, 1916–1921.

——. *De caelo et mundo*. Edited by Paulus Hossfeld. Münster: Aschendorff, 1971.

——. *Alberti Magni de vegetabilibus libri VII*. Edited by Hermann Stadler and Karl Jessen. Berlin: Georg Reimer, 1867.

——. *De mineralibus*. Edited by Dorothy Wyckoff. Oxford: Clarendon, 1967.

——. *Opera omnia*. Edited by Auguste Borgnet. 38 vols. Paris: Louis Vives, 1890–1899.

——. *Super Matthaeum*. Edited by Bernhardus Schmidt. Münster: Aschendorff, 1987.

Arnau de Vilanova. *Epistola de reprobacione nigromantice ficcionis*. Edited by Sebastià Giralt. Barcelona: Universitat de Barcelona—Fundació Noguera, 2005.

——. *Speculum medicine*. Edited by Michael R. McVaugh. Barcelona: Universitat de Barcelona —Fundació Noguera, 2018.

Augustine. *S. Aurelii Augustini Opera omnia*. Edited by Franco Monteverde. Roma: Città Nuova, 2010.

Avicenna. *Avicenna latinus: Liber de anima, IV–V*. Edited by Simone van Riet. Leuven: Peeters / Brill, 1968.

——. *Canon*. Venice: Luca Antonio Giunta, 1527.

——. "*Translatio libri Avicennae De viribus cordis et medicinis cordialibus Arnaldi de Villanova*." Edited by Kristin Elizabeth Peterson. PhD. diss., Harvard University, 1993.

Bacon, Roger. *Opera quaedam hactenus inedita*. Vol. 1, *I. Opus tertium. II. Opus minus. III. Compendium philosophie*. Edited by John S. Brewer. London: Longman, Green, Longman, and Roberts, 1859.

——. *Opera quaedam hactenus inedita*. Vol. 2, *Communia naturalium I et II*. Edited by Robert Steele. Oxford: Clarendon, 1905.

Bacon, Roger. *Opera quaedam hactenus inedita*. Vol. 5, *Secretum secretorum cum glossis et notulis. Tractatus brevis et utilis ad declarandum quedam obscure dicta fratris Rogeri*. Edited by Robert Steele. Oxford: Clarendon, 1920.

———. *Opus maius*. Edited by John Henry Bridges. 3 vols. Oxford: Clarendon, 1897–1900.

———. *Part of the Opus tertium of Roger Bacon*. Edited by A. G. Little. Aberdeen: Aberdeen University Press, 1912.

Bohak, Gideon, and Charles Burnett. *Thabit ibn Qurra* On Talismans *and Ps.*-Ptolemy On Images 1–9. *Together with the* Liber prestigiorum Thebidis *of Adelard of Bath*. Florence: SISMEL—Galluzzo, 2021.

Chartularium Universitatis Parisiensis. Edited by Henri Denifle and Émile Chatelaine. Paris: Université de Paris, 1889–1897.

Pietro d'Abano. *Conciliator differentiarum philosophorum et medicorum*. Venice: Luca Antonio Giunta, 1565.

———. "El *De venenis* de Pietro d'Abano. Estudio preliminar, edición crítica y traducción." Edited by Alba Aguilera. PhD. diss., Universitat Autònoma de Barcelona, 2018.

Siger de Brabant. *Quaestiones in metaphysicam*. Edited by Armand Maurer. Leuven: Publications universitaires—Béatrice-Nauwelaerts, 1983.

The Speculum astronomiae *and Its Enigma: Astrology, Theology, and Science in Albertus Magnus and His Contemporaries*. Translated by Paola Zambelli. Dordrecht: Kluwer, 1992.

Thomas Aquinas. *The Letter of Saint Thomas Aquinas: De occultis operibus naturae ad quemdam militem ultramontanum*. Edited by Joseph B. McAllister. Washington: Catholic University of America Press, 1939.

———. "Opera spuria." In *Opuscula omnia*. Vol. 5. Edited by Pierre Mandonnet. Paris: Lethielleux, 1927.

———. *Quaestiones disputatae*. Vol. 2. Edited by P. Bazzi. Turin: Marietti, 1965.

William of Auvergne. *Opera omnia*. Paris: François Muguet, 1674.

Secondary Sources

Burnett, Charles. "Adelard, Ergaphalau and the Science of the Stars." In *Adelard of Bath: An English Scientist and Arabist of the Early Twelfth Century*. Edited by Charles Burnett, 133–45. Warburg Institute Surveys and Texts 14. London: The Warburg Institute, 1987.

Delaurenti, Béatrice. "La fascination et l'action à distance: Questions médiévales (1230–1370)." *Médiévales* 50 (2006): 137–54.

———. "Pietro d'Abano et les incantations: Présentation, édition et traduction de la *differentia* 156 du *Conciliator*." In *Médicine, astrologie et magie entre Moyen Âge et Renaissance: Autour de Pietro d'Abano*. Edited by Jean-Patrice Boudet, Franck Collard, and Nicolas Weill-Parot, 39–106. Florence: SISMEL—Galluzzo, 2013.

———. *La puissance des mots. Virtus verborum: Débats doctrinaux sur le pouvoir des incantations au Moyen Âge*. Paris: Cerf, 2007.

Draelants, Isabelle. "The Notion of 'Properties': A Tension Between Sciencia and Ars in Medieval Natural Philosophy and Magic." In *The Routledge History of Medieval Magic*. Edited by Sophie Page and Catherine Rider, 169–86. London: Routledge, 2019.

Fanger, Claire. "Things Done Wisely by a Wise Enchanter: Negotiating the Power of Words in the Thirteenth Century." *Esoterica* 1 (1999): 97–132.

Federici Vescovini, Graziella. *Medioevo magico: La magia tra religione e scienza nei secoli XIII e XIV*. Turin: UTET, 2008.

——. "Pietro d'Abano e l'astrologia-astronomia." *Bollettino del Centro internazionale di storia dello spazio e del tempo* 5 (1986): 9–28.

French, Roger, and Andrew Cunningham. *Before Science. The Invention of the Friars' Natural Philosophy*. Aldershot: Scholar, 1996.

Giralt, Sebastià. "The Astrological Works Attributed to Arnau de Vilanova: The Question of Their Authenticity." In *Geomancy and Other Forms of Divination*. Edited by Alessandro Palazzo and Irene Zavattero, 397–420. Florence: SISMEL—Galluzzo, 2017.

——. "*Proprietas*: Las propiedades ocultas según Arnau de Vilanova." *Traditio* 63 (2008): 327–60.

Hackett, Jeremiah. "Roger Bacon on Astronomy-Astrology: The Sources of the *Scientia Experimentalis*." In *Roger Bacon and the Sciences. Commemorative Essays*. Edited by Jeremiah Hackett, 175–98. Leiden: Brill, 1997.

——. "Roger Bacon On *Scientia Experimentalis*." In *Roger Bacon and the Sciences. Commemorative Essays*. Edited by Jeremiah Hackett, 277–315. Leiden: Brill, 1997.

Klaassen, Frank. *The Transformations of Magic: Illicit Learned Magic in the Later Middle Ages and Renaissance*. University Park: Pennsylvania State University Press, 2013.

Maurer, Armand. "Between Reason and Faith: Siger of Brabant and Pomponazzi on the Magic Arts." *Mediaeval Studies* 18 (1956): 1–18.

McVaugh, Michael R. "The Development of Medieval Pharmaceutical Theory." In Arnau de Vilanova, *Opera medica omnia*. Vol. 2, *Aphorismi de gradibus*. Edited by L. Garcia-Ballester, J. A. Paniagua, and Michael R. McVaugh, 1–136. Barcelona: Universitat de Barcelona, 1975.

Paravicini Bagliani, Agostino. *Le Speculum astronomiae une énigme? Enquête sur les manuscrits*. Florence: SISMEL—Edizioni del Galluzzo, 2001.

Paschetto, Eugenia. *Pietro d'Abano, medico e filosofo*. Florence: Vallecchi, 1984.

Sannino, Antonella. "*Nigromantia secundum physicam, nigromantia imaginum*: Arte e scienza in Guglielmo d'Alvernia." In *La magia naturale tra Medioevo e prima età moderna*. Edited by Lorenzo Bianchi and Antonella Sannino, 81–130. Florence: SISMEL—Galluzzo, 2018.

Sturlese, Loris. "Intelletto acquisito e divino. La dottrina filosofica di Alberto il Grande sulla perfezione della ragione umana." *Giornale critico della filosofia italiana* 23, no. 2 (2003): 161–89.

Véronèse, Julien. "L'Ars notoria au Moyen Âge et à l'époque moderne. Étude d'une tradition de magie théurgique (XIIe–XVIIe siècle)." PhD. diss., Université Paris X–Nanterre, 2004.

Weill-Parot, Nicolas. *Les "images astrologiques"au Moyen Âge et à la Renaissance: Spéculations intellectuelles et pratiques magiques (XIIe-XVe siècle)*. Paris: Champion, 2002.

——. *Points aveugles de la nature: La rationalité scientifique médiévale face à l'occulte, l'attraction magnétique et l'horreur du vide (XIIIe–milieu du XVe siècle)*. Paris: Belles Lettres, 2013.

Wilcox, Judith and John Riddle, "Qusta ibn Luqa's Physical Ligatures and the Recognition of the Placebo Effect, with an Edition and Translation." *Medieval Encounters* 1, no, 1 (1995): 1–50.

WITCHCRAFT AND WEATHER

THE PROBLEM OF MAGICAL CONTROL OF THE WEATHER

CAROLINA ESCOBAR-VARGAS

LET ME FIRST pose a simple question: did people in the Middle Ages believe that the weather could be controlled through magic? As with anything involving magic and its definitions, the answer is not straightforward. Attitudes towards the possibility of magically manipulating the weather varied widely in the medieval period, ranging from acceptance to disbelief and outright condemnation. These attitudes shifted in response to changing social structures and evolving systems of belief, which influenced the context within which texts and events were interpreted. When discussing the central question, it is essential to highlight that the idea of weather manipulation through magic is closely tied to the concept of demons and their ability to alter the weather at will, given their unique physical nature. If it was deemed theologically possible for demons to control the weather, then the question moves on to humans and their relationship with demons. Could humans manipulate or propitiate demons to alter the weather? Were purported magicians simply deceived by demons into believing they could control the weather, or were they being instrumentalized by demons themselves? These questions will be explored in this article to evaluate the changing attitudes towards weather magic during the Middle Ages.

In his influential work, *The Etymologies*, Isidore, the seventh-century bishop of Seville, devotes an entire chapter to describing various magical practices and practitioners from classical authorities.[1] Although Isidore does not include weather magic in his typology, he does mention that magicians, commonly referred to as *maleficus* by the general public due to the severity of their crimes, can "agitate the elements, disturb the minds of people, and slay without any drinking of poison, using the violence of spells alone."[2] Isidore's use of the term *concutiunt*, which means to shake, agitate violently, and shatter in association with *elementa*, leaves the possibility of weather manipulation open. If magicians can shatter the weather, the suggestion of weather magic becomes

1 Isidore, *Etymologies*, trans. Barney et al. For the Latin text see: Isidore of Seville, *Etymologiarvm*.

2 Isidore, *Etymologies*, trans. Barney et al.; "Hi et elementa concutiunt, turbant mentes hominum, ac sine ullo veneni haustu violentia tantum carminis interimunt." Isidore, *Etymologiarvm*, 8.9.9.

Carolina Escobar-Vargas is an Associate Professor of Medieval History at the Universidad Nacional de Colombia, Sede Medellin. She is the co-author, alongside Anne Lawrence-Mathers, of *Magic and Medieval Society* (2014), and has published on issues relating to magic in the Central Middle Ages, Geoffrey of Monmouth and most recently on the distinctions between perceived notions of fiction and reality in the Middle Ages in chronicle material.

plausible. However, Isidore does not clearly spell out the connection between magic and weather manipulation in *The Etymologies*.

Other mentions of the weather in the *Etymologies* are limited to a typology of the weather in Book 13, where natural causes are ascribed for its changing nature, and to forecasting through sign interpretation. For instance, the flight of a fish called the *mill-ago* over water can be interpreted as a sign of changing weather.[3] Isidore also briefly mentions how constellations and their rising can indicate weather conditions.[4] Due to the limited evidence available in the *Etymologies*, it is difficult to determine if weather manipulation was believed to be possible in the early Middle Ages, and by whom. However, Isidore's mention of *malefici*, who can "agitate the elements," suggests the possibility of weather manipulation through magic.

The Bible indicates that God has the ability to modify the weather as he pleases. In Exodus 9:22–26, when Moses confronts Pharaoh and his magicians, Jannes and Jambres, God sends hail, thunder, lightning, and fire as the seventh plague to Egypt, causing chaos and destruction everywhere except in the land where the Israelites were.

> 22. And the Lord said to Moses: Stretch forth thy hand towards heaven, that there may be hail in the whole land of Egypt upon men, and upon beasts, and upon every herb of the field in the land of Egypt. 23 And Moses stretched forth his rod towards heaven, and the Lord sent thunder and hail, and lightnings running along the ground: and the Lord rained hail upon the land of Egypt. 24 And the hail and fire mixt with it drove on together: and it was of so great bigness, as never before was seen in the whole land of Egypt since that nation was founded. 25 And the hail destroyed through all the land of Egypt all things that were in the fields, both man and beast: and the hail smote every herb of the field, and it broke every tree of the country. 26 Only in the land of Gessen, where the children of Israel were, the hail fell not.[5]

The passage demonstrates that the weather is under God's control and is part of the natural system he created. As evident from the Exodus text, God can change the weather as a manifestation of his anger or to display his power and wonder. Nevertheless, did people in the Middle Ages believe other entities, such as demons, could alter the weather? Could they manipulate it to harm human beings or out of malice?

Early patristic authors, Augustine in particular, believed that if permitted by God, demons could manipulate the elements to tempt and torment humanity. This ability was partly due to their nature. In his *City of God*, quoting Apuleius, Augustine describes demons as: "animal in genus, passive in soul, rational in mind, aerial in body, and eternal in time."[6] According to Apuleius's analysis, their eternal nature is unique to them and the gods. Their animal nature and rationality of mind are shared with humans and the

---

3 Isidore, *Etymologies*, trans. Barney et al.; Isidore, *Etymologiarvm*, 12.6.36.

4 Isidore, *Etymologies*, trans. Barney et al.; Isidore, *Etymologiarvm*, 3.74.5.

5 Douay-Rheims English Translation of the Vulgate Bible: https://vulgate.org/ot/exodus_9.htm.

6 Augustine, *City of God*, ed. Dyson; Augustine, *De civitate Dei*, 8.16.

gods, while their passiveness of soul is shared only with humans. Their aerial nature is theirs alone. This unique nature enables them to manipulate the creation in ways that are beyond human capabilities.[7]

However, according to Augustine, this should not be seen as a quality to be admired, and demons should definitely not be considered worthy of divine honour. Augustine is unsurprisingly harsh in his stance on demons, stating: "But how much less worthy are these aerial animals of divine honour, who are rational only so that they may be miserable, who are passive only so that they may suffer, and who are eternal only so that their misery may have no end!"[8] Furthermore, in Book 10, chapter 21, he goes on to discuss: "the Power Delegated to Demons for the Trial and Glorification of the Saints," where he asserts:

> At certain appointed and foreordained times, indeed, power has been granted to the demons, so that they may incite the men whom they possess to give vent to their enmity against the City of God. Such tyrannical demons do not only receive sacrifice from those who offer it willingly, but also extort it by violent persecution from the unwilling.[9]

Due to the nature of demons, the medieval Church believed they could manipulate creation in ways that humans could not. They could use this power to test and torment humanity. However, it remains unclear whether, in the early Middle Ages, Church writers believed that demons could manipulate the weather to harm humans or whether they thought weather magic was possible.

According to a Carolingian tract by Agobard of Lyon entitled *De grandine et tonitruis*, people in the area of Lyon and northeast of present-day France blamed those whom they called the *tempestarii* for causing destructive rain and hailstorms.[10] The *tempestarii* were believed to cause these storms either to damage a neighbour's field or to aid the so-called aeronauts from Magonia in stealing crops. Agobard strongly criticises these beliefs, branding as liars and false witnesses anyone who claimed to know of either the *tempestarii* or the Magonians. He accuses them of taking from God through their false testimony.[11]

Agobard firmly believed that only God could create and control the weather, as it was an expression of his almighty power. He supported this claim with biblical analy-

---

7 Augustine, *City of God*, ed. Dyson, 8.16–19.

8 Augustine, *City of God*, ed. Dyson; Augustine, *De civitate Dei*, 8.16.

9 Augustine, *City of God*, ed. Dyson; Augustine, *De civitate Dei*, 10.21.

10 The Latin text can be found in Agobard of Lyon, *Opera Omnia* and in Agobard of Lyon, *Liber contra insulam*, Patrologiae Latina 104. For a modern translation into English, see Lewis, "Agobard of Lyons." A partial translation is also present in P. E. Dutton, *Carolingian Civilization: A Reader*. For more on Agobard's *De grandine et tronitus*, see Bailey, "Magic and Disbelief"; Dutton, "Thunder and Hail"; Meens, "Thunder Over Lyon"; and Jolivet, "Agobard de Lyon."

11 "And whoever adheres to something that is not, not only draws back from the One Who created him, but also from the very thing that was created." Cited from Lewis, "Agobard"; Agobard, *De grandine*, col. 149.

sis, citing the passage in Exodus where hail and rain were brought to Egypt as the seventh plague of God, as well as examples from the psalms.[12] Agobard regarded those who believed in the nonsense of Magonia and the *tempestarii* as ignorant of God's power. In his view, the weather should inspire either fear at the wrath of a just God who punished idolaters or wonder and amazement at his omnipotent power.

However, Agobard acknowledged that, due to God's inscrutable nature, he might allow demons to tempt good people and torment both good and evil people, as seen in the case of Job. Nevertheless, Agobard did not pursue this line of argument in his tract. Instead, he finished by comparing the belief in the *tempestarii* to another widely held belief of the time, the so-called Beneventan complot, which involved a group of Beneventans spreading an impossible amount of poison powder throughout Carolingian lands.[13] Agobard's tract expressed scepticism towards superstitions such as the *tempestarii*, highlighting the Christian error and apparent superstition of such beliefs, much like the *Canon Episcopi*. This influential legal text was first recorded in the early tenth century

12 "Therefore, because every liar is an advocate of falsehood, and every advocate of falsehood is a false witness, acting against the truth, we may see now whether those who say that a divine work is accomplished by a human agent are upheld by any authority. Now, in Holy Scripture the place where hail is first mentioned is found among the plagues by which Egypt was struck; for this in fact is the seventh plague of Egypt." (Exodus 9:18): '*Behold, I will cause it to rain tomorrow at this same hour, an exceeding great hail: such as hath not been in Egypt form the day that it was founded until this present time.*' In these words, the Lord said that He Himself, not some human, would send hail on the next day—certainly not Moses or Aaron, who were righteous and men of God, nor Jamnes or Mambres, the Egyptian enchanters, who are recorded as the Pharaoh's magicians, whom the apostle said resisted Moses (cf. 2 Timothy 3:8), and thus they also oppose the truth. For indeed, as has been written, using Egyptian incantations and certain mysteries, they stretched out their staffs one at a time in the presence of the Pharaoh and the staffs were turned into serpents, although Aaron's staff devoured theirs (cf. Exodus 7:11–12). And they turned water into blood, and brought forth frogs from rivers, although they were not able to stop the frogs, as Moses did through the command of the Lord that they remain only in the river. But when it came to gnats, and the magicians were able to do nothing thereafter, they said the finger of God was against them and they attempted nothing further of that kind. Certainly, if any man had been able to unleash hail, Jamnes and Mambres would have unleashed it, since they turned water into blood and brought forth frogs from rivers, while those who are called 'storm-makers' are unable to do these things." Cited from Lewis, "Agobard"; Agobard, *De grandine*, cols. 149–50.

13 "A certain stupidity was spread a few years ago, when some cattle died, so that people said that Grimaldus, the Duke of Benevento, had sent men with powder that they sprinkled through the fields and mountains, meadows and springs—because he was hostile to the most Christian Emperor Charles, and cattle died from this sprinkled powder. We have heard of, and seen, many men seized for this reason, some of them struck down and slain, but most of them tied to boards, thrown into the river, and killed. And, what is truly amazing, the very ones who were seized would give evidence against themselves, saying that they had such a powder and they had sprinkled it. For thus the devil, when his power was received into them by the secret and righteous justice of God, was able to enter them to such an extent that they became false witnesses against themselves to the point of death. And neither instruction nor torture nor death itself deterred them from daring to speak this falsehood against themselves." Cited from Lewis, "Agobard"; Agobard, *De grandine*, col. 158.

by Regino of Prüm in his canonical collection and denounced women who believed they flew at night alongside the pagan goddess Diana.[14]

Is Agobard the only one who disbelieves in the magic displayed by the *tempestarii*? Were the *tempestarii* ever classified as a type of magical practitioner in later works? Another example of a well-defined classification system can be found in the writings of twelfth-century philosopher and cleric John of Salisbury. While serving the archbishops of Canterbury, and before he himself became the bishop of Chartres, John wrote a critique of court life that was dedicated to Thomas Beckett, then the right-hand man of Henry II and later the archbishop of Canterbury. In chapter 9 of the first book of his *Policraticus*, written in 1159, John begins by stating that "Long ago the Christian Fathers condemned those who practiced the more demoralizing forms of legerdemain, the art of magic, and astrology because they realized that all these arts, or rather artifices, derive from unholy commerce between men and demons."[15] From the outset, the focus is on the sinister relationship that could link humans and demons, which characterizes the magical arts. In chapter 10, John asserts that:

> Magicians do indeed exist, and are so-called because of the magnitude of their incantations, for they by God's grace, cause the elements to shudder, destroy the identity of things, often predict the future, cloud the minds of men, send dreams, and so far as that goes, by the violence of their charms slay them.[16]

Expanding on the Isidorian text, John of Salisbury not only quotes but also adds and modifies, emphasizing that magicians not only make the elements tremble, cloud men's minds, and kill with their charms, but also have the power to destroy the essence of things, foretell the future and induce dreams. With respect to weather magic, just as Isidore did, John leaves the possibility of weather manipulation open by using the term *concutiunt* in association with *elementa*.[17] When the time comes to create a detailed typology, John continues to add and modify. In addition to Isidore's list of *incantatores* (enchanters), *arioli* (wizards), *aruspices* (soothsayers), *phycii* (diviners), *mathematici* (astrologers), *horoscopi*, *salissatores*, *sortilegi* (fortune tellers), *auguri* and *necromantii* (necromancers), he includes *imaginarii*, and *specularios* (crystal-seers) from the Bible, *vultivoli* and *coniectores* (dream-interpreters) from classical authorities (primarily Virgil and Quintilian), and even contributes his own category with *chiromantici* (palmists), which is the first time this term appears in a medieval Latin source.[18] If John had known about the *tempestarii*, he most likely would have included them in his list, as he did with *imaginarii*, *specularios*, *vultivoli*, and especially *chiromantici*. This addition indicates that

14 A full translated version of the *Canon Episcopi* can be found in: Kors and Peters, *Witchcraft in Europe*. For more on the *Canon Episcopi*, see Halstead, "'They Ride on the Backs of Certain Beasts"; Lawrence-Mathers and Escobar-Vargas, *Magic and Medieval Society*.

15 John of Salisbury, *Frivolities of Courtiers*, 1.9.49; John of Salisbury, *Policraticus*. 1.9.

16 John of Salisbury, *Policraticus*, 1.10.

17 John of Salisbury, *Policraticus*, 1.10.

18 John of Salisbury, *Policraticus*, 1.12.

John was willing to incorporate contemporary practices into his classification system and not just those found in classical authoritative texts. However, if he had been aware of the *tempestarii*, not including them might suggest his rejection of them in a manner similar to Agobard's argument, although this is highly unlikely. Even though he studied in Chartres, there is no guarantee that John would have been familiar with Agobard's work or the Carolingian belief about the *tempestarii* in the area around Lyon. John's lack of interest in weather magic raises the question of whether there any instances of weather magic or its practitioners in other twelfth-century sources.

A prominent place to look for weather magic is in the famous narrative by Geoffrey of Monmouth, the *Historia Regum Britanniae*. This seminal work, written in the 1130s, claims to fill a long-standing gap in the history of England, running from its foundations at the hands of the mythical hero Brutus to the arrival of the Anglo-Saxons in the seventh century, as described by Bede. As such, the *Historia* is a seminal narrative leading to the widely accepted story of Arthur, his forefathers, and, of course, the famous Merlin.

As a *vates*, a term reminiscent of pagan prophets, Merlin does not perform any sort of weather manipulation in the *Historia*, nor do any of the magicians that appear at various points in the narrative.[19] The closest the narrative gets to any sort of clear interaction with heavenly bodies and sublunary spheres comes in the form of Merlin's interpretation of a rare comet in the sky that foretells the birth of Arthur and his lineage.[20] Similarly, in the absence of Merlin, Arthur has access to members of a college of stargazers, who are only mentioned in passing.[21] Thus, there are no instances of weather manipulation in the narrative, be it divine or demonic.

However, in another fabulated chronicle, purporting to record the life of a legendary historical conqueror and ruler, the *Res Gestae Alexandri Macedonis*, we find another infamous magician, Nectanebus. The *Res Gestae* is a keystone to both the historical and literary traditions of Alexander. In this narrative, Nectanebus is the legendary Egyptian ruler who fathered Alexander the Great in the guise of a dragon. Unlike the *Historia*, the *Res Gestae* was not written in the twelfth century; it is associated with the name of Julius Valerius Alexander Polemius, a fourth-century translator into Latin of a Greek narrative by Pseudo-Callisthenes, providing a romanticized biography of Alexander the Great.

The *Res Gestae* was widely copied during the Middle Ages, mainly in an abridged version that transmitted the story of Nectanebus, as found in the Epitome published by Julius Zacher in 1867. It appears alongside the *Historia Regum Britanniae* in no fewer than nine manuscripts, all but one dating from the twelfth and thirteenth centuries. Of Nectanebus, we read:

> Of all these Nectanabus was proved to have been the wisest, since he could accomplish with words what others did by force of arms. Finally, worldly elements were prepared for him in such a way that, when fear of war hung over

19 For the references to Merlin as a *uates* see: Geoffrey of Monmouth, *History*, 171 and 187. For additional instances of magic in the *Historia*, see Escobar-Vargas, "El Marco."

20 Geoffrey of Monmouth, *History*, 179.

21 Geoffrey of Monmouth, *History*, 211.

> him, he would go deep into the recesses of his royal palace, all alone, and take a basin with him. While he was filling this with pure spring-water, out of wax he would fashion a likeness of a boat and put in it human images. When all these things began to float, soon they appeared to be in motion and to live. He also used an ebony wand and spoke incantations by which he called on gods above and below, and so he contrived to have the boat submerged in the basin. As a result it would happen that all his actual enemies would be submerged in the sea along with the sinking of the wax figures. And so for a long time he was secure in power over his kingdom.[22]

There are several intriguing aspects to this narrative. While Nectanebus's use of magic ensures the peaceful existence of his kingdom, a positive outcome, this is not unusual given the pagan setting and origins of the narrative. However, Nectanebus's use of water magic hints at his ability to manipulate the elements, resulting in disastrous consequences for enemy ships that rise against him. He seems to introduce additional elements to his magic, employing wax images that operate under the principles of what would later be called "sympathetic" magic. This element exemplifies the *vultivoli* of Virgil and John of Salisbury. Above all, Nectanebus is male, privileged, and potentially highly educated, and his magic displays elaborate and expensive ritual elements. These features will become significant below when compared to later depictions of weather magic in other types of sources. So, are there any additional instances of weather magic from the later medieval period?

The *Picatrix* is a tenth-century Arabic magical treatise that describes several magical operations for manipulating the weather.[23] Originally written in Arabic, the *Picatrix* was translated into Hebrew and then Castilian ca. 1256 in the court of Alfonso X. Finally, it was translated into Latin not long after.[24] The treatise consists of four books, each containing about a dozen chapters of a heterogenous nature and it is wide-ranging in scope. One of the most prominent features of the Picatrix is its emphasis on astrological magic, which involves harnessing the power of the planets and stars to achieve specific effects on the physical world; thus, the appearance of weather magic here is not surprising. Indeed, as proposed by Attrell and Porreca, two among the fourteen categories they have identified as objectives in *Picatrix* rituals are agriculture and the "elements/properties of matter" category. This category comprises "rituals that attempt to control the raw materials that were thought to make up the material universe, i.e., the four elements and their primary effects on human activities: air in terms of storms and weather; earth and fire in terms of how they interact with each other; and water in terms of precipita-

22 DeAngeli, "Julius Valerius," 121. For the Latin text, see Iulius Valerius, *Res Gestae*.

23 A modern edition can be found in *Picatrix*, trans. Attrell and Porreca. For the Latin edition, see *Picatrix, The Latin Version*, ed. Pingree. For more on the *Picatrix*, see Pingree, "Ghaya and the Picatrix,"; Boudet, Caiozzo and Weill-Parot, *Images et magie*; Saif, *The Arabic Influences*; Avner, "Travelling"; Boudet and Coulon, "La version arab."

24 Pingree, "Ghaya and the Picatrix," 27, Alejandro García Avilés, "La magie." For more on the circulation of the Picatrex see Weill-Parot, "*Images corporeiformes*."

tions, flooding, and related effects."[25] The treatise thus provides several instructions on how to manipulate or prevent damage from the weather, including hail, rain, storms, and wind.

For instance, Book 4, chapter 7 (On What Is Found Concerning the Art of Magic in the "Chaldean Agriculture," Which Abubaer Abenvaxie Translated from the Chaldean Language into Arabic), introduces several examples of how to protect crops from potentially harmful weather events. First, it provides a detailed example of how to inscribe specific symbols on a piece of wood to defend vines from poor weather:

> A sage whom we have named elsewhere (namely Zeherith) cites the nineteen experiments written out below. The first is for defending vines from poor weather. Take a marble or wooden tablet, and inscribe images of vines and grapes upon it—do this between the twenty-second day of October and the fourth of December (that is, any day out of these); place this tablet thus prepared in the middle of the vines. This image is proven to defend vines from bad weather.[26]

Similarly, it offers a straightforward yet potentially expensive method of protecting crops from hailstorms, requiring a considerable number of people and a sufficient amount of silk:

> When clouds approach looking like they might carry hail and one wishes to defend crops from the hailstorm, assemble many associates, some of whom should carry silk in their hands and some should go to the field carrying nothing. Make them throw the silk bit by bit toward the clouds, and make the others who are without silk walk around clapping their hands and palms. Make everyone keep shouting in a loud voice like farmers do when they want to drive off birds and evil beasts. Make them do this many times. Make sure that those associates be even in number; the more numerous they are, the better. This has been tested and found to be very true.[27]

Yet another simple method to disperse a storm involves the use of an expensive steel mirror and loud shouting.[28] However, in contrast, this same chapter provides details on a sophisticated and complex operation to create a magical talisman capable of controlling the winds, demons, the living and the dead. This operation involves creating a mirror-shaped talisman using gold and silver, inscribing it with powerful names, and suffumigating it with a woman's hair, incense, and each of the seven bodily substances (blood, semen, saliva, ear wax, tears, excrement, and urine) of man:

> In a book published by the wise Geber, I found this written for producing a storm and very many other things. Make a mirror out of gold or gilded silver,

25 *Picatrix*, trans. Attrell and Porreca, 18.

26 *Picatrix*, trans. Attrell and Porreca, 255–56; *Picatrix, The Latin Version*, ed. Pingree, 210.

27 *Picatrix*, trans. Attrell and Porreca, 254; *Picatrix, The Latin Version*, ed. Pingree, 209.

28 *Picatrix*, trans. Attrell and Porreca 254; *Picatrix, The Latin Version*, ed. Pingree, 209.

> [210] and suffumigate it with hair from a woman's comb, and anoint it with your semen. Next, suffumigate it with hairs from her clothes. After having bathed, look into the mirror, and in it have her likeness appear, then yours immediately (or yours first, then hers). This was tested by a man called Ptolomy of Babylon. Three Indian sages found it in Egypt and proved that such a mirror must be made when the Moon is conjoined with Jupiter and gilded or polished while the Moon is with Venus. I wish to reveal to you how to make this mirror and how to use and guard it (because it affects all humankind). Temper the mirror with living and natural blood, suffumigate it, then write the names of the seven stars, their seven figures, and the names of the seven angels and the seven winds upon it. The names of the seven stars are these: 'ZOHAL, MUSTERI, MARRECH, XEMZ, ZOHARA, HOTARID, and ALCHAMAR.' These symbols should be drawn in a circle around the outer edge:
>
> 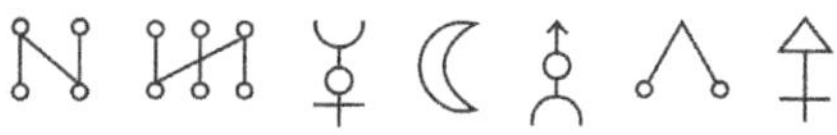
>
> These are in a circle. Next, write the names of these seven angels on the inside of the polished and gilded circle: 'CAPTIEL, SATQUIEL, SAMAEL, RAPHAEL, ANAEL, MICHAEL, and GABRIEL.' When this is done, write the names of the seven winds on the unpolished part; these are the winds of power, whose names are: 'BARCHIA, BETHEL, ALMODA, HAMAR, BENABIS, ZOBAA MARRACH, FIDE ARRACH, and SAMORES MAYMON ACZABI.' Then suspend the mirror in silk for seven days above water, and suffumigate it. Suspend it from a bramble branch. Suffumigate it for three nights with pleasant incenses (better yet with the ones found in the book of Moses). If you gaze into that mirror and guard it well, know that through it you will bring together men, winds, spirits, demons, the living, and the dead. All shall be obedient to you and heed your command. Proceed such that there is some of each of man's seven properties in the suffumigation (namely, blood, semen, saliva, ear wax, tears of the eyes, excrement, and urine). Suffumigate with those things, and instruct the winds of your desires; they shall enact your will. Guard this, and heed everything I have said. You will thereby have power over winds, humans, and demons, and you will do what you wish. When you are washed and clean, call them; they will come to you obediently. Do this above a basin or any clean vessel full of water. There you will behold the fulfillment of what you sought.[29]

Beyond the complex operations that require frequent access to costly materials and specialized knowledge for weather control, the *Picatrix* also suggests relatively simpler methods, such as prayers to obtain protection from hazardous weather. For example, in Book 3, chapter 7 (*On the Attraction of Planetary Powers; How We May Speak with Them;*

29 *Picatrix*, trans. Attrell and Porreca, 254–55. Note that the symbols have been taken from the Latin edition of the text as they were not available in the translation: *Picatrix, The Latin Version*, ed. Pingree, 209–10.

How an Effect Is Divided Between the Planets, Images, Sacrifices, Prayers, Suffumigations, and Words; and the Conditions of Heaven Necessary to Each of the Planets), a protective prayer to Jupiter is provided:

> There are, however, others who pray to Jupiter without suffumigation so that by his power they might be saved from a storm at sea. Rasis said in his book of metaphysics:
>
> For evading danger at sea, turn yourself toward Jupiter sitting in mid-heaven, and speak: 'God hails you, O noble planet, splendid, precious, and honoured star! In you God placed power and spirits for doing good, giving form to the bodies of the universe that themselves enter into divine law and life, helping those who sail at sea and saving their lives. I ask you through the strength that God has placed in you that you grant me your light and spirit by which I will be saved. Wash and purify the sins of my nature such that my senses and my spirit be enlightened that I may know and understand.'
>
> If your work is done accordingly, you should see the appearance of a burning candle before you. If you do not see it, know that your work was done incorrectly. Repeat it until you see this burning candle, and then what you seek shall be.[30]

Apart from various instructions on how to create special objects to ward off destructive weather events, specific details on the production of magical talismans to prevent or call upon rain during times of need can be found throughout Book 2 (*The Second Book Begins Wherein Stands a General Discussion on the Heavens' Signs, the Motion of the Eighth Sphere, and Their Effects in This World*).[31] However, the most detailed and complex instructions on how to prepare a talisman against the negative effects of rain, hail, and snow can be found in Book 3, chapter 10 (*On the Demonstration of the Planetary Spirits' Compounds; Reducing Damage from Rituals and Effects; the Wonders of Magic and Foods, Suffumigations, Ointments, and Fragrances That the Operator of the Planetary Spirits Must Use; the Effects Proper to the Planets and the Effects that Operate Unseen*). Notably, the reference to stones in this section is intricately tied to the personas of Alexander and Aristotle, introducing a distinct political context. This sets the section apart from the examples discussed earlier, where the manipulation of weather via magical means was predominantly situated within an agricultural framework. These instructions involve manipulating melted metals, various organic plant and animal-based ingredients, minerals, and the problematic use of human blood. Additionally, the process is strengthened through ritualistic operations that involve the use of names of power and complex astrological knowledge, referred to in the text as "the works of Perfect Nature":

> The second stone is named Helemetiz. This stone is recommended against rain, hail, and snow. When any of these happen, raise this stone with your right hand

---

30 *Picatrix*, trans. Attrell and Porreca 161; *Picatrix, The Latin Version*, ed. Pingree, 120.

31 See for example *Picatrix*, trans. Attrell and Porreca, 114, 121, 122, 123; *Picatrix, The Latin Version*, ed. Pingree, 74, 80–81, 81, 82.

> toward the heavens, and you will be safe. This stone is tawny in colour. Its composition is this: take 4 oz. of hellebore, and liquefy it in the fire with white wolfsbane. When it is liquefied, add 4 oz. of silver and 4 oz. of lead. When all things have been liquefied together, lift it from the fire, and work it with the powers of the spirits. Take bones from the hands and feet of a pig, which are well-cleaned from flesh and nerves, then cook them well in brine. Once sufficiently cooked, lift them from the fire, and let them dry. Pulverize and liquefy them with mandrake and chalk in an earthenware vase, well-sealed with goldsmith's luting—that is, place first in that vase one part of chalk and mandrake, then on top of it another portion of bone dust in turn until the vase is filled. Liquefy these over a dung fire for one night. Afterward, remove the vase from the fire, and allow it to cool. Grind these things into a powder. Toss a small amount of red and clear arsenic on top of it. Grind them up again with human blood sprinkled from a vein. Grind them up for an entire day, then set them aside for use. Once these things have been accomplished, melt the first substance upon which, little by little, should be thrown this latter substance until they are well-blended. When this is done, remove it from the fire, and allow it to cool because you will find it tawny in colour. Work this stone into an appropriately-sized, spherical shape on a lathe. Subsequently, work with the words and operations that we have stated above on the works of 'Perfect Nature.' If you see rain, snow, hail, and thunder anywhere and if you want to remove them from your area, speak those words that we have stated before, and raise your right hand holding the stone toward the heavens. Everything will settle. This is the stone composed from immaterial powers and spirits.[32]

Overall, the Picatrix contains a variety of techniques for manipulating the weather by combining physical actions and verbal recitations. Notably, the text provides minimal guidance on preventing or controlling thunder and lightning. While many of the topics covered fall within the purview of astrologers and learned magicians, some of the suggested methods may not appear as advanced or scholarly to theologians. For instance, one approach involves instructing a menstruating woman to throw herself naked onto the ground with her legs raised toward an approaching storm cloud to protect a field or harvest from hail.[33] Several of the examples discussed here are situated for application within an agricultural context; however, consideration is given to its potential application within political settings. It is noteworthy, however, that there is a relatively limited usage of weather-magic in texts on learned and ritual magic up to the thirteenth century.

---

32 *Picatrix*, trans. Attrell and Porreca 190. For the ritual of "perfect nature," see *Picatrix*, trans. Attrell and Porreca, 150–52; *Picatrix, The Latin Version*, ed. Pingree, 147. Chapter 8 of Book 4 also mentions mixed stones from the river Algeriche that, when rubbed together, can cause rain to fall into the river and continue as long as they are rubbed. *Picatrix*, trans. Attrell and Porreca, 263; *Picatrix, The Latin Version*, ed. Pingree, 218–19.

33 *Picatrix*, trans. Attrell and Porreca, 264; *Picatrix, The Latin Version*, ed. Pingree, 220.

This makes the late-medieval association of weather magic with witchcraft extremely interesting. Late-medieval sources often portray practitioners of weather magic in a negative light, depicting them as malicious, evil or demonic. References to weather manipulation by demons are found in inquisitorial manuals and later chronicles, drawing upon established scholastic discourses. In his third lecture on Job's first trial, which can be found in his *Expositio super Iob ad litteram*, thirteenth-century theologian Thomas Aquinas settles the question of whether demons can manipulate the weather by considering if "demons can bring about turbulence in the air, can stir up the winds, and can make fire fall from heaven."[34] Aquinas concludes that with God's permission, demons can indeed alter the weather, as "corporeal nature is still born to obey spiritual nature, as far as local movement is concerned"[35] and,

> whatever then can be done only with local motion, can be done by not only the good, but also the wicked angels from their natural power, unless prohibited by divine power. The winds the rains and other like disturbances in the atmosphere come about only from the motion of the vapours released from the earth and the water. Thus the natural power of a demon is sufficient to procure these things. However, sometimes they are prohibited from this by divine power so that they are not permitted to do everything which they can do naturally. Nor is this contrary to what is said in Jeremiah, 'Are there any among the false gods of the nations which can give rain?' (14:22). For it is one thing that the rain takes place by natural cause and this is the office of God alone who orders natural causes to this; it is another thing to use artificially those natural causes ordered by God to rain to produce rain or wind sometimes in an almost extraordinary way.[36]

According to Aquinas, weather falls under God's exclusive control, and only He possesses the authority to alter it. Nevertheless, demons, with God's permission, are believed to have the capacity to manipulate weather. The evidence indicates that theologians and chroniclers held the view that such manipulations could occur through a demonic pact forged between demons and humans. This also suggests the potential for demons to act out of malice in their role as testers of souls. Furthermore, there is a discernible surge in interest in this matter emerging from theological and legal circles during the later Middle Ages.

In the fifth book of the *Formicarius*, fifteenth-century theologian and religious reformer Johannes Nider discusses *maleficis* and their deception.[37] The book takes the

---

34 Aquinas, *Expositio*.

35 Aquinas, *Expositio*, 1.3.

36 Aquinas, *Expositio*, 1.3.

37 Nider, *Formicarius*, 5.4. A modern edition is available as: Nider, *Des sorciers* and partially in *L'imaginaire*, ed. Ostorero et al. For more on Nider and the *Formicarius*, see Nighman, "The *Manipulus*"; Galbreth, "Nider and the Exemplum"; Bailey, *Battling Demons*; Bailey, "From Sorcery"; and Bailey, "The Disenchantment."

form of a dialogue between a student named Piger and a theologian. It explores the question of whether demons and their disciples can perform harmful acts such as lightning strikes and hailstorms under the heading: "demons and their disciples can perform such *maleficia* by means of lightning, hailstorms, and the like, which some doubt."[38] The theologian builds upon Aquinas's teachings to assert that, with God's permission, "demons can induce a perturbation of the air, shatter the winds, and make fire rain from the sky."[39] Nider includes both demons and their disciples in performing such acts of *maleficia*. The weather is thus manipulated through an unsanctioned and repulsive relationship between humans and demons, causing harm to human beings.[40]

Nider's views differ from those of Agobard of Lyon, who showed disbelief in the ability of the *tempestarii* to control the weather. In another work, the moral treatise *Preceptorium divine legis*,[41] where he discusses magic and sorcery, Nider gives an example of how a *malefica* evinces her pact with a demon by appearing to cause rain after dipping a broom in water:

> Regarding this, it will be discussed later. However, these things are not immediately done by *maleficis* themselves. Rather, demons who made a pact with the *maleficis* from the beginning of the world and during the time of ancient idolatry, know immediately what effect they should procure according to the intention of the *maleficis*. For example, when a *malefica* dips a broom in water to make it rain, the broom itself does not cause the rain. Instead, it is the demon who sees this and has power over all corporeal things, and over the air, winds,

38 Nider, *Formicarius*, 5.4.10. "But winds and rains and other disturbances of the atmosphere can arise from the movement of vapours dissolved from the earth and water; hence, for the production of such things, the natural power of a demon is sufficient." Nider, *Formicarius*, 5.4.12.

39 Nider, *Formicarius*, 5.4.12.

40 Nider, *Formicarius*, 5.4.22 "When the judge Peter wanted to capture the aforementioned Stadelein through his servants, so great a tremor was struck into their hands and bodies, and such a foul stench entered their nostrils, that they almost despaired of daring to attack the malefactor. To them the judge said, 'Attack the wretched man without fear, because the power of public justice will destroy all the strength of his wickedness,' and thus the outcome or effect proved the truth of the matter. The same judge gave this example: 'When I had captured Stadelein, who had greatly damaged the earth with hail and famine, and had devastated many places with lightning, I asked the defendant about the truth, to which, after the fourth pull of the cords, he first gave me this answer: 'I can easily bring hail, but I am not able to harm at will, only those who are deprived of God's help; those who protect themselves with the sign of the cross will not perish by my lightning.' To which the judge replied, 'How do you proceed to raise storms and hail?' The defendant answered, 'First we implore the prince of all demons in the field with certain words, that he may send someone designated by us to strike him, then we come to a certain demon, in some field we sacrifice a black chick, throwing it high into the air, where it obeys the demon who took it, and immediately it raises the air, not always in places designated by us, but by permission of the living God, throwing hail and lightning.' The judge added a third question, 'Can such storms raised by you and by demons be remedied by some means?' He replied, 'They can, by these means, namely: I adjure you, hail and winds, by the three divine nails of Christ that pierced his hands and feet, and by the four holy evangelists, Matthew, Mark, Luke, and John, to descend in dissolved form into the water'."

41 The Latin text can be found in: Nider, *Preceptorium*.

> and clouds, that can immediately procure and cause such things if God permits. The *maga* gives a sign with the broom, but it is the demon who acts and procures the rain through his power, whom the *maga* serves in bad faith, and has surrendered to his services or to others.[42]

The notion of a demonic pact causing weather disturbances is explored in the infamous fifteenth-century *Malleus maleficarum*. In a chapter discussing methods of sorcery, the text outlines how sorceresses can cause bad weather,[43] adding to examples of witches stirring up hailstorms throughout the book. This chapter builds upon Nider's *Formicarius*, 5.4, which in turn elaborated on Aquinas's discussion of Job. It states that demons and their followers are capable of causing acts of sorcery, including the stirring up of lighting, hailstorms, and rainstorms:

> with God's permission the demons are able to cause a disturbance of the air, to stir up winds, and to make fire fall from heaven [...] since wind and rain and other such disturbances of the air can be made through the mere movement of vapours released from the earth and air, the natural virtue of a demon is sufficient to cause such events.[44]

The argument follows the same line of argument as before: God justly inflicts the evils committed in the world as a result of humanity's sins. However, demons prefer to harm humans in cooperation with sorcerers, and due to their nature: "they know how to attach active to passive elements both in the air and around the fiery sphere on occasions when they are given permission by God and cause fire to fall from heaven or lightning bolts to strike."[45] This theoretical discussion is then followed by anecdotal evidence, initially linked to the *Formicarius*, where an accused person confronted by a judge provides testimony about their manipulation of the weather:

> first in the field we use certain words to beseech the Prince of All Demons to send one of his subordinates to strike the person indicated by us. Then, when a certain demon comes, we sacrifice a black rooster to him at a crossroads by casting it up into the air. Having accepted it, the demon obeys and immediately stirs up a breeze. Yet he does not always cast the hailstorms and lighting bolts

---

42 Nider, *Preceptorium*, 1.11.16.22. For a different translation of this passage, see Bailey, "The Feminization." On this passage see also, Bailey, "The Disenchantment" and Bailey, "From Sorcery."

43 "The method by which they stir up hailstorms and rainstorms and also make lightning strike humans and domestic animals." Institoris and Sprenger, *Hammer*. For the Latin text, see Institoris and Sprenger, *Malleus Maleficarum*, 2.15. See also, Broedel, *Malleus Maleficarum*. For additional examples of witches impacting the weather see the literature included in Ostorero, *Le diable au sabbat* and Ostorero and Véronèse, *Penser avec les demons*.

44 Mackay, *Hammer*, 380–81; Institoris, *Malleus*, 2.15.

45 Mackay, *Hammer*, 381; Institoris, *Malleus*, 2.15.

> into the places intended by us, but does so according to the permission of the Living God.[46]

Here, the contrast with previous depictions of weather magic is striking. Unlike Nectanebus, this male practitioner appears uneducated and unprivileged. The elements of his ritual evoke images of *superstitio* and *maleficium*, i.e., perverse necromancy, rather than sophisticated water divination. It is more akin to the depiction of the *tempestarii*, who were ridiculed by Agobard of Lyon centuries earlier. However, the text does not ridicule this male practitioner; instead, the exemplum is meant to be taken seriously. It also serves to illustrate the genuine and significant danger posed by demons and their accomplices, even to the simplest of people.

A second anecdote follows about two proven witches: Stafus, who resided in Berne, and his disciple, Hoppo. A barrage of typical accusations against *malefici* is brought forwards, including weather manipulation, as they:

> knew how, whenever they wished, to bring dung, hay or grain or anything at all from a neighbour's field to their own without anyone seeing, how to cause very strong hailstorms, and harmful breezes as well as lightning bolts, how to cast toddlers walking along the waters in the sight of their parents into the water without anyone seeing, how to bring about barrenness in humans and domestic animals, how to reveal concealed things to others, how to cause harm in objects and bodies in any way at all, sometimes how to kill whomever they wished with a strike of lighting and to cause many other baneful things, where and when God's justice permitted these things to happen.[47]

We are far removed from Isidore's stripped-down definition of *malefici* and Agobard's purported disbelief, as well as from Pseudo-Callisthenes' story of whole invading armies being stopped by manipulating the elements with a magic bowl, an ebony staff, and detailed waxen figurines. These two *malefici*, Stafus and Hoppo, can cause all sorts of harm to their neighbours, including precise weather manipulation, such as striking lightning in a specific location, which is a novelty thus far. They do this so they can steal or damage crops in the fields. This exemplum brings the reality of weather magic to the present, the mundane, the common, and the familiar, removing it from the realm of literary fantasy and historical and theological complexity.

The final case study in this chapter is particularly significant in emphasizing the points made, especially as both practitioners involved are women, unlike in previous examples. The incident in question was caused by "a very savage hailstorm [that] was stirred up, and for a distance of one mile it crushed the produce, crops and vineyards to such an extent that two years later the harvest in the vineyards was hardly judged to be plentiful."[48] This level of destruction is comparable to the seventh plague in Egypt

46 Mackay, *Hammer*, 382; Institoris, *Malleus*, 2.15.

47 Mackay, *Hammer*, 382; Institoris, *Malleus*, 2.15.

48 Mackay, *Hammer*, 383; Institoris, *Malleus*, 2.15.

attributed to God. As a response to such strange and harmful events, an inquisition was conducted, potentially by Institoris, one of the two men credited with the composition of the *Malleus*, which resulted in the detention of Agnes, a bathkeeper, and Anna of Mindelheim.

Under "light" torture, Agnes was asked if she knew anything about the hailstorm incident. Although she had refused to confess anything under duress, she apparently answered freely, describing an encounter in her house where a demon summoned her at noon and instructed her to bring water from the open country. When she asked what the demon wanted to do with the water, he replied that he wished to make it rain. Agnes went through the city gate and found the demon standing under a tree. She was then told to dig a small hole and pour water into it, which she did while stirring the water with her finger in the name of the devil and all other demons. The water disappeared, and the devil took it up into the air. The delay between the rising of the water and the hailstorm lasted until she arrived home. Both Agnes and Anna confessed to the same thing and were condemned to be burned to ashes.[49]

After reading this account, it becomes clear that women accused of sorcery were believed to have the power to manipulate the weather and cause harm. The demons are portrayed as the ones in control, while the sorceresses are merely carrying out their orders using simple materials like water and a finger. There is no sophisticated bowl or ebony staff involved here, nor any reference to a magical ring or sophisticated amulet. It is clear that the power of the demons alone is enough to stir up the elements. The passage concludes by stating: "let these facts suffice, though actually, the number of events that could be cited about the infliction of such acts of sorcery is virtually countless."[50] Additionally, the text explains that lighting strikes can occur without the involvement of sorceresses, but evidence suggests that they have caused them. The passage concludes by asserting that since sorceresses (*maleficae*) can cause lightning bolts as easily as hailstorms, any uncertainty regarding their ability to manipulate the elements should be dispelled.[51] The text thus supports the belief that these events were widespread and removes any doubt about the ability of sorceresses to manipulate the weather and cause harm.

The *Malleus Maleficarum* is not the only source to cite examples of weather manipulation by so-called witches or *malefici*. In a fifteenth-century Brut, or *Chronicle of England*, there is an entry for the year 1441 that describes how Eleanor, the wife of Humphrey of Gloucester, the uncle and guardian of the young Henry VI, is accused of using magic against the king.

---

49 Mackay, *Hammer*, 383–85; Institoris, *Malleus*, 2.15.

50 Mackay, *Hammer*, 385; Institoris, *Malleus*, 2.15.

51 "without the cooperation of the sorceresses. Nonetheless, it has been found [...] that sorceresses have caused them [...]. Reason also lends its support since they can cause lightning bolts as easily as they can hailstorms. Hence all uncertainty is removed." Mackay, *Hammer*, 386; Institoris, *Malleus*, 2.15.

The charges brought against Eleanor include a conspiracy with a clerk named Roger Bollingbroke, by which "certeyn clerkes, and women þat ar called 'wicches,' had made theire operacion and theire craft to destroy men and women, or whom they list, vnto deth by theire fals craft and worching."[52] The chronicle describes Roger as "hir Clerk, a Nigromancier, by the deuels crafte and ymaginacion in his worching."[53] Under duress, Roger confesses to the use of "ymages of siluer, of wexe, and of oþer metalles, and swerdys, with many oþer dyuers instruments of this fals craft of Nigromancy and the devels powere."[54] These instruments are shown to both Roger and the duchess to extract a confession from her, which, according to this version of the chronicle, is given. Other accomplices are imprisoned, and some even die there, such as the canon Thomas Southwell. The infamous witch of Eye, Margery Jourdemayne, who was a relapsed witch with a past incarceration for black magic, is charged with high treason and burnt at the stake. After Bollingbroke is hanged, the duchess is convicted, imprisoned and sentenced to submit herself to public penance. She is also made to offer a taper at various churches around London after barefoot processions.[55]

The episode both opens and closes with violent disturbances of the weather in the form of hailstorms. According to this version of the chronicle, the enquiry begins after it hailed, rained, and there was great lightning. The people were aghast and afraid of the tempest and thought that wicked fiends and spirits "arered out of helle by coniuracion" were trying to harm the king who had just passed the city. Similarly, after Eleanor's humiliation but before she is imprisoned in Peel Castle in the Isle of Man, "when she was brought first out of Westminster, þere was such wedryng of thonder, lightnyng, hayll and rayne, þat the peple were sore adredde and agast of the grete noyse and hydous of þe weder, at soddenly was doon and shewed þere at theire passage at þat tyme."[56]

This episode presents a second testimony on weather magic and its connection to witchcraft in the fifteenth century. It illustrates how wealthy merchants in fifteenth-century London, the purported authors of the chronicle, were willing to believe in a plot to harm the king involving weather manipulation. This demonstrates a significant shift in attitudes since Agobard's scepticism towards the *tempestarii*, as theologians, inquisitors, and the affluent elite of the late Middle Ages are far removed from the superstitious peasants that Agobard criticized in his work *De grandine et tronitruis*.

Based on the evidence examined, it appears that during the Middle Ages, there was growing acceptance amongst the learned of the possibility of manipulating the weather through magic. The methods varied, with some requiring the services of a highly edu-

52 *Brut*, ed. Brie, 477–88. Other contemporary sources of the anecdote do not include a reference to weather magic, see for example: *A Chronicle of London*, ed. Nicolas and Tyrell and *Chronicle of the Grey Friars*, ed. Nichols. See also: Griffiths, "The trial"; Ralley, "Stars"; Carey, *Courting Disaster*; "Astrology"; Petrina, *Cultural Politics*; North, *Horoscopes*.

53 *Brut*, 478.

54 *Brut*, 478.

55 *Brut*, 478–82.

56 *Brut*, 482.

cated and sophisticated male practitioner with access to significant resources and exotic materials. Chronicle accounts, like the *Brut,* suggest belief that the elements, including the air, responded to the presence of demonic activity. Thus, weather magic increasingly served as a reminder of the dangers posed by demons to humanity due to their malice and the harm that could result from consorting with them. Here, attitudes shifted, with disbelief giving way to belief in the physical reality of weather manipulation through magical means. This serves as evidence of the many fears and anxieties that came to characterize theological and inquisitorial discourse by the end of the Middle Ages.

Bibliography

Primary Sources

Agobard of Lyon. *Liber contra insulam uulgi opinionem de grandine et tonitruis.* Edited by Jacques Paul Migne. Patrologiae cursus completus. Series Latina 104. Paris: Migne, 1864.

——. *Opera Omnia.* Edited by L. Van Acker, 3–15. Corpus Christianorum Continuatio Mediaevalis 52 Turnhout: Brepols, 1981.

Augustine. *The City of God Against the Pagans.* Edited by R. W. Dyson. Cambridge: Cambridge University Press, 2013.

——. *De civitate Dei Libri XXII.* Edited by Bernard Dombart and Alfons Kalb. Stuttgart: Teubner, 1993.

The Brut, or The Chronicles of England. Edited by F. W. D. Brie. Early English Text Society 136. Vol. 2. London: Kegan Paul, Trench, Trübner, 1908.

Chronicle of the Grey Friars of London. Edited by John Gough Nichols. London: Camden Society, 1852.

A Chronicle of London from 1089 to 1483 Written in the Fifteenth Century, and for the First Time Printed from MSS. In the British Museum. Edited by Nicholas Harris Nicolas and Edward Tyrell. London: Richard Taylor, 1827.

Geoffrey of Monmouth. *The History of the Kings of Britain.* Edited by Michael D. Reeve and translated by Neil Wright. Woodbridge: Boydell, 2009.

L'imaginaire du Sabbat. Edition critique des textes les plus anciens (1430 c.–1440). Edited by Martine Ostorero, Agostino Paravicini Bagliani, and Kathrin Utz Tremp. Cahiers Lausannois de'Histoire Médiévale, 26. Lausanne: Université de Lausanne, 1999.

Institoris, Henricus, and Jacobus Sprenger. *The Hammer of Witches. A Complete Translation of the* Malleus Maleficarum. Translated by Christopher S. Mackay. Cambridge: Cambridge University Press, 2009.

Institoris, Heinricus, and Jakob Sprenger. *Malleus Maleficarum.* Nuremberg: Koberger, 1494. https://collections.nlm.nih.gov/catalog/nlm:nlmuid-9413083-bk.

Isidore of Seville. *Etymologiarvm Sive Originvm Libri XX.* Edited by W. M. Lindsay, Oxford: Oxford University Press, 1911.

——. *The Etymologies of Isidore of Seville.* Edited and translated by Stephen A. Barney, W. J. Lewis, J. A. Beach, and Oliver Berghof. Cambridge: Cambridge University Press, 2006.

Iulius Valerius Alexander Polemius. *Res Gestae Alexanderi Macedonis.* Edited by Michela Rosellini. München: De Gruyter, 2004.

John of Salisbury. *Frivolities of Courtiers and Footprints of Philosophers, Being a Translation of the First, Second and Third Bookds and Selections from the Seventh and Eighth Books of the Policraticus of John of Salisbury*. Edited by Joseph B. Pike. New York: Octagon, 1972.

——, *Policraticus I-IV*. Corpus Christianorum Continuatio Mediaevalis 118. Edited by Katherine S. B. Keats-Rohan. Turnhout: Brepols, 1993.

Kors, Alan Charles, and Edward Peters. *Witchcraft in Europe, 400–1700, A Documentary History*. Philadelphia: University of Pennsylvania Press, 2001.

Lewis, W. J. "Agobard of Lyons (9th Century): On Hail and Thunder." *Internet Medieval Sourcebook*. Edited by Paul Halsall. https://sourcebooks.fordham.edu/source/agobard-onhailandthunder.asp (accessed May 10, 2024).

Nider, Johannes. *Des sorciers et leurs trumperies, La Fourmillière Livre V*. Edited and translated by J. Céard. Grenoble: Millón, 2005.

——. *Formicarius*. Edited by G. Colvener. Douai: 1602.

——. *Preceptorium divine legis*. Milan: Giovanni Antonio di Onate, 1487. https://archive.org/details/ita-bnc-in2-00000911-001/page/n8/mode/2up (accessed May 10, 2024).

Picatrix, The Latin Version of the Gāyat Al-Hakīm. Edited by David Pingree. London: The Warburg Institute, 1986.

Picatrix. A Medieval Treatise on Astral Magic. Translated by Dan Attrell and David Porreca. University Park: The Pennsylvania State University Press, 2019.

Thomas Aquinas. *Expositio super Iob ad litteram. Commentary on the Book of Job 1.3*. Edited by The Aquinas Institute. https://aquinas.cc/la/en/~Job; translated by Brian Mullady, edited and html-formatted Joseph Kenny. Lander: The Aquinas Institute for the Study of Sacred Doctrine, 2016, https://isidore.co/aquinas/SSJob.htm (accessed May 10, 2024).

Secondary Sources

Avner, Ben-Zaken. "Travelling with the Picatrix: Cultural Liminalities of Science and Magic." In *Religious Individualisation (Historical Dimensions and Comparative Perspectives)*. Edited by Martin Fuchs, Antje Linkenbach, Martin Mulsow, Bernd-Christian Otto, Rahul Bjørn Parson, and Jörg Rüpke. 1033–106. München: De Gruyter, 2020.

Bailey, Michael D. *Battling Demons. Witchcraft, Heresy, and Reform in the Late Middle Ages*. University Park: The Pennsylvania State University Press, 2003.

——. "The Disenchantment of Magic: Spells, Charms, and Superstition in Early European Witchcraft Literature." *American Historical Review* 111, no. 2 (April 2006): 383–404.

——. "The Feminization of Magic and the Emerging Idea of the Female Witch in the Late Middle Ages." *Essays in Medieval Studies* 19 (2002): 120–34.

——. "From Sorcery to Witchcraft: Clerical Conceptions of Magic in the Later Middle Ages." *Speculum* 76, no. 4 (October 2001): 960–90.

——. "Magic and Disbelief in Carolingian Lyon." In *Civilizations of the Supernatural: Witchcraft, Ritual, and Religious Experience in Late Antique, Medieval, and Renaissance Traditions*. Edited by Fabrizio Conti, 177–20. Budapest: Trivent, 2020.

Boudet, Jean-Patrice, and Jean-Charles Coulon. "La version arab (*Ghāyat al-ḥakīm*) et la version latine du *Picatrix*." *Cahiers de recherches médiévales et humanistes* 33 (2017): 67–101.

Boudet, Jean-Patrice, Anna Caiozzo, and Nicolas Weill-Parot. *Images et magie: Picatrix entre Orient et Occident*. Paris: Champion, 2011.

Broedel, Hans Peter. *The* Malleus Maleficarum *and the Construction of Witchcraft. Theology and Popular Belief*. Manchester: Manchester University Press, 2003.

Carey, Hilary M. "Astrology at the English Court in the Late Middle Ages." In *Astrology, Science and Society: Historical Essays*. Edited by P. Curry, 41–56. Woodbridge: Boydell Press, 1987.

——. *Courting Disaster. Astrology at the English Court and University in the Later Middle Ages.* London: Macmillan, 1992.

DeAngeli, Edna S. "Julius Valerius' Account of the Birth of Alexander: Text and Translation." In *John Gower's Literary Transformations in the* Confessio Amantis*: Original Articles and Translations*. Edited by Peter G. Beidler, 119–41. Washington: University Press of America, 1982.

Dutton, Paul Edward. *Carolingian Civilization: A Reader.* Peterborough: Broadview, 1993.

——. "Thunder and Hail Over the Carolingian Countryside." In *Agriculture in the Middle Ages*. Edited by D. Sweeney, 111–37. Philadelphia: University of Pennsylvania Press, 1995.

Escobar-Vargas, M. Carolina. "El Marco de la Historia: El Papel de la Profecía en la *Historia Regum Britanniae* de Geoffrey de Monmouth." *Lingüística y Literatura* 68 (2015): 83–105.

Galbreth, Beatrice. "Nider and the Exemplum—A Study of the *Formicarius*." *Fabula* 6, no. 1 (1964): 55–72.

Griffiths, Ralph A. "The Trial of Eleanor Cobham: An Episode in the Fall of Duke Humphrey of Gloucester." *Bulletin of the John Rylands Library* 51, no. 2 (1969): 381–99.

Halstead, Chris. "'They Ride on the Backs of Certain Beasts': The Night Rides, the *Canon Episcopi*, and Regino of Prüm's Historical Method." *Magic, Ritual and Witchcraft* 15, no. 3 (Winter 2020): 361–85.

Jolivet, Jean. "Agobard de Lyon et les faiseurs de pluie." In *La méthode critique au Moyen Âge*. Edited by Mireille Chazan and Gilbert Dahan, 15–25. Turnhout: Brepols, 2006.

Lawrence-Mathers, Anne, and Carolina Escobar-Vargas. *Magic and Medieval Society*. London, Routledge, 2014.

Means, Rob. "Thunder Over Lyon: Agobard, the *tempestarii* and Christianity." In *Paganism in the Middle Ages: Threat and Fascination*. Edited by Carlos Steel, John Marenbon, and Werner Verbeke, 157–66. Leuven: Leuven University Press, 2012.

Nighman, Chris. "The *Manipulus florum*, Johannes Nider's *Formicarius*, and Late Medieval Misogyny in the Construction of Witches Prior to the *Malleus maleficarum*." *The Journal of Medieval Latin* 24 (2014): 171–84.

North, John D. *Horoscopes and History*. London: The Warburg Institute, 1986.

Ostorero, Martine. *Le diable au sabbat. Littérature déonologique et sorcellerie (1440–1460)*. Florence: SISMEL-Edizioni del Galluzzo, 2011.

Ostorero, Martine and Julien Véronèse, eds. *Penser avec les demons. Démonologues et demonologies (XIIIe-XVIIe siècles)*. Florence: SISMEL—Galluzzo, 2015.

Petrina, Alessandra. *Cultural Politics in Fifteenth-Century England, the Case of Humphrey, Duke of Gloucester.* Leiden: Brill, 2004.

Pingree, David. "Between the *Ghaya* and the *Picatrix*. I: The Spanish Version." *Journal of the Warburg and Courtauld Instittutes* 14 (1981): 27–56.

Ralley, Robert. "Stars, Demons and the Body in Fifteenth-Century England." *Studies in History and Philosophy of Biological and Biomedical Sciences* 41 (2010): 109–16.

Saif, Liana. *The Arabic Influences on Early Modern Occult Philosophy*. Basingstoke: Palgrave Macmillan, 2015.

THE BOUNDARIES OF MAGIC AND MEDICINE IN MEDIEVAL THEOLOGY

VICTORIA BURNS-PRICE

IN THE MEDIEVAL period the seemingly disparate disciplines of medicine and magic were actually closely linked with one another, in practice if not always in theory. Furthermore, across the wide timescale that makes up the Middle Ages, both medicine and magic as independent concepts went through significant changes and developments. There were many reasons for this, largely rooted in the phenomenon of the twelfth-century renaissance and the widespread translation of Greek and Arabic texts. The re-emergence of "natural philosophy" led to renewed interest in where ideas like magic and medicine were placed within this wider philosophical network. Similarly, the definitions of both magic and medicine shifted. Ecclesiastical and secular authorities sought to define and control these disciplines for both theoretical and juridical reasons. However, the resulting theoretical restrictions did not always align with the actual practices that individuals were undertaking in the real world, and there were many instances in medieval society where medicine and magic merged into one another. Equally, the definitions which emerged were not only increasingly complex and contradictory, but also allowed individual interpretation—especially in the case of practices which were new and not easy to categorize.

This topic has featured in much modern scholarship within a range of contexts. Iolanda Ventura, for instance, has written a significant body of work considering the role of botany and herbals in medieval medical practice.[1] In the realm of magic, Catherine Rider discusses the relationship between magic and medicine in a number of publications. Most notably, her 2011 article, "Medical Magic and the Church in Thirteenth-Century England," which considers how the Church defined "magical" cures, and to what extent charms and talismans were accepted as medicine.[2] Rider's 2006 book, *Magic and Impotence in the Middle Ages*, looks at the very specific practice of magically-caused impotence, a major concern for canon lawyers and theologians due to its potential impact on the sacrament of marriage.[3] Lea Olsan has written extensively on the use of charms and how they compare to, or are distinct from, Christian prayers, in both *The Marginality of Charms in Medieval England* (2013), and her *Charms and Prayers in Medi-*

1 Most recently, Ventura, Hunt, and Mayer, "Plants and Medicine," in *A Cultural History of Plants*, vol. 2.

2 Rider, "Medical Magic and the Church."

3 Rider, *Magic and Impotence.*

Victoria Burns-Price is a freelance university tutor specializing in medieval magic, currently teaching with the University of Oxford's Continuing Education Department.

eval Medical Theory and Practice (2003).[4] More recently, Olsan co-contributed a chapter to the 2019 text, *The Routledge History of Medieval Magic*, alongside Peter Murray Jones, titled "Medicine and Magic," which provides a thorough overview of the history and development of medical magic and how this compared to formalized medicine.[5]

Building on this scholarship, this chapter will further explore the complex and shifting boundary between magic and medicine. It will demonstrate that there are examples in both formal and informal practices where what some considered to be legitimate medical or religious practices were deemed unacceptable by others due to perceived associations with unknown forces. A central focus will be on changes over time, especially in canon law, which laid out the theoretical and practical stance of the Church. Specific texts which shall be used in this chapter include the works of Isidore of Seville and Augustine of Hippo, as well as of the foundational scholar in the field of canon law, Gratian. The main argument will be that practices involving the use of natural substances proved particularly problematic and thus are of special interest for historians.

Medieval medicine was an evolving discipline, as the chapter in this volume by Anne Jeavons demonstrates, which progressed as knowledge from the classical and Islamicate worlds became accessible. In the early medieval period formal medicine was largely based on the little Greek knowledge that survived.[6] The available texts outlined, amongst other things, the theory of the four humours.[7] An excess or lack of any of these four humours was considered a likely cause of illness, and the cure was often to try to rebalance the body utilizing the relevant elements and natural substances. The consensus of medical historians is that the twelfth century was a turning point for the availability of medical texts. Consequently, medicine moved from being a skilled trade (termed *medicina*) to a form of philosophy worthy of research and formal education in the newly developed universities (*physica*).[8] The universities of Bologna, Paris, Montpellier, and Oxford all developed medical faculties between the twelfth and fifteenth centuries. This development led to a formalized curriculum based upon set texts.

This narrative concerns medicine as it was understood by the educated and wealthy elite and practised by educated individuals who had access to copies of key texts. However, medicine was a requirement throughout society, regardless of education or wealth, and so other practitioners were also active who provided cheaper, more accessible services. Monks sometimes made their medical knowledge available to the wider community.[9] In other instances, individuals relied on orally-transmitted

4 Olsan, "The Marginality of Charms"; Olsan, "Charms and Prayers."

5 Jones and Olsan, "Medicine and Magic."

6 Vol. 1 of Isidore of Seville, *Etymologiarum*, ed. Lindsay; Hippocrates et al., *The Aphorismes of Hippocrates*.

7 Jouanna, *Greek Medicine from Hippocrates to Galen*, ed. van der Eijk, 335.

8 Wallis, ed., *Medieval Medicine: A Reader*, xxii.

9 See Hammond, "Physicians in Medieval English Religious Houses."

remedies.[10] In conclusion, the types of medical knowledge and healing accessible across the social spectrum were disparate, and perceived links to magical activities were more likely to be problematic amongst the cures used by the poorer members of society, as shall be explored below.

Medieval magic is a difficult concept to define. Most of the medieval theologians who considered the topic relied on the writings of Church Fathers who focussed primarily on the struggle with classical paganism. Augustine was a prolific writer, but perhaps his main contribution to ideas of magic in the medieval period was his insistence that magic was demonic. Augustine firmly asserts that magic is superstitious, a category into which pagan religions also fall, and that pagan gods are actually demons.[11] Continuing this logic, he concludes that all magic is indeed reliant on demons. This view was echoed by Isidore of Seville, who also demonstrates another belief held by early theologians, that magic was primarily varying forms of divination. This can be seen in his *Etymologiae* which comprises a list of different types of divination such as *necromantii*, *geomantiam*, *hydromantiam*, *æromantiam*, *pyromantiam*, *arioli*, *haruspices*, *augures*, *auspices*, *astrologi*, *mathematici*, *genethliaci*, *horoscopi*, *sortilegi*, and *salisatores*.[12] Later definitions of magic remained heavily reliant on those of the Church Fathers. Hugh of St. Victor's *Didascalicon*, produced in the 1130s, reproduces Isidore's list of magical practices, suggesting that divination was the main concern up until this time.[13] Similarly, Peter Lombard's *Sententiarum* refers back to Augustine and states that: "The magic arts are made powerful by the devil's strength and knowledge, strength and knowledge which was given to him by God either to deceive the wicked, or to warn or train the good."[14] In the twelfth century there was even debate amongst theologians and lawyers as to whether magic was real, what it could achieve if it was, and how much that necessarily concerned the Church.[15] By the thirteenth century, the discussions of magic in theological works were becoming more prominent and lists of practices associated with demonic intervention were longer and more complex. The intricacies of important practices using natural substances are the central issue for this case study.

10 See Rider, "Medical Magic and the Church"; Rider, "Lay Religion and Pastoral Care."

11 Augustine, *De doctrina Christiana*, ed. and trans. Green, bk. 8, chaps. 16, 18.

12 Isidore of Seville, *Etymologiarum*, bk. 8, chap. 9, §§1–4, 1:347.

13 *The Didascalicon of Hugh of St. Victor*, ed. and trans. Jerome Taylor, bk. 6, chap. 15, 154.

14 Peter Lombard, *Sententiarum*, ed. Migne, II.7.6, 665: "Magicæ artes virtute et scientia diaboli valent, quæ virtus et scientia est ei data a Deo, vel ad fallendum malos, vel ad monendum vel ad exercendum bonos."

15 The famous tenth-century *Canon Episcopi* which is used by later texts, such as the fifteenth-century *Malleus Maleficarum*, to reinforce the danger magic posed, actually declares that women accused of night flights to meet with the Devil are completely deceived by demonic forces and are not travelling anywhere or performing any of the things they are accused of, except in their own minds.

Natural Substances

The use of plants, animal parts, and stones has long been linked with medicinal practice. However, in the medieval period the use of natural items was also associated with the supernatural and could be utilized for calling upon both divine and demonic powers.[16] Indeed, at times, the very same substances and activities were understood by some to be using natural powers and by others to be tapping into the demonic. It is common to associate the use of natural substances with the wider populace as such practices often use commonplace materials and are theoretically available to anyone. However, expensive and often illustrated manuscripts frequently included instruction on medical uses of gemstones or rare ingredients, indicating that natural remedies, albeit more exotic ones, were also being used by the wealthy and educated.[17] The activities discussed below are therefore relevant to a cross-section of society. The main form of evidence we have in relation to these practices is textual. Manuscripts describing plants, animals, and stones, alongside their properties and uses, date back to antiquity and continued to be produced throughout the medieval period. These are classified as herbals, bestiaries, and lapidaries respectively.

The concept of utilizing plants for medicinal purposes is an ancient one. The Ebers Papyrus, dating from the sixteenth century BCE and currently held in the University of Leipzig, demonstrates the interest in the subject in Egypt, while the Mesopotamians documented the medicinal properties of some plants in the seventh century BCE, as seen in tablets held by the British Museum.[18] Herbals date back to the first century BCE with the *De materia medica* of Dioscorides being an early example.[19] The purpose of such texts was to list the known medical properties of plants for reference. Similarly, bestiaries listing animals alongside their appearance and characteristics also developed from classical predecessors. Early bestiaries came to include Christian religious allegory. A notable example is the third-century anonymous *Physiologus*. This text was widely distributed across medieval Europe, surviving in hundreds of manuscript copies.[20] Alongside the *Etymologiae* of Isidore of Seville, it became the basis for most medieval bestiary texts.[21] However, in one later group many of the allegorical elements disappeared and details of animals emphasized medical uses of body parts. This approach drew upon the *De animalibus* of Albertus Magnus, written ca. 1250. This was originally a commentary on the work by Aristotle by the same name but developed into an influen-

---

16 For discussion of the complexities arising from this, see Sebastià Giralt, chapter 7 above.

17 The fact that there are many practices that cross the social divide warrants its own discussion, but there is not room here to do it justice.

18 London, British Museum, no. 46226, ca. 7th century BCE clay tablet: https://www.britishmuseum.org/collection/object/W_1881-0706-688 (accessed May 10, 2024).

19 Stannard, "Medieval Herbals," 23.

20 Surviving manuscripts include Bern, Burgerbibliothek, MS 318 (ninth century); Oxford, Bodleian Library MS Auct. T. 2. 23 (tenth century); London, British Library, MS Royal 6 A XI (twelfth century), and BL MS Sloane 278 (thirteenth century).

21 For helpful studies see Hassig, ed., *The Mark of the Beast.*

tial work in its own right. The lapidaries listed different stones and their properties and again they originated in classical works, such as sections of Pliny the Elder's *Naturalis historia*. Richard Kieckhefer picks out *De lapidibus* by Bishop Marbode of Rennes, an eleventh-century Latin text which describes the features and properties of sixty stones, as a particularly popular example.[22] Further respectability was given by Albertus Magnus, in his *De mineralibus*. Many of the entries are focussed on describing the physical aspects of the stones in question, but some have detailed explanations of their medicinal properties as well. These texts provide convincing evidence that individuals believed in, and used, the power of nature for healing and protection.

A popular herbal text throughout the medieval period was the *Herbarium* of Pseudo-Apuleius, dating from the fifth century CE, of which over sixty medieval manuscript copies survive.[23] The *Herbarium* is devoted to the description of plants, including their physical appearance, properties, and uses. One example is the mandrake, which can be used in different forms, such as juice from the leaves or powdered root, to cure ailments including headache, sleeplessness, earache, gout, insanity, and nerve spasms.[24] In the realm of bestiaries, physical descriptions of animals were accompanied by details of their behaviours. For example, most describe how tigers can be tricked by using mirrors in order to steal their cubs.[25] Another influential text is the *Liber medicinae ex animalibus*, written in the fourth century by Sextus Placitus. This focuses on medicinal uses of animals, such as consuming pickled dogs to protect against pain.[26] Other texts, however, emphasize the concept of the marvellous, and detail mythical animals like manticores, phoenixes, and unicorns.[27] Turning to consideration of stones, Bishop Marbode of Rennes' *De lapidibus* provided important medical information.[28] *Memphitis*, for example, can be used to numb pain if ground up and applied to injuries while *aetites* are stones which have both a masculine and feminine version and, when used together, can aid with childbirth. Sapphires are described as useful for the curing of headaches and sores, as well as for their ability to encourage prayers and restore God's peace, marking their place within both medical and religious observance. Similarly, Matthew Paris' thirteenth-century *Liber additamentorum*, which lists the gems and rings held by

---

22 Kieckhefer, *Magic in the Middle Ages*, 103.

23 Interestingly, there are four surviving copies of the text in the Old English vernacular, often titled the *Old English Herbarium*, demonstrating both its widespread use and its interest for those outside of formal Latin teaching. See Van Arsdall, *Medieval Herbal Remedies*. The British Library (hereafter BL) holds MSS Cotton Vitellius C III, Harley 585, Sloane 1975 and Harley 6258 B, all from the eleventh and twelfth centuries. MS Cotton Vitellius C III is the only extant illustrated version of the *Old English Herbarium* and is available fully digitized on their website. See also Collins, *Medieval Herbals*, 65.

24 Van Arsdall, *Medieval Herbal Remedies*, 133.

25 See for instance the rhyming bestiary in Oxford, Bodleian Library, MS Canon Ital 38.

26 Stewart, "The Mediaeval Bestiary and Its Textual Tradition," 66.

27 London, BL, MS Royal 12 F XIII includes a manticore (fol. 24v) and a unicorn (fol. 10v).

28 Marbode, bishop of Rennes, *Libellus de lapidibus preciosis*, VII, 16.

St. Albans Abbey in Hertfordshire, includes reference to a stone used for protection in childbirth.[29]

The application of herbs, animal parts, and stones in a medical setting might therefore seem to have been a straightforward affair. However, the use of plants was a concern to Church authorities. There is reference to such activities in the twelfth-century *Decretum* of Gratian, who states clearly that the gathering of herbs under certain circumstances (for example, under a full moon while reciting an incantation) is contrary to the teachings of the Church.[30] Significant concern regarding the use of natural substances reappears in the works of Bonaventure in the thirteenth century, who declares that the Devil works his power through such items.[31] A case can be made that users of natural items might be unaware of the theological complexities surrounding these activities and assume that natural substances have innate properties that can legitimately be utilized through medical means for the purposes of healing. Without being well-versed in theological writings such users would perhaps know that sage can be used to cure headaches, as described in the *Compendium medicinae* of Gilbertus Anglicus, but simultaneously be unaware of Gratian's concern around how the herbs in question were gathered.

However, in other examples the inconsistency surrounding the legitimacy of certain practices is more explicit. For example, given the medical and religious credentials sapphires have been bestowed in *De lapidibus*, it is all the more interesting that the text also lists *necromantia* among its powers, a practice firmly understood as being within the realm of magic throughout the medieval period. Indeed, sapphires are not the only gem associated with necromancy and magic in this text, and diadochos is another.[32] Other magical gems include toadstones, which supposedly came from the head of a toad and were thought to be useful as an antidote to poison, and which were often incorporated into jewellery. The use of animals was also, at times, complicated. The example given above from the *Liber medicinae ex animalibus*, regarding the use of dogs in a remedy against pain, was a complicated treatment. The first-born pup had to be killed soon after its birth, before being cleaned, pickled, and consumed. If this was done, it was promised that the recipient would not feel pain at any time. This is more reminiscent of complex magical practices rather than straightforward medical remedies. Some authoritative figures, including Albertus Magnus and William of Auvergne, made a case for "natural" magic.[33] While acknowledging that certain phenomena did not have an easily explainable basis in religion or science, they refuted that this meant that they were definitively demonic as a result. Other theologians, including Albertus Magnus' own student Thomas Aquinas, largely argued against this concept and argued that anything which demon-

29 BL, MS Cotton Nero D I, fol. 146v.

30 Gratian, "Decretum," ed. Friedberg, Part 2, C. 26 q. 5, at 1028.

31 Bonaventura, *Commentaria Sententiarum*, bk. 2, dist. 7 pt. 2 art. 2 q.3, 2:205.

32 Marbode, bishop of Rennes, *Libellus de lapidibus preciosis*, XLVI, 38.

33 See Giralt, above; and Lawrence-Mathers and Escobar-Vargas, *Magic and Medieval Society*, 53.

strates a power beyond what is reasonably expected is magic and all magic is demonic.[34] The complexities of these arguments and their largely unresolved nature are considered at length in Sebastià Giralt's chapter in this book.[35]

As Giralt explains, the reframing of Greek philosophical principles within the Christian worldview led to a new understanding of the created world within theological circles. Some theologians began to argue that there was a unifying structure within which all creation existed and that as a result seemingly disparate phenomena were actually interconnected. Natural philosophy, or natural magic, sought to understand these connections and, furthermore, sought to use them to advantage. In this area, too, we can find examples where the boundaries between medicine and magic begin to break down.

One of the largest and most prolific disciplines within the new learning of the twelfth century was astrology. This was a complex field and could be used for a wide variety of applications, in which the theoretically firm boundary between *magica* and *medicina* was blurred or disappeared altogether.[36] It was considered a legitimate way to diagnose medical issues and prescribe cures, especially through its integration with the theory of the four humours. As well as being associated with a season and an element, each of the humours was also associated with specific planetary bodies. However, certain forms of astrology were strongly associated with demonic magic and condemned. The casting of birth horoscopes for medical reasons might be acceptable, but they could also be considered an example of divination which, by claiming to know the future, undermined the key concept of free will. Such claims were also impossible, as only God and his prophets can truly know the future, so were, in fact, the result of demonic deception. This made astrological practices the subject of intense discussion.

While Isidore of Seville's *Etymologiae* lists astrology as a form of divination, medieval theologians were less clear on this taxonomy. Aquinas and Bonaventure were unequivocal in their belief not only that "divination" was not possible, but that it was a demonic deception: "[some] foreknowledge is not properly called divination; as when a doctor predicts a healthy future or an astrologer predicts an eclipse or rain, or other such things [...] in these things which have been observed by all, he [Lombard] does not call it divination [...] but divination is strictly of those things which have no settled cause: indeed to foreknow this is for God alone, and it is through the usurpation of his acts that those who strive to predict the future are called *divini*."[37] Nevertheless, the same theologians saw some forms of astrology as legitimate. Aquinas stated: "Astrologers are not able to foretell events, unless the cause may be traced back to the movements of the

34 Aquinas, *Summa theologica*, 2a2ae q.96.

35 See chapter by Sebastià Giralt in this volume.

36 See chapter by Anne Lawrence-Mathers in this volume.

37 Aquinas, *Scriptum super Sententiis*, lib. 2 dist. 7 q. 2 art. 2: "Eorum præcognitio non proprie dicitur divinatio; ut quando medicus prædicit sanitatem futuram, et astrologus eclipsim vel pluviam, et aliquod huiusmodi [...] in illis quæ omnibus nota sunt, nullus dicit divinationem esse [...] sed divinatio proprie est eorum quæ causas determinatas non habent: hæc enim præcognoscere, solius Dei est, a cujus actus usurpatione, divini vocantur qui futuris prænuntiandis intendunt" (https://aquinas.cc/la/en/~Sent.II.D7.Q2.A2.C.4).

stars [...] as for instance the transmutations which occur in the body such as tempers, barrenness, plague, and the like."[38]

A common application of astrological knowledge was in medicine. The Zodiac Man, a diagram which aligned the signs of the zodiac with their corresponding body parts, is found in many surviving medical manuscripts. As the planetary rays impacted material substances on Earth, this included the human body. Noting the appropriate signs and the planets (if any) in them could then help physicians to diagnose and treat various ailments. This was considered standard medical practice and was widely accepted. Indeed, the Zodiac Man survived to the end of the medieval period and beyond. Such a diagram is included in copies of the *Kalendarium* of John Somer, a fourteenth-century astronomer, alongside tables of eclipses of the sun and moon. The same information is found in printed almanacs into the seventeenth century.[39]

This idea of a systemic connection between the human body, the illnesses which affect it, and the cures to counteract them, links back to concepts within natural philosophy which suggested that the human body and its connections with the wider physical world were worthy of philosophical study. Accordingly, some educated practitioners of what was condemned as magic by the Church argued that they were not utilizing demonic powers to access the occult, but natural powers. While it has been demonstrated that a single, coherent definition of magic for the whole of the medieval period across the social spectrum is an impossibility, broadly speaking the Church increasingly considered any occult activity where the outcome could not be easily explained by practical experience to be utilizing demonic powers and therefore condemned it as magic. Theologians like William of Auvergne and Albertus Magnus, as described above, debated this, arguing that it was possible to access occult, but natural powers. Such distinctions were particularly important, and particularly complex, in the case of medical astrology.

This only really emerged in the twelfth century and was therefore being navigated by the authorities in Western Europe for the first time. It was never condemned outright. Indeed, the widespread and long-lived career of the Zodiac Man has already been discussed. However, in other instances the Christian authorities declared that astrology's tenets were too far removed from genuine scientific knowledge to be acceptable. These practices were defined as astral magic. Astral magic was a set of highly ritualistic practices which involved attempts to harness the powers of the celestial bodies by using ceremony, astrological images and fumigations. *Picatrix*, a text translated into Latin in the thirteenth century, outlines such practices in great detail.[40] While its practitioners claimed that they were calling on the natural powers of the planets (or in some cases claimed they were calling on divine, angelic beings), it was condemned as an overtly demonic activity akin to necromancy. Generally speaking, astral magic aside, the use to which an astrological activity was put, together with any additional

38 Aquinas, *Scriptum super Sententiis*, lib. 2 dist. 7 q. 2 art. 2.

39 See Lawrence-Mathers, "The Hours and the Almanac"; Curth, *English Almanacs*.

40 For the Latin text see *Picatrix, The Latin Version*, ed. Pingree. For a modern English translation see *Picatrix*, trans. Attrell and Porreca.

objects or words required, were of most interest to the authorities when deciding on its acceptability.

Finally, alchemy, another discipline drawn from Arabic learning which emerged in the twelfth century and involved study of natural substances, also had some medical applications. Alchemy was accepted as a branch of natural philosophy which was concerned with the study of the material world and the quest to understand its secrets. The ultimate goal of alchemy was the *magnum opus* which would produce the philosopher's stone, also known as the elixir of life. While this was thought to be able to turn base metal to gold and provide immortality, it was also considered able to operate as a panacea, curing all known ills. However, the Church authorities were less concerned about alchemy, largely leaving its condemnation to the secular authorities, who focused on fraudsters. It was also the case that study of alchemy was so demanding and so frequently unsuccessful that it was never much used in medical practice.[41]

Spoken and Written Word

Like the powers of the celestial bodies, language, both written and spoken, was also a complicated area, which was believed to interact with the qualities of natural substances. Prayer could be used to connect with the divine while curses could call upon demonic magic to harm innocents. Legitimate medical practice largely did not rely on language, but there was a crossover between medical applications and both religion and magic. The use of the written word in medicine took many forms which can be classified as prayers on one hand and charms on the other. Well-known prayers called on divine power for help and protection and were completely acceptable. Charms, on the other hand, can be differentiated from prayers as they are not directly calling on divine help and are instead aimed at the illness or injury itself, or the afflicted individual, and calling for their recovery.[42] Praying in times of need, such as significant illness or injury, was not unusual or unacceptable. Praying to ward off danger and to ask for protection either daily or before a significant event was also commonplace and not considered un-Christian by the Church. Examples of such prayers include loricas, so-called after the Latin word *lorica* meaning armour or breastplate, which were part of the medieval Irish monastic tradition and were specifically for protection. Surviving loricas include those of St. Patrick and St. Fursey.[43] Charms, however, could cross into the realm of magic. The distinction between the two could be difficult to ascertain and, for those not well educated in theology, it would be easy to undertake what was believed to be a prayer, but which the Church would identify as a charm. If the "prayer" was not directed to God directly, for exam-

41 See Newman "Medieval Alchemy."

42 Karen Jolly discusses charms and their relationship to Christian prayers in Jolly, "Anglo-Saxon Charms in the Context of a Christian World View."

43 Which survive in manuscripts BL MSS Egerton 93 and Add. 30512 respectively.

ple, but to the illness or afflicted body part then that was not considered acceptable and would classify as a charm.[44]

A formula in the Old English medical text known as *Lacnunga* to help against "elf-shot" (a sharp, stabbing pain), ends with a reference to God, but not a direct appeal for divine help, and would by no means be considered a prayer by later authorities. The Church judged that if the "prayer" is not calling to God directly then it is not using divine power. If it is not using divine power, then the understanding of where the words got their power from was limited to the demonic and therefore magic. Other charms were much more overt, and it was unlikely that individuals using them would not be aware that they were probably outside the realm of legitimate religious practice. Charms of this kind can often be found in early medieval medical texts, often as a form of remedy rather than an example of formal medicine. However their use continued into the late medieval period, as Catherine Rider and Lea Olsan have shown. Two examples provided by Olsan span the medieval period, the tenth-century *Bald's Leechbook* and the fifteenth-century *Liber medicinarum*.[45] *Bald's Leechbook* is an early collection of medical remedies while *Liber medicinarum* is a medical text written by John Arderne, an English surgeon. That both of these texts include examples of charms demonstrates long lived nature of these practices, as well as the fact that they were utilized by both herbalists and medical physicians alike.

The use of language is one of the areas with the strongest crossovers between the realms of magic, medicine, and religion. Medicine could not utilize language in itself but language was considered representative of power, whether divine or demonic. When utilized correctly, language could be used to call upon the divine and ask for assistance. However, it could also be used to tap into occult, demonic powers which were dangerous magic. The technicalities of how the language was used made all the difference to how an observer might categorize it, whether as religion or magic. Despite the apparent demarcations between prayers and magic, legitimate medical texts by reputed physicians such as John Arderne still included "charms" within their wider portfolio of medical knowledge.

It is therefore important to consider exactly how these elements were used. In some cases, components of an activity would be completely acceptable individually, but when combined they became magical and therefore outside of Christian teaching. For example, using a certain plant for its medicinal properties was, as seen above, acceptable medical practice. However, if plants or stones, or even written prayers, were tied to the body to aid the healing process the object in question became a ligature, something which was specifically banned by Augustine as being superstitious: "Indeed, to this type belong all ligatures and remedies which the discipline of medicine also condemns, which they name either in incantations or in things known as characters, or in the practice of suspending of certain things, and tying them or even, in some way, mak-

44 Kieckhefer, *Magic in the Middle Ages*, 69–70.

45 See Olsan, "Charms and Prayers in Medieval Medical Theory and Practice."

ing them dance […]."[46] Elsewhere, Augustine associated superstition with magic more explicitly: "That is superstitious which is instituted by humans and pertains to the making and worshipping of idols or the worshipping of creation, or part of it, just as if it were God, or which pertains to consultations and certain pacts whose meaning is agreed and sealed with demons, such as the efforts of the magical arts […]."[47] By the medieval period, superstitious and pagan practices were linked closely to demons and therefore magic. Natural remedies or prayers for healing which would be acceptable in many circumstances could become magical if they were used as ligatures. Related complications applied to the category of amulets. These were wearable objects which utilized the powers of natural products to provide protection. In this form they were considered overtly magical and were used to access occult powers to achieve their desired ends. However, wearing a religious symbol to achieve the same results, warding off evil or bringing protection, was an accepted and commonplace practice. Clearly it was possible for some objects to combine both identities, and this issue of combining sources of power raises important questions.

We have already seen that Gratian was concerned if actions and prayers were combined in particular ways. For example, if herbs were collected while a prayer was recited this was moving into the territory of the occult and the magical, despite the fact that collecting herbs and reciting prayers were individually acceptable. An example can be found in the *Lacnunga*, which includes a translation of Pseudo-Apuleius' *Herbarium*. It recommends that a verbal formula is sung while herbs are prepared and applied to the patient. The formula in question references Woden, an interesting inclusion for such a text in itself. This concern from canon lawyers could be due to the strong link between chants, or written words, and demonic magic. Magic was thought to be based on a formal pact between the practitioner and the demon. There are many examples of this pact as a written document and many stories of the pact often refer to a written version, for example, Caesarius of Heisterbach in the thirteenth century describes magicians with the pact hidden under their skin.[48] The use of chants in ritualistic magic, or as part of a ritual to summon a demon, also strengthens this association. Bonaventure's *Commentary* describes chants and words in connection with demons: "Such chants are vain and pernicious and are not offered to the devil because he is charmed by these, but [he is charmed] in the making of heretics."[49] While these examples are separate to the descriptions of charms there is a link between the concepts. If words were calling on divine power, it was generally acceptable, unless used alongside other practices. However, if

46 Augustine, *De doctrina Christiana*, ed. and trans. Green, bk. 2, chap. 20, 90–93. The application of prayers in this way can be seen in Olsan, "The Marginality of Charms in Medieval England," 135.

47 Augustine, *De doctrina Christiana*, ed. and trans. Green, bk. 2, chap. 20, 92–93.

48 Ceasarius of Heisterbach, *Dialogus Miraculorum*, ed. Strange, dist. 5, chap. 18, 1:297: "Respondit iterum daemon: Cyrographa mea, in quibus hominia mihi ab eis facta, sunt conscripta, sub ascellis suis inter pellem et eamem consuta conservant, quorum beneficio talia operantur, nec ab aliquo laedi poterunt."

49 Bonaventurae, *Commentaria*, bk. 2, dist. 7 pt. 2 art. 2 q.3, 2:205: "Omnia talia carmina vana sunt et perniciosa; nec facit diabolus quia in illis delectetur, sed in infidelitate facientium."

they were calling on "angels" by name, which theologians argued were probably actually demons, or unnamed forces it got more complicated and strayed into the territory of magic.

The context of a practice was also key to the perception of what powers it was calling upon. A common religious practice during the medieval period was the use of votive offerings at shrines to implore saints and other divine powers to provide healing. This had been a common practice in antiquity and the use of *ex votos*, offerings given in exchange for a prayer answered, continued into the Christian world. These items were often made of wax, or sometimes metal, and depicted something related to the prayer, often a body part which required healing. At Exeter Cathedral the tomb of Bishop Edmund Lacy, who died in the mid-fifteenth century, was often presented with wax models of limbs in an attempt to call on the saint to intercede on their behalf and provide divine healing.[50] Usually, the votive offering would take the form of the healthy body rather than in its afflicted state. This link between a visual representation of a desired outcome and achieving it is also present in medieval magic.

The concept of "sympathetic magic," introduced by James Frazer in his nineteenth-century work *The Golden Bough*, was dependent on this idea. Sympathetic magic denotes magical practices which relied on depicting or emulating the desired result to draw on the magic in question. This was not one consistent set of practices undertaken by a particular societal group, rather it is a modern term given to any form of magic reliant on emulation via visual or performative means. Examples include the use of what came to be called in English "poppets." An early example may be evidenced in a deed of ca. 963–975 transferring ownership of land at Ailsworth (Northamptonshire) to the Bishop of Winchester. The land had previously been owned by, and confiscated from, a woman convicted of using pins in a 'hidden instrument' to cause harm to a neighbour.[51] Similarly, Matteuccia Francisci was a female practitioner of love magic who was tried in 1428. The records of that trial include accusations that she provided her clients with wax images of hearts which could be burned to incite desire.[52] The use of models or images is present in both cases here, but in the context of a votive offering, calling on divine powers, it was acceptable, whereas outside of this context the assumption is that it must be calling on demonic powers. It is possible that a differentiation can be drawn between an offering, which remains whole as a gift, and an image being used as a tool. The poppet doll and wax hearts are manipulated and ultimately destroyed to achieve their aims, whilst the votive offerings remain unharmed.

---

50 Webb, *Pilgrimage in Medieval England*, 71.

51 Whitelock, ed., *English Historical Documents: Volume I, c. 500–1042*, 562–63.

52 Kieckhefer, *Magic in the Middle Ages*, 59.

Conclusion

There are many reasons for the complications around the boundary between the disciplines of medicine and magic, as this chapter has shown. The introduction of new learning in the twelfth century led to problematic concepts such as astrology and alchemy emerging in the Latin West which, at least as far as Church law was concerned, straddled legitimate science and demonic magic. One of the main reasons for the difficulty in establishing clear boundaries between acceptable medicine and unacceptable magic was the disconnect between common practices, such as charms or the use of natural substances, and the official terminology of the Church. Many individuals utilizing these practices were likely to have only limited knowledge of the complexities of theological teachings, and to be unaware that their seemingly innocuous actions were possibly tapping into demonic powers. Likewise, the Church authorities and theological scholars had a limited understanding of the beliefs and practices of the wider populace. When these two spheres came together, there was therefore a clash between perceived medicine and perceived demonic magic. Examples of this include individuals tying medical remedies or healing prayers to afflicted body parts believing this would focus their healing powers, but in fact creating a ligature which was understood as superstitious at best, but magical at worst, by the Church.

Already complex definitions of categories were sometimes adapted to accommodate this; but specific activities might also be harshly categorized in order to eliminate them. Augustine's lists of "superstitious" provide examples of this, as does Gratian's judgement against gathering herbs while reciting prayers. In some cases, educated individuals knew that their activities were likely to be condemned and so attempted to justify their actions as belonging to an acceptable category, as in the example of astral magic. The differentiator between acceptable and unacceptable was sometimes so subtle that judgements depended on perceived intentions rather than the action itself. In such cases, the same action could be interpreted as a devout religious practice or demonic magic. Similarly, some theologians, such as William of Auvergne or Albertus Magnus, advocated for a natural magic, whereas others, following Augustine, rejected any such blurring of categories.

A final issue is that sometimes the actions themselves were of less concern than the perceived sources of their effects. For example, the same type of cure could be classified as medical, religious, or magical depending on the underlying power understood to be at work, whether natural, divine, or demonic. The differing uses of stones and herbs outlined above demonstrate this. The impact of lingering pagan remedies and oral traditions, such as the persistence of charms in medical texts from Bald's *Leechbook* in the Anglo-Saxon period through to the *Liber Medicinalum* by John Arderne in the fifteenth century, is also significant. This chapter has argued that all three areas must be considered in conjunction if the shifting borders and apparent contradictions are to be properly understood. Such an approach is important for an informed understanding of a much-debated topic, even if full agreement is as unlikely to be reached as in the medieval period itself.

Bibliography

Manuscripts and Archival Material

Bern, Burgerbibliothek, MS 318
Oxford, Bodleian Library, MS Auct. T. 2. 23
London, British Library, MS Add. 30512
London, British Library, MS Cotton Nero D I
London, British Library, MS Cotton Vitellius C III
London, British Library, MS Egerton 93
London, British Library, MS Harley 585
London, British Library, MS Harley 6258 B
London, British Library, MS Royal 6 A
London, British Library, MS Royal 12 F XIII
London, British Library, MS Sloane 278
London, British Library, MS Sloane 1975
London, British Museum, no. 46226

Primary Sources

Augustine. *De doctrina Christiana*. Edited and translated by R. P. H. Green. Oxford: Clarendon, 1995.

Bonaventura. *Commentaria in Quatuor Libros Sententiarum Magistri Petri Lombardi*. Vols. 1-4 of *Opera Omnia*. Quaracchi: Collegium S. Bonaventurae, 1882.

Ceasarius of Heisterbach [Caesarius Heisterbacensis Monachi Ordinis Cisterciensis]. *Dialogus Miraculorum*. Edited by Josef Strange. 2 vols. Cologne: Heberle, 1851.

Gratian. "Decretum." In *Corpus Iuris Canonici*, vol. 1. Edited by Aemilius Friedberg. Graz: Akademische Druck- und Verlagsanstalt, 1959. Available at www.columbia.edu/cu/lweb/digital/collections/cul/texts/ldpd_6029936_001/index.html (accessed February 6, 2023).

Hippocrates, Johan van Heurne, Leonhart Fuchs, and Galen. *The Aphorismes of Hippocrates, Prince of Physitians with a Short Comment on Them Taken out of Those Larger Notes of Galen, Heurnius, Fuchsius, &c.: With an Exact Table Shewing the Substance of Every Aphorisme*. London: for Humphrey Moseley, 1655.

Hugh of St. Victor. *The Didascalicon of Hugh of St. Victor*. Edited and translated by Jerome Taylor. New York: Columbia University Press, 1961.

Isidore of Seville. *Etymologiarum sive originum, libri XX*. Edited by W. M. Lindsay. 2 vols. Oxford: Oxford University Press, 1911.

Lombard, Peter. *Sententiarum Libri Quatuor*. Edited by Jacques-Paul Migne. Patrologiae cursus completus. Series Latina 192. Paris: Migne, 1855.

Marbode of Rennes. *Libellus de lapidibus preciosis*. Vienna: Hieronymus Vietor, 1511. https://archive.org/details/LibellusDeLapidibusPreciosis/marbode-b-lapidibus-1511-RTL015154-LowRes/page/n15/mode/2up?q=saphiri> (accessed February 6, 2023).

Picatrix, The Latin Version of the Gāyat Al-Hakīm. Edited by David Pingree. London: The Warburg Institute, 1986.

Picatrix. A Medieval Treatise on Astral Magic. Translated by Dan Attrell and David Porreca. University Park: The Pennsylvania State University Press, 2019.

Thomas Aquinas. *Scriptum Super Sententiis*. Edited by The Aquinas Institute. https://aquinas.cc/la/en/~Sent.I.

——. *The Summa Theologica of St. Thomas Aquinas*. 2nd (rev.) ed. London: Burns, Oates, and Washbourne, 1920.

——. *Summa theologiae*. Translated by Fathers of the English Dominican Province. New York: Benziger, 1947–48. The Aquinas Institute. https://aquinas.cc/la/en/~ST.I. Also at www.newadvent.org/summa.

Whitelock, Dorothy, ed. *Volume 1: c. 500–1042*. Vol. 1 of *English Historical Documents*. 2nd ed. London: Routledge, 1996.

Secondary Sources

Collins, Minta. *Medieval Herbals: The Illustrative Tradition*. London: British Library, 2000.

Curth, Louise Hill. *English Almanacs, Astrology and Popular Medicine, 1550–1700*. Manchester: Manchester University Press, 2007.

Frazer, James, *The Golden Bough*. Vol. 1, *The Magic Art and the Evolution of Kings 1*. Third ed. 12 vols. Cambridge: Cambridge University Press, 2012. First published 1890 in 2 vols. And 2nd ed. *The Golden Bough: A Study in Magic and Religion*.

Hammond, E. A. "Physicians in Medieval English Religious Houses." *Bulletin of the History of Medicine* 32, no. 2 (1958): 105–20.

Hassig, Debra, ed. *The Mark of the Beast: The Medieval Bestiary in Art, Life and Literature*. London: Routledge, 1999.

Jolly, K. L., "Anglo-Saxon Charms in the Context of a Christian World View." *Journal of Medieval History* 11, no. 4 (1985): 279–93.

Jones, Peter Murray, and Lea T. Olsan. "Medicine and Magic." In *The Routledge History of Medieval Magic*. Edited by Sophie Page and Catherine Rider, 299–311. London: Routledge, 2019.

Jouanna, Jacques. *Greek Medicine from Hippocrates to Galen: Selected Papers*. Edited by Philip van der Eijk, translated by Neil Allies. Leiden: Brill, 2012.

Kieckhefer, Richard. *Magic in the Middle Ages*. Cambridge: Cambridge University Press, 1997.

Lawrence-Mathers, Anne. "The Hours and the Almanac in Tudor England." In *Women and Writing c. 1340–c. 1650*. Edited by Anne Lawrence-Mathers and Philippa Hardman, 34–61. Woodbridge: York Medieval Press, 2010.

Lawrence-Mathers, Anne, and Carolina Escobar-Vargas. *Magic and Medieval Society*. London, Routledge, 2014.

Newman, William R. "Medieval Alchemy." In *The Cambridge History of Science*. Edited by David C. Lindberg and Michael H. Shank, 385–403. Cambridge: Cambridge University Press, 2013.

Olsan, Lea T. "The Marginality of Charms in Medieval England." In *The Power of Words: Studies on Charms and Charming in Europe*. Edited by James Kapaló, Éva Pócs, and William Ryan, 135–64. Budapest: Central European University Press, 2013.

——. "Charms and Prayers in Medieval Medical Theory and Practice." *Social History of Medicine* 16, no. 3 (2003): 343–66.

Rider, Catherine, "Lay Religion and Pastoral Care in 13th-Century England: The Evidence of a Group of Short Confession Manuals." *Journal of Medieval History* 36, no. 4 (2010): 327–40.

——. "Medical Magic and the Church in Thirteenth-Century England." *Social History of Medicine* 24, no. 1 (2011): 92–107.

——. *Magic and Impotence in the Middle Ages*. Oxford: Oxford University Press, 2006.

Stannard, Jerry. "Medieval Herbals and Their Development." *Clio Medica* 9, no. 1 (1974): 23–33.

Stewart, Patricia. "The Mediaeval Bestiary and Its Textual Tradition." PhD diss., (University of St. Andrews, 2012.

Van Arsdall, Anne. *Medieval Herbal Remedies: The Old English Herbarium and Anglo-Saxon Medicine*. London: Routledge, 2002.

Ventura, Iolanda, Tony Hunt, and Johannes Gottfried Mayer. "Plants and Medicine." In *A Cultural History of Plants*, edited by Annette Giesecke and David Mabberley. Vol. 2, *In the Post-Classical Era*. Edited by Alain Touwaide, 101–18. London: Bloomsbury, 2022.

Wallis, Faith. *Medieval Medicine: A Reader*. Toronto: University of Toronto, 2010.

Webb, Diana, *Pilgrimage in Medieval England*. London: Hambledon, 2000.

BETWEEN NATURAL AND DEMONIC?

ONOMANTIC DIVINATION IN THE LATER MIDDLE AGES

JOANNE EDGE

> "Now I will demonstrate Pythagoras's figure. Within it you will likely enough find everything that you ask, whether it goes well or ill."[1]

THE GERMAN COURTIER and physician Johannes Hartlieb (ca. 1410–1468) wrote his *Namenmantik* sometime in the 1430s or 1440s. It is a relatively long vernacular treatise on the different forms of name-number divination—onomancy—that Hartlieb brought together in one place. In this work, Hartlieb describes five different sorts of onomantic tables, those of Pythagoras, Ptolemy, Plato, Aristotle, and Haly Abbas, and takes the reader through the vast array of different things that onomancy can be used to predict.[2] This was not the only occult topic Hartlieb wrote about in this period—he also produced texts on chiromancy (divination by lines on the hand), geomancy (divination from interpreting dots and lines drawn in the sand or on paper) and lunar divination. Educated in medicine at Padua, graduating in 1439, Hartlieb would later go into the service of several noblemen: beginning with Albert VI, duke of Austria, then Dukes Albrecht III and Sigmund of Bavaria–Munich. All the noblemen Hartlieb was in service to had an interest in or were affected by the occult in some way—for example, Albert III of Bavaria–Munich's mistress (perhaps even his first wife), Agnes Bernauer (ca. 1410–1435), had been executed for sorcery.

A decade or two later, in 1456, Hartlieb wrote another tract, this time for his patron, the Margrave Johann of Brandenburg-Kulmbach (1406–1464), entitled *The Book of All Forbidden Arts*. Johann was nicknamed "The Alchemist" because he took such an interest in the art of transmuting base metals into gold. Far from a treatise explaining how to conduct various divinatory practices, Hartlieb's book is an unequivocal condemnation of all occult practices, listing each one as he goes. This is what Hartlieb has to say here about onomancy:

1 Hartlieb, *Namenmantik*, trans. Pope, fol. 131v.

2 Hartlieb, *Namenmantik*, trans. Pope, fols. 130r–135v.

Joanne Edge is a historian and palaeographer, who completed her undergraduate and postgraduate work at the University of London. She is currently a Postdoctoral Research Fellow at the University of Edinburgh. She would like to thank Ben Pope for his translation of Hartlieb's *Namenmantik*, Seb Falk for his useful and encouraging comments on the first draft of this chapter, and the volume's editors and an anonymous peer-reviewer for their support and feedback. This chapter is a synthesis of the arguments in the first two chapters of Edge, *Onomantic Divination*.

> There are other books having to do with such calculation, such as the books of Pythagoras, who gives many letters and figures, and for each there are certain numbers; by means of these one determines who will win, which is surely a superstition. Further, one of these books, also ascribed to Pythagoras, teaches which of two spouses will die sooner. The same book has caused frequent and serious conflict between married couples, which is the source of great pity and lament. Esteemed prince, you should not allow that in your princedom when Your Grace encounters it. For according to holy Scripture, each person should prevent such sin as he can prevent, and one who does not do so is guilty of that sin. That is what the teacher Datus writes.[3]

Given he had written an entire treatise on this form of divination, it is not surprising that Hartlieb accurately describes two forms of onomancy that circulated in late medieval manuscripts in this passage—this form of divination often claimed to predict the winner in a duel or fight, and which of two spouses might die sooner. Therefore, as a younger man, and maybe even while a student at Padua, Hartlieb had written a treatise uncritically demonstrating a plethora of ways in which one might predict future events via onomancy. But as an older courtier in the service of noblemen, he wrote a book of advice for one of his patrons which unequivocally condemned a wide range of magical and divinatory practices, including a specific condemnation of onomancy. As Richard Kieckhefer points out, there are several possible reasons for this: he may of course have changed his mind as an older man about the dangers of such practices. Or, he may simply have been producing the sorts of texts necessary and relevant to the circumstances he was in. Another, in my opinion less convincing, option is that one or both of these attributions to Hartlieb are spurious.[4] But this precise sort of seeming *volte face* from Hartlieb, for whatever reason, is a good illustration of the liminal place occupied by onomantic divination in the later Middle Ages. On one hand, onomancy could be viewed as acceptable practice, suitable for a physician, for example, to use. On the other, it might be seen as illicit divination, antithetical to Christianity. This chapter will place this nuance in the wider context of late medieval theology and natural philosophy.

Divination—the prediction of future events or obtaining hidden knowledge via a codified interpretation of signs—both in the medieval Latin West and across time and place, is a practice that has been historically rather neglected. Individual texts and methods of divination have been the subject of articles and book chapters, and the work of scholars such as Charles Burnett have been invaluable in understanding the phenomenon at hand. A multi-authored, double volume handbook, *Prognostication in the Medieval World*[5] appeared in 2021, the output of a years-long research consortium at the University of Erlangen. It is worth pointing out here that prognostication is the general

3 Hartlieb, "Book of All Forbidden Arts," in Kieckhefer, ed. and trans., *Hazards of the Dark Arts*, 51. The figure of "Datus" has not been identified.

4 The argument in these first two paragraphs is a summing up of that in Kieckhefer, trans. and ed., *Hazards of the Dark Arts*, 4–6.

5 Heiduk, Herbers, and Lehner, eds., *Prognostication in the Medieval World*.

prediction of future events. Divination sits in a sub-category of prognostication and is based specifically on the interpretation of signs. While a much-welcomed contribution to the field, what is surprising is that this huge volume fails to properly categorize and discuss, even in the chapter on the mantic arts, one of the most popular forms of divination in the later Middle Ages—onomancy. Onomancy, extant in various forms in manuscripts in the medieval West throughout the Middle Ages essentially operates by assigning numbers to the names of particular individuals, doing some calculations and usually also adding some astrological data, dividing the sum to reveal a remainder, which is then used to predict some future event in the life of the said individual. Often this question was "will I live or die?," "which of these two people will win a duel?" or "will a fugitive be found?" It could also be used to predict which of a married couple might die first, or the sex of an unborn child. Onomancies in their various forms are extant in some 65 manuscripts produced in Britain in the period 1150–1500 alone.[6] Onomancy was one of the most popular forms of divination that circulated in the later Middle Ages, along with geomancy, based on manuscript attestations.

Onomancy, then, was popular in late medieval literate society—but looking at it from a modern perspective it seems childish, like a game many of us might have played as children. However, delving into medieval natural philosophical tracts on the problem of universals demonstrates how seriously the potential power of numbers and names was taken in the Middle Ages. As the history of divination in the Latin West cannot be separated from that of magic—essentially, both were condemned together as being antithetical to the Christian religion and working via demonic power since the late Roman Republic—one might expect onomancy to always be viewed through a condemnatory lens. However, theologians and natural philosophers at the University of Paris, beginning with William of Auvergne (d. 1249), began to postulate a theologically acceptable category of natural magic. This included things like the hidden powers of magnets, the spontaneous generation of frogs and toads, and other natural processes that were unknown but nevertheless a part of God's wonderful creation.[7]

What I want to do here is show that there was sufficient nuance created by three factors for onomancy to be *potentially* viewed as an acceptable practice in the later Middle Ages. The first is the linking in condemnatory discourse of magic and divination since the earliest beginnings of Christianity; the second is the lively debate in natural philosophical and theological circles over the problem of universals; and the third is the tentative creation of the category of natural magic the thirteenth century. This, of course, does not mean all copyists and readers of onomancy saw it that way—and I have not come across any medieval commentary on onomancy explicitly linking it to natural magic—but simply that enough subtlety had been introduced to natural philosophical discourse to allow for this interpretation. We will begin, however, with a brief discussion of the sorts of onomantic texts that circulated in manuscripts in the later Middle Ages.

---

6 Edge, *Onomantic Divination.*

7 On natural magic see Page, *Magic in the Cloister*, 31–33 and Draelents, "Notion of Properties." See also, Sebastià Giralt above (chap. 7 of this volume).

Onomancy: Forms and Functions

Three main forms of onomantic divination are extant in manuscripts produced in England in the period 1150–1500—in Latin, Middle English, and Anglo-Norman. The most popular is the *Sphere of Life a Death*—a figure (usually round), with every number between one and thirty placed inside it, within three columns and bisected horizontally. It is accompanied by written instructions which could take the form of a long piece of prose, a short poem, or something else. This text is usually included next to the figure. The *Sphere* can be used to get a binary yes/no answer, and it most commonly claims to predict the life or death of a sick person. To use it you take the name of the sick person, and you use the table within or next to the figure to assign a specific number to each letter of their name. You then add this into a grand total. Then, you take the number of the day of the moon on which they first fell ill (this is any number between one and thirty) and also the planetary number of the day of the week (these are almost always listed with the *Sphere* figure too). You add these three subtotals into a grand total and divide by thirty (or sometimes twenty-nine). The remainder is then sought in the centre of the device. If in the top half, the person will live/the answer is good, if in the bottom, the person will die/the answer is bad. The three columns indicate whether recovery or death will be quick, intermediate or slow.[8] The *Sphere* was translated into Latin from Greek as early as 805 CE—the first extant copy is dated to 798–805, now surviving in Cologne.[9] The early medieval *Sphere* circulated mainly in a computistical context, that is with texts and figures of time-reckoning used to calculate Christian feasts such as the date of Easter. A similar argument to the one I make here can be made for early medieval onomancy in the Latin West—that is, the *Sphere*—occupying a legally liminal space between acceptable and unacceptable. After all, it is found almost solely in a monastic context along with important items of timekeeping for the Christian calendar, but at the same time, general condemnations of divination had been in circulation since Christianity's beginning.[10]

The second form of onomancy found in later medieval manuscripts pits two numbers against each other, and has been called the *Victorious and Vanquished*. It answered questions such as "which of a married couple will die first?" It is first attested in Latin translation in the Eadwine Psalter produced ca. 1160 at Canterbury, and therefore is almost certainly a product of the twelfth-century translation movement of scientific texts from Greco-Arabic into Latin, since it circulated in the Arabic version of Pseudo-Aristotle's *Secret of Secrets*. This worked by onomantically adding up the totals for the two names to be pitted together and working out the answer based on which remainder number "beat" the other, as outlined above. This was obviously immediately less useful to a practising doctor than the *Sphere* and so it was also possible to work out life or

8 On the *Sphere of Life and Death*, see Edge, "Licit Medicine." See also Giralt, in this volume.

9 Cologne, Erzbischöfliche Diözesan- und Dombibliothek, MS 83 II, fol. 218v. I owe this reference to David Juste.

10 For an excellent discussion on the potential liminality of divination and other unorthodox practices in the earlier Middle Ages see van Rhijn, *Leading the Way to Heaven*, 211–40 (chap. 7).

death by pitting the name of the sick person against the number of the day of the moon for which the calculation is made—i.e. any number between one and thirty.[11]

The third type of onomancy present in later medieval manuscripts are those in the *Alchandreana* corpus. The *Alchandreana* was a set of fairly elementary astrological texts attributed to a probably legendary astrologer called Alchandreus, which also included onomancy. These astrological onomancies are methods of working out a client's birth data—the lunar mansion and planet under which they were born. Some *Alchandreana* manuscripts also contained onomantic texts which claimed to work out which of a married couple would die first, whether a woman was a prostitute, the sex of an unborn baby or whether or not a rumour was true—the answer to which was based on whether the remainder was odd or even.[12] The *Sphere of Life and Death, Victorious and Vanquished,* and *Alchandreana* onomancies, then, are the main forms of onomantic divination present in late medieval manuscripts. They are found often together in "prognostic sections" within manuscripts[13] or separately copied into blank pages; they were present in manuscripts intended for physicians, students, monks, and the aristocracy. Onomancy, and the sort of questions it claimed to answer, had mass appeal among literate people in late medieval England.

Magic and Divination: Intertwined Histories

The history of magic and divination in the Middle Ages cannot be discussed separately, because since at least the late Roman Republic (146–31 BCE), the two had been inextricably linked as unacceptable. With the advent of Christianity, the early Church Fathers, particularly Augustine (354–430 CE), sought to fuse theology with the ancient wisdom of the Greeks and Romans. In discussing divination, Augustine made it clear in his *City of God* that it was unacceptable for Christians to take part in because it went against the idea of man's free will; the concept of divine providence; and also that it always, whether you knew it or not, operated via the power of demons.[14] Such was his interest in the topic that Augustine even wrote a separate short treatise, *On the Divination of Demons*, explaining precisely how demons were able to wield such power.[15]

Augustine's thinking would be influential for centuries to come, being repeated and modified by theologians such as Isidore of Seville (ca. 560–636), John of Salisbury (1115–1180) and Thomas Aquinas (1225–1274). Although divination was its own definable category, it was nevertheless discussed and condemned both alongside and as part of the category of magic. Importantly, Isidore's categorization of magi in his *Etymologiae* encompassed a wide range of unorthodox ritual practitioners, including diviners[16]—a

11 On the *Victorious and Vanquished*, see Burnett, "The Eadwine Psalter," 143–46.

12 On the onomancies in the *Alchandreana* corpus see Juste, *Les Alchandreana primitifs*, 206–16.

13 Coined in Chardonnens, *Anglo-Saxon Prognostics*, 25.

14 Augustine, *City of God*, ed. Dyson, bk. 2, chap. 24, v. 9, at 84–86 and 198–203.

15 Augustine, *De divinatione daemonum*, ed. Zycha, 599–618.

16 See Klingshirn, "Isidore of Seville's Taxonomy," 59–90.

categorization that was repeated by John of Salisbury five centuries later.[17] After all, if both essentially operated via the power of demons and were antithetical to Christianity, why did it matter whether magic and divination were separate phenomena? This is important to bear in mind as we go along: divination and magic were to those condemning them inextricably linked, no matter what their differences might actually be.

Despite the fact that the descriptions of a lot of forbidden practices listed in condemnations of magic and divination might read like literary tropes, with no connection to the texts and practices that actually circulated in the Middle Ages,[18] onomancy was itself specifically condemned several times. Most significantly, it was denounced in Gratian's *Decretum*, a work of the 1140s that attempted to synthesize all decretals of canon law from the beginnings of Christianity to the time of writing. This meant there were a lot of conflicting decrees within Gratian, of course, but this censure is quite clear:

> [They must not] by certain numerical values of letters, and of the moon, inquire into the life or death of the sick, or future prosperity or adversity, by Pythagorean necromancy.[19]

Building on Gratian, and after the Fourth Lateran Council of 1215, when renewed efforts were made to equip parish priests to educate their communities, pastoral manuals began to be written, and several survive in multiple copies. One of these, the extremely popular *Summa Confessorum* of Thomas of Chobham (ca. 1160–ca. 1230) repeated the condemnation in Gratian verbatim.[20] Much later, the printed manual of Alexander Carpenter (fl. 1429), entitled *Destructorium viciorum* which was very popular in the fifteenth and sixteenth centuries, also repeated the censure in Gratian. Thus, condemnations of divination and onomancy circulated in the later Middle Ages as part of pastoral instruction.

A Universal Problem: Names and Numbers

What's in a name? This question, part of a much bigger debate on the problem of universals, had been on the minds of writers and thinkers since at least the time of Plato (428–348 BCE). On the topic of names as universals, the sorts of questions philosophers both before and after the advent of Christianity asked might be "do all people with the same name share some sort of common essence?" and "are those who give names somehow inspired to choose in accordance with some unknowable universal shared characteristic of the named?" Essentially, they were asking *if names exist in and of themselves.*

---

17 Escobar-Vargas, "Magic, Technology and New Categories of Knowledge," 60.

18 On this standardized list of practices and its transmission to the Middle Ages, see Veenstra, *Magic and Divination*, 105 and 154–59; for a more positive view of this list as reflective of actual practice see Bailey, *Fearful Spirits*, 28–34.

19 "[...] sive per quosdam numeros litterarum, et lunae, per Pitagoricam nigromantiam egrotantium vitam vel mortem, vel prospera vel adversa futura inquirunt [...]." Gratian, "Decretum," ed. Friedberg, Part 2, C. 26 q. 7. c. 16, at 1045.

20 Thomas of Chobham, *Summa Confessorum*, 7.5.11a, ed. Broomfield, 485. On the popularity of Chobham's manual see Rider, "Medical Magic and the Church," 94.

Opinions on this varied from person to person. Writing his *Contra Celsum* in the third century, the early Church Father Origen (ca. 184–ca. 254 CE) had quite a lot to say on the topic of names:

> Now if by a special study we could show the nature of powerful names, some of which are used by Egyptian wise men, or the learned men among the Persian magi, or the Brahmans, or Samanaeans among the Indian philosophers, and so on according to each nation, and if we could establish that so-called magic is not, as the followers of Epicurus and Aristotle think, utterly incoherent, but, as the experts in these things prove, is a consistent system, which has principles known to very few; then we would say that the name Saboath, and Adonai, and all the other names that have been handed down by Hebrews with great reverence, are not concerned with ordinary created things, but with a certain mysterious divine science that is related to the Creator of the universe. It is for this reason that when these names are pronounced in a particular sequence which is natural to them, they can be employed for certain purposes; and so also with other names in use in Egyptian which invoke daemons who have power only to do certain particular things; and other names in Persian which invoke other powers, and so on with each nation. So also the names of daemons upon earth, which have possession of different localities, will be found to be related to the languages used in each respective locality and nation. A man, then, who has grasped a more profound understanding of these matters, even if only to a small extent, will take care to apply names correctly in their respective connexions, some in one case, some in another; lest he should be like those who mistakenly apply the name of God to lifeless matter, or degrade the name of goodness from the first cause or from virtue and beauty to the level of blind wealth and to the harmony of flesh and blood and bones that exists when we are in good health and vigour, and to supposed nobility of birth.[21]

Origen makes two important points about names in this passage: firstly, names are divinely inspired; and secondly, men must understand and use names in a correct fashion. There was nothing arbitrary about them at all from the perspective of this early Christian.

In the seventh century, Isidore of Seville wrote his *Etymologiae*, which sought to explain the etymology of all things in the mundane world. This is what Isidore had to say about the origin of Old Testament names:

> Many of the early humans take the origin of their names from conditions specific to them. Their names were imparted to them prophetically in such a way that they concord with their future or their previous conditions.[22]

21 Origen, *Contra Celsum*, 1:24, trans. Chadwick, 23–24.

22 Isidore of Seville, *Etymologies*, trans. Barney et al., vol. 2, 6.1, p. 162.

On Adam's naming of Cain, he went on to say: "Cainan means 'lamentation' or 'possession of those,' for as Cain means 'possession,' so the derivative name, which is Cainan, forms 'possession of those'."[23] Although he was discussing Old Testament names specifically, Isidore promoted the idea that given names were divinely inspired and therefore much more than arbitrary designators.

One of the most important figures in the pre-university cathedral schools, Peter Abelard (1097–1142), writing his *Glosses on Porphyry* at the very beginning of the twelfth century, contributed to the universal debate over nouns:

> Yet any names of any existing things, insofar as is in their power, generate understanding rather than opinion, since their inventor meant to impose them in accordance with certain natures or characteristics of things, even if he did not know how to think out the nature or characteristic of the thing.[24]

Although talking here about general nouns, Abelard's point can just as easily be applied to the names of individuals. His basic point is that names are inspired, whether the person doing the naming is aware of it or not. About two hundred years after Abelard, John Duns Scotus (ca. 1266–1308), scholar, theologian, and philosopher active at both Paris and London, took a somewhat more nuanced stance on the nature of names:

> [...] signifying presupposes understanding in the sense that everything signified has already been understood, without which a spoken utterance would not have been imposed on it. But after it is imposed, an utterance can signify that to which it was imposed, even though it is [subsequently] understood by no one.[25]

John Buridan (ca. 1300–ca. 1358), French priest and theologian, based his theory of names on the method by which they are applied to individuals:

> [...] concerning the terms 'Socrates' and 'Plato' I say that they are truly and properly individual terms, for the name 'Socrates' was imposed on this man by means of pointing [to him], as for example [by saying that] let this boy be named by the proper name 'Socrates.' For that name imposed in this way cannot apply to anybody else, except as a result of a new imposition, but there will be equivocation.[26]

The debate on the proper nature of names, then, carried on after the twelfth-century translation movement of Aristotelian texts into Latin. Theologians took different viewpoints on the topic but the fact they continued to debate meant that ideas about names as universals, and to what extent they were inspired versus arbitrary signifiers, remained

---

23 Isidore of Seville, *Etymologies*, trans. Barney et al., vol. 2, 6.1, p. 162.

24 Abelard, "Glosses on Porphyry," ed. and trans. Spade, 46.

25 Duns Scotus, *Quaestiones in libros Perihermenias Aristotelis*, q. 3, ad. 4, ed. Andrews et al. Translation in Cameron, "Meaning," 349.

26 Buridan, "Quaestiones in Porphyrii Isagogen 9," ed. Tatarzynski, 162. Translation in Gyula Klima, *John Buridan*, 86. Reproduced in Cameron, "Meaning," 351.

current in theological discourse. So, both antique and medieval sources pointed towards a strong current of belief about the nature of names from a variety of perspectives—Christian, magical, natural—and this debate adds to the idea of onomancy occupying a liminal state between licit natural magic and illicit demonic divination.

Another universal problem that had been ongoing since Plato was that of numbers. Platonic thought held that numbers were the building-blocks of nature: numbers existed outside of abstract descriptors. The only Platonic text available to the Church fathers and early medieval theologians was the *Timaeus* which had been subject to a partial translation and commentary by Chalcidius in the fourth century CE. *Timaeus*, written in the form of a monologue, was all about the physical nature of the universe, and is full of references to number as the basic unit of nature. In the section titled *On Numbers* this is what Chalcidius's commentary had to say:

> By all accounts, then, the origin of numbers is found to be the most ancient, while the beginnings or principles of numbers themselves are unity and duality, since they are clearly the origins of other numbers. By this line of reasoning we reach the conclusion that soul, being composed of a double Being and two-fold nature, in harmony with the potency of numbers, and vivifying the celestial bodies and living beings that possess the faculty of reason and scientific knowledge, has the capacity to know all the things from the combination of whose potencies it itself consists.[27]

Despite Chalcidius's commentary on the *Timaeus* being the only Platonic text to circulate in Latin before the twelfth century, Platonic ideas were nevertheless promulgated in this time via other means. For example, the *Introduction to Arithmetic* of the Neopythagorean Nichomachus of Gerasa (ca. 60–ca. 120 CE) stated:

> All that has by nature with systematic method been arranged in the universe seems both in part and as a whole to have been determined and ordered in accordance with number, by the forethought and the mind of Him that created all things; for the pattern was fixed, like a preliminary sketch, by the domination of number pre-existent in the mind of the world-creating God, number conceptual only and immaterial in every way, but at the same time the true and the eternal essence, so that with reference to it, as to an artistic plan, should be created all these things, time, motion, the heavens, the stars, all sorts of revolutions.[28]

The early Church Fathers wove together Platonic number theory with scriptural writings. Augustine, in Book 11 of his *City of God* discusses the perfection of the number six in relation to God's creation of the world in six days, as well as the importance of number to the study of the Bible:

27 Chalcidius, *On Plato's Timaeus*, trans. Magee, 207.

28 Nichomachus, *Introduction to Arithmetic*, Intro. 1.6.1, trans. D'Ooge. Quoted in Schrenk, "God as Monad," 5.

> I have thought it appropriate to call these things briefly to mind here in order to demonstrate the perfection of the number six, which is, as I have said, the first number to be exactly made up of the sum of its parts; and in this number of days God finished His work. We must not overlook the science of number, therefore, which, in many passages of Holy Scripture, is found to be of great value to the diligent student. Not without reason is it said in praise of God, 'Thou has ordered all things in number, and measure, and weight."[29]

Augustine's contemporary Macrobius (fl. ca. 400 CE), in his commentary on Cicero's *Dream of Scipio*, stated:

> The monad, the beginning and end of all things, yet itself not knowing a beginning or ending, refers to the supreme God, and separates our understanding of him (the One, without number) from the number of things and powers following [...] It is also that Mind which, unaware of the changes of time, is always in one time, the present [...] Then, too, by giving a little thought to the matter, you will find the monad refers to the Soul. Indeed, the Soul is free from contamination with anything material, owing itself only to its Creator and to itself, and being endowed with a single nature.[30]

For Augustine and Macrobius, then, the number one—*monad*—was inextricably linked to both God and the human soul.

A further early Christian, the Roman aristocrat and martyr Boethius (ca. 480–524 CE), writing in the decades after Augustine and Macrobius, is best known for his *De consolatione philosophiae*, written in in 523 while Boethius was a prisoner of Theoderic. However, another one of his works exerted huge influence over number theory, *De institutione arithmetica*. Chapter 2 is entitled *Concerning the substance of number*, and follows Nichomachus of Gerasa:

> From the beginning, all things whatever which have been created may be seen by the nature of things to be formed by reason of numbers. Number was the principal exemplar in the mind of the creator. From it was derived the multiplicity of the four elements, from it were derived the changes of the seasons, from it the movement of the stars and turning of the heavens.[31]

The interest of Christian thinkers in number theory did not end with Boethius. The theologians working at the cathedral schools of the eleventh century and the burgeoning universities of the twelfth developed the concept of numbers as key to events in the Old Testament. Like Macrobius and Augustine, Thierry of Chartres (d. ca. 1150), identified

---

29 Augustine, *The City of God*, bk. 11, ed. Dyson, 490–91.

30 Macrobius, "Commentary on the Dream of Scipio," trans. Stahl, 1.8–9, Quoted in Schrenk, "God as Monad," 6.

31 Boethius, "De Institutione Arithmetica," trans. Masi, 75–76.

God with the monad.[32] And this is how Hugh of St. Victor, in his *De arca noe morali* written in the late 1120s described the dimensions of Noah's Ark:

> But the fact that the length of the ark is six times its width and ten times its height provides us with an allegorical figure for the human body in which Christ appeared, for it is itself His body. For the length of a body from crown to heel is six times its width from one side to the other, and its height moreover is ten times its thickness through from back to front. So if you measure a recumbent man when he is lying down quite flat, his length from head to foot is six times his width across from right to left or left to right, and ten times his thickness from the ground. Six is the number of times that fifty goes into three hundred, and there are six periods in the three ages of the world. Again, three hundred signifies faith in the Trinity, or because of the [Greek] letter Tau, of which the numerical value is 300, and which still retains the shape of the cross among the Syrians, it signifies the cross. Fifty denotes the remission of sins, thirty the measure of the age of the fullness of Christ.[33]

In *De arca noe morali*, then, the Ark was made according to precise measurements that corresponded numerically with Christ and the Cross. Thus, the argument that numbers were to a greater or lesser extent "real," and not abstract, was a strong current in early and high medieval philosophy—and these ideas and debates did not ebb with the twelfth-century translation movement. In the thirteenth century, the so-called "Oxford Platonism" movement,[34] whose members included Robert Grosseteste (1175–1253), Roger Bacon (1220–1292) and Robert Kilwardby (ca. 1215–1279) all defended numbers as having real existence.[35] Thus, the idea of numbers as more than mere concepts remained prevalent in scholastic circles until the end of the Middle Ages and beyond.

The Concept of Natural Magic in the Thirteenth Century

A key turning point happened in the decades either side of 1200, when a good portion of the new Latin translations of Aristotle and other philosophical materials had been completed and circulated rapidly. The nascent universities—especially Paris—enabled a huge attempt to incorporate newly-available Aristotelian texts and ideas into existing frameworks of knowledge. The increased interest in the properties of creatures and substances in Western thought, fused with newly-translated Arabic medical ideas about transformations and effects, meant that new ideas about natural magic overlapped with—and can be seen as a category of—natural philosophy.[36] Beginning in the twelfth century, Petrus Alfonsi (1062–1140), Dominicus Gundisalvi (ca. 1115–1190)

32 Schrenk, "God as Monad," 8.

33 Hugh of St. Victor, *Selected Spiritual Writings*, trans. Squire, 66–67.

34 Weisheipl, "Albertus Magnus and the Oxford Platonists," 124–39.

35 Silva, "Albert the Great on Mathematical Quantities," 1192.

36 Draelants, "Notion of Properties," 169.

and Daniel of Morley (ca. 1140–ca. 1210) and Michael Scot (1175–ca. 1232) discussed a category, conceived differently in each case, of the natural sciences called *nigromancia* which, according to Scot, was "the science which is concerned with the properties of things." *Nigromancia* was first used in Toledan translation circles as a translation of the Arabic *sihr*, meaning "magic," which had no direct translation in Latin. Why this term was adopted and persisted is probably due to Isidore of Seville's seventh-century words, "in Greek *nekros* means a dead man, and *manteia* means divination" which were copied and repeated down the centuries. This led to a confusion between *necros* ("dead" in Greek) and *nigram* ("black" in Latin) to signify a form of ancient divination to revive and interrogate the dead, or through the use of blood from dead bodies. So due to this complex confusion and semantic association, *nigromancia* became, through Alfonsi, Gundisalvi, Morley, and Scot, the name of a category that dealt with the natural properties of things—although where it sat within the competing divisions of knowledge heralded by Latin, Greek, and Arabic ways of classifying knowledge varied.[37]

One of the first scholars to call this new discipline "natural magic" was William of Auvergne (d. 1249), who became Bishop of Paris in 1228. What is immediately interesting about William is that he admits to, as a young man, dabbling in occult ritual magic in his *Magisterium Divinale et Sapientiale* of the 1230s. This aimed to fuse ancient philosophical reason with Christian revelation.[38] Crucially, in the final part of his *Magisterium* entitled "De Universo," William formulated the category of "natural magic" as an acceptable category of natural philosophy, using the term *magica* or *magia naturalis*. In this category were things like the spontaneous generation of frogs and animal instincts, which he contrasted to the illusions of demons. The source of power here is central to my argument—William makes it clear that natural magic operates via God as part of his Creation.[39]

As part of this debate on natural magic, the use of astrological images in some contexts was defended in the *Speculum Astronomiae*, written in the thirteenth century. Surviving in some sixty manuscript copies, the *Speculum* has been attributed by Paola Zambelli and others to Albert the Great (ca. 1200–1280), Master at the University of Paris. However, this authorship has been contested–Bruno Roy, following the work of David Pingree, argued that Richard Fournival (1201–ca. 1260), philosopher and royal surgeon, might be the author. More recently, Augusto Paravinci Bagliani pointed to the Italian astrologer and university master Campanus de Novara (ca. 1220–1296) as its creator.[40] Whatever the case, there is no firm evidence for authorship in any of the surviving manuscripts precisely because the author deliberately chose to remain anonymous—perhaps unsurprisingly, given the nature of the treatise. This is what the *Speculum* says about differences between permitted astrological images and forbidden demonic ones:

37 Draelants, "Notion of Properties," 176–78.

38 Marrone, "William of Auvergne on Magic in Natural Philosophy," 743.

39 Page, *Magic in the Cloister*, 31. See also, Giralt above (chap. 7 of this volume).

40 For a useful discussion of the scholarship relating to the authorship of the *Speculum Astronomiae*, see Burnett, Review of *Le "Speculum Astronomiae"*, 1364–66.

> This wisdom, then, is divided into two parts. The first [part] is introductory and is concerned with the principles of [astrological] judgements. But the second part is fulfilled in the exercise of making judgements; and this [second part] is further divided into four sections. The first is concerned with revolutions [of the years]; the second with nativities; the third with interrogations; [and] the fourth with choosing favourable hours—to which that section which deals with images is subjoined, of which it is said; 'the most sublime part of astronomy is the science of images'. But those cursed necromantic books on images, illusions and characters, rings and sigils are associated with this part [of the science] because they [i.e. the necromancers] borrow certain astronomical observations for themselves for the purpose of simulation in order to render themselves [as] slightly credible. By the will of God, I will disclose their poison in what follows [...].[41]

For the *Speculum*'s author, then, astrological images were not *de facto* problematic. The issue arose when astrological images were incorporated into forbidden magic spells and rituals, often in an attempt to make something demonic look acceptable. This is an essential point.

Thus, certain practices labelled illicit divination in canon law *might* now fit into the new scholastic concept of natural magic as postulated in the thirteenth century. But this completely depended on the perspective of the reader who might come across such a device. The debate on universals, which encompassed both names and numbers, was taking place at the same time as this new category of natural magic was postulated in exactly the same scholastic settings. So, it would depend on whether or not the reader saw names and numbers, the constituent operative elements of onomancy, as "substances" which had quintessential natural properties, or simply as signifiers.

Conclusion

Onomancy was a form of divination, and divination was condemned along with magic in discourse since at least the late Roman Republic. Unlike many divinatory items that were first translated into Latin in the twelfth century, forms of onomancy are present in manuscripts in the early medieval Latin West. Divination and magic were one and the same to many of those who condemned these practices as all operating by the power of demons. At the same time, Platonic debates on universals, including those on the power of names and numbers were lively in Christian theology, from the time of the earliest Church Fathers. The influential figure of Augustine of Hippo set the tone for the early Middle Ages on magic and divination, and on the power of names and numbers. Divination was not permissible, because, like magic, it operated via the power of demons. Names and numbers, to some degree, were "real." God was the *monad* or single unit; the number six was also very important as the number of days it took God to create the world.

41 *The* Speculum astronomiae *and Its Enigma*, trans. Zambelli, 223.

It was in the thirteenth century that conceptual frameworks began to shift. The new translations of Aristotelian and Islamic texts of natural philosophy and the occult led a series of Parisian masters—William of Auvergne, the author of the *Speculum Astronomiae*, Thomas Aquinas—to postulate different ways of thinking about magic and divination. The category of "natural magic" was proposed. While I have not come across any specific examples of onomancy being described as a form of natural magic, I contend that this new way of thinking about natural properties, combined with the intertwined history of magic and divination and the powerful debate on universals in medieval philosophy, meant that it was possible to see onomantic divination as operating on the basis of natural properties, linking it with the concept of natural magic. If you followed Platonic reasoning, numbers and names existed to some degree and were "real" outside of being abstract signifiers—they were part of God's creation. At the same time, it was equally possible to believe that onomancy was unacceptable divination which operated via the power of demons, as the strictures against all forms of magic and divination continued and intensified until the end of the Middle Ages.

Bibliography

Manuscripts

Cologne, Erzbischöfliche Diözesan- und Dombibliothek, MS 83 II.

Universitätsbibliothek Heidelberg, Cod. Pal. germ. 832 = Johannes Hartlieb. *Namenmantik* (the *Heidelberger Schicksalsbuch*). Translated by Ben Pope.

Primary Sources

Abelard, Peter. "Glosses on Porphyry." In *Five Texts on the Mediaeval Problem of Universals: Porphyry, Boethius, Abelard, Duns Scotus, Ockham*. Edited and translated by Paul Vincent Spade. Indianapolis: Hackett, 1984.

Augustine. *The City of God Against the Pagans*. Edited by R. W. Dyson. Cambridge Texts in the History of Political Thought. Cambridge: Cambridge University Press, 1998.

——. *De divinatione daemonum*. Edited by Joseph Zycha. In Corpus Scriptorum Ecclesiasticorum Latinorum 41. Prague: Tempsky, 1900.

Boethius. "De Institutione Arithmetica." In *Boethian Number Theory: A Translation of the De Institutione Arithmetica (with Introduction and Notes)*. Translated by Michael Masi. Amsterdam: Rodopi, 1983.

Buridan, John. "Quaestiones in Porphyrii Isagogen 9." In Jan Buridan, *Kommentarz do Isagogi Porfiriusza*. Edited by R. Tatarzynski, 111–95. Warsaw: Przeglad Tomistyczny, 1986.

Calcidius. *On Plato's Timaeus*. Translated by John Magee. Cambridge, MA: Harvard University Press, 2016.

Duns Scotus, John. *Quaestiones in libros Perihermenias Aristotelis*. Edited by R. Andrews, G. Etzkorn, G. Gál, R. Green, T. Noone, R. Plevano, A. Traven and R. Wood. Washington, DC: Franciscan Institute, 2004.

Gratian. "Decretum." In *Corpus Iuris Canonici*, vol. 1. Edited by Aemilius Friedberg. Graz: Akademische Druck- und Verlagsanstalt, 1959.

Hugh of St. Victor. *Selected Spiritual Writings of the Revered Twelfth-Century Mystic.* Translated by Aelred Squire. London: Faber and Faber, 1962.

Isidore of Seville. *The Etymologies of Isidore of Seville.* Edited and translated by Stephen A. Barney, W. J. Lewis, J. A. Beach, and Oliver Berghof. Cambridge: Cambridge University Press, 2006.

Kieckhefer, Richard, ed. and trans. *Hazards of the Dark Arts: Advice for Medieval Princes on Witchcraft and Magic.* University Park: Pennsylvania State University Press, 2017.

Macrobius. *Commentary on the Dream of Scipio.* Translated by William Harris Stahl. New York: Columbia University Press, 1952.

Nichomachus of Gerasa. *Introduction to Arithmetic.* Translated by Martin D'Ooge. University of Michigan Studies, Humanistic Series 16. New York: MacMillan, 1926.

Origen. *Contra Celsum.* Translated by Henry Chadwick. Cambridge: Cambridge University Press, 1965.

The Speculum astronomiae *and Its Enigma: Astrology, Theology, and Science in Albertus Magnus and His Contemporaries.* Translated by Paola Zambelli. Dordrecht: Kluwer, 1992.

Thomas of Chobham. *Summa Confessorum.* Edited by F. Broomfield. Louvain: Nauwelaerts, 1968.

Secondary Sources

Bailey, Michael D. *Fearful Spirits, Reasoned Follies: The Boundaries of Superstition in Late Medieval Europe.* Ithaca: Cornell University Press, 2013.

Burnett, Charles. "The Eadwine Psalter and the Western Tradition of the Onomancy in Pseudo-Aristotle's Secret of Secrets." *Archives d'Histoire Doctrinale et Littéraire du Moyen Âge* 55 (1988): 143–46. Reprinted in Burnett, Charles. *Magic and Divination in the Middle Ages: Texts and Techniques in the Islamic and Christian Worlds.* Variorum Collected Studies Series 557. Aldershot: Ashgate, 1996.

——. Review of *Le "Speculum Astronomiae," une énigme? Enquête sur les manuscrits,* by A. P. Bagliani. *Speculum* 78, no. 4 (2003): 1364–66.

Cameron, Margaret. "Meaning: Foundational and Semantic Theories." In *The Oxford Handbook of Medieval Philosophy.* Edited by John Marenbon, 342–62. Oxford: Oxford University Press, 2012.

Chardonnens, Lázsló Sándor. *Anglo-Saxon Prognostics, 900–1100: Study and Texts.* Leiden: Brill, 2007.

Draelants, Isabelle. "The Notion of Properties: Tensions Between *Scientia* and *Ars* in Medieval Natural Philosophy and Magic." In *The Routledge History of Medieval Magic.* Edited by Sophie Page and Catherine Rider, 169–86. Abingdon: Routledge, 2019.

Edge, Joanne. "Licit Medicine or 'Pythagorean Necromancy?' The 'Sphere of Life and Death' in Late Medieval England." *Historical Research* 87, no. 238 (November 2014): 611–32.

——. *Onomantic Divination in Late Medieval Britain: Questioning Life, Predicting Death.* Woodbridge: Boydell and Brewer, 2024.

Escobar-Vargas, Maria Carolina. "Magic, Technology and New Categories of Knowledge in the Central Middle Ages." *Reading Medieval Studies* 41 (2015): 53–66.

Heiduk, Matthias, Klaus Herbers, and Hans-Christian Lehner, eds. *Prognostication in the Medieval World: A Handbook.* 2 vols. Berlin: De Gruyter, 2020.

Juste, David. *Les Alchandreana primitifs: Étude sur les plus anciens traités astrologiques latins d'origine arabe (Xe siècle).* Leiden: Brill, 2007.

Klima, Gyula. *John Buridan.* Oxford: Oxford University Press, 2009.

Klingshirn, William E. "Isidore of Seville's Taxonomy of Magicians and Diviners." *Traditio* 58 (2003): 59–90.

Lemay, Richard. "The Teaching of Astronomy in Medieval Universities, Principally Paris in the Fourteenth Century." *Manuscripta* 20, no. 3 (1976): 199–202.

Marrone, Steven P. "William of Auvergne on Magic in Natural Philosophy and Theology." In *Was ist Philosophie im Mittelalter? Qu'est-ce que la philosophie au moyen âge? What is Philosophy in the Middle Ages? Akten des X. Internationalen Kongresses für Mittelalterliche Philosophie der Société Internationale pour l'Etude de la Philosophie Médiévale, 25. bis 30. August 1997 in Erfurt*. Edited by Jan A. Aertsen and Andreas Speer, 741–48. Berlin: De Gruyter, 2012.

Page, Sophie. *Magic in the Cloister: Pious Motives, Illicit Interests, and Occult Approaches to the Medieval Universe*. University Park: Pennsylvania State University Press, 2013.

Rhijn, Carine van. *Leading the Way to Heaven: Pastoral Care and Salvation in the Carolingian Period*. London: Routledge, 2022.

Rider, Catherine. "Medical Magic and the Church in Thirteenth-Century England." *Social History of Medicine* 24, no.1 (2011): 92–107.

Schrenk, Lawrence P. "God as Monad: The Philosophical Basis of Medieval Theological Numerology." In *Medieval Numerology: A Book of Essays*. Edited by Robert L. Surles, 3–10. New York: Garland, 1993.

Silva, Marco Aurélio Oliveira da. "Albert the Great on Mathematical Quantities." *Revista Portuguesa de Filosofia* 73, no. 3 (2017): 1191–1201.

Veenstra, Jan R. *Magic and Divination at the Courts of Burgundy and France: Texts and Contexts of Laurens Pignons "Contres les devineurs" (1411)*. Leiden: Brill, 1997.

Weisheipl, James A. "Albertus Magnus and the Oxford Platonists." *Proceedings of the American Catholic Philosophical Association* 32 (1958): 124–39.

LATE-MEDIEVAL BRONTOLOGIES

POPULAR SUPERSTITION OR ASTROLOGICAL MEDICAL GUIDE?

JANET WALLS

IN THE LATE Middle Ages, the vagaries of the weather were thought of as having a defined place in God's creation and yet being extremely hard to predict in detail and with accuracy. Given the importance of meteorological phenomena for economically, medically, and politically crucial aspects of medieval life it is not surprising that they were included in several short, predictive texts, now grouped under the name of "prognostics" and offering advanced knowledge of various sorts. These texts, and especially examples from the early medieval period, have been the subject of increasing interest among scholars.[1] They foretell the future using a variety of methods, some triggered by weather events themselves, such as wind, or thunder. The latter are known as brontologies and are found in surviving manuscripts from across early medieval Europe. However, this chapter will demonstrate both that brontologies continued in use to the end of the medieval period and that they held an important place amongst the resources used by professionals such as medical practitioners in the fourteenth and fifteenth centuries.

In brontology, thunder events are used as the markers for prognostication. It was known in England in the early and High Middle Ages, but few examples survive from that time,[2] whereas, sixty-six texts have been found in a variety of late-medieval English manuscripts, written in Middle English, Latin or combinations of both. These were found in volumes focused on medicine, rather than estate management. Moreover, brontologies grew in number and variety at this time, suggesting active interest rather than mere copying from exemplars. Importantly, this was happening at times of already challenging weather, pandemics and political unrest, which might have led to a rejection of such venerable forms of prediction; and yet in the case of brontologies the reverse was true. This chapter will investigate their contexts in late-medieval England and the evidence they provide for concepts of a relationship between human health and the natural world.

1 For example, Chardonnens, *Anglo-Saxon Prognostics*; Cesario, "Weather Prognostics"; Heiduk, Herbers, and Lehner, *Prognostication in the Medieval World*.

2 Chardonnens, *Anglo-Saxon Prognostics* has ten text editions: 247–69.

Janet Walls is a doctoral research student at the University of Reading working on the survival of brontologies in late-medieval manuscript compilations, who has published on brontology and regimens of health in *Reading Medieval Studies*.

Translations from Latin and translations and transcriptions from Middle English (where necessary) are supplied close to their original form, using the transcription conventions below.[3] Where any modern punctuation has been added to original texts to clarify meaning this was kept to a minimum.

Brontology Manuscript Contexts

Certain groups, such as merchants, doctors and surgeons (the latter two groups practising at diverse levels and offering various specialisms) were growing in power and influence at the time brontology was appearing in manuscripts of astrological medicine. In astrological medicine, planetary influences were believed to be active upon individuals at any given time, affecting them physically, mentally, and in their ability to succeed in business. The foreknowledge of events provided by prognostics, understood in the context of beliefs about the powers and effects of the planets, was invaluable to their professions. Therefore, astrological medicine provided an armoury of knowledge for practitioners of all sorts, differing from medical astrology in its practical application of humoral theory. Fully trained physicians, who would have studied for at least six years, were expected to be able to use tools such as planetary tables and to understand the Ptolemaic models for planetary movements upon which the tables were based, as well as being familiar with an increasing body of purely medical texts. Chaucer's description of a successful physician sums up both the knowledge and the high fees associated with such individuals.[4] For the majority who could not afford the personal attentions of highly trained physicians, who were thin on the ground anyway,[5] prognostics offered much faster (if less personal) insight into coming climatic and health-related factors and outcomes.

This was aided by increased book acquisition among lay people in the fifteenth century, with examples of groups of guild acquaintances choosing and writing out their own copies, or even versions, of material and sharing them amongst themselves.[6] This is one explanation for composite manuscripts, made up of separate booklets bound together, in the wider study. Significantly, these people were seldom estate owners, but town-based individuals whose success lay in their professional standing and reputation, such

3 Transcription conventions used in this chapter:

- þ used as the single thorn symbol for "th."
- ʒ yogh character used by scribes to represent sounds "g," "gh," or "y."
- ( ) parentheses signify expanded abbreviations.
- · indicates an original *punctus* representing a pause, also used to identify numbers in texts.

4 See the description of the Physician, in "The General Prologue" to Chaucer's *Canterbury Tales*, ed. Benson, Fragment 1, lines 411–44.

5 There were forty Oxford University medical students throughout the fourteenth century, fifty-four during the fifteenth century, and fifty-nine graduated from Cambridge over the whole period from 1300 to 1499, see Rawcliffe, *Medicine and Society*, 108.

6 Barron, "What Did Medieval London Merchants Read?," 62–63.

as fishmonger William Walworth, died 1383, owner of a personal library, whose brother was a clerical lawyer from Oxford and canon of York.[7] The scribes or compilers of medical and scientific volumes had the connections to acquire these texts from such university contexts and amalgamate them into personalized textbooks and reference guides, often using very good quality materials. One example is California, San Marino, Huntington Library, MS HM 1336,[8] written for Robert Taylor of Boxford by Simon Wysbech, a student of canon law at Cambridge University, which features a brontology with astrological medicine. Another example is Cambridge, Trinity College, MS R.14.52, which bears the monogram of John Vale, secretary and factor to Sir Thomas Cook.[9]

The Manuscript Witnesses

The sixty-six brontology texts mentioned above are located in fifty English manuscripts, the earliest of which are from the first half of the fourteenth century, whilst the majority are from the fifteenth century. Although all but a handful deal with astronomy and astrology somewhere in the manuscript, twenty-five were selected for close study of their application of these sciences to humoral medicine and brontology, in a number of individualized ways, the most developed examples being compound medical prognostics. To illustrate this, seven manuscripts with detailed groupings of astrological medical texts and brontology are discussed in this chapter, in an approximate chronological order.[10] The first five of these are noteworthy because they each amalgamate brontology with astrological material into one compound text in different styles and combinations. The other two manuscripts are examples of multiple brontology texts. In the first five manuscripts the purposes of amalgamation may have been to create a convenient reference tool for a practitioner, but the needs and interests of individual practices dictated the final forms. The earliest, London, British Library, MS Sloane 282,[11] has a prognostic derived from the disposition of the calendar month, itself conflated with the relevant zodiac period:

> in mense ianuarii sol dicitur in aquario quiritur tunc maxime habundant ague cum moratur in isto signo[12]

---

7 Further examples of merchants who willed personal libraries to their heirs, dating from the mid-fourteenth century onwards; Henry Graspays, London fishmonger, d. 1348, William Bristow, London cordwainer, d. 1367, and the following aldermen (senior city officials): Walter de Berneye, mercer, d. 1377/9, Richard Lyons, vintner, d. 1381, William Kyng, draper, d. 1393/4, from Barron, "What Did Medieval London Merchants Read?," 60–61.

8 San Marino, Huntington Library, MS HM 1336 (*olim* Phillipps MS 6883).

9 Cambridge, Trinity College, MS R.14.52, fol. 1r; Hicks "Case of Sir Thomas Cook," 82–96.

10 Precise dating of many of these manuscripts is very difficult as dates are seldom given within them, so this often relies on palaeography or the date ranges of calendars, when present, or the inclusion of texts with known publication dates.

11 Sloane 282, s. xiv^{ex}.

12 Sloane 282, fol. 85v.

(In the month of January when the sun is said to be in Aquarius it is said that at this time especially people will die of much ague in this sign.)

This is combined with a brontology by the same method:

Si tonitru(um) sit in hoc signo. magne pluvie erunt per loca . et terror erit filiis ho(min)im . Venti . eo anno gen(er)abu(n)t tussi(m) et scabiem et una p(er)s hominu(m) incipiet contendere et illa conte(n)cio magna erit in seculo.

(If it thunders in this sign there will be heavy rain in places and there will be fear among people. Wind will cause the cough and the scab in that year and one nation will start a conflict and it will be a major conflict throughout the century.)

In Oxford, Bodleian Library, MS Bodley 591,[13] the compound text begins with a St. Paul's Day weather prognostic predicting good or bad weather for the year from the weather on the feast of the Conversion of St. Paul (January 25). Next, a zodiac nativity notes how a person born at that time will be affected by the dispositions of the sign, "Quando natus est in Aquario nechligens erit" (when they are born in Aquarius they will be lazy). Then the text continues with a months-brontology and a prognostic from the disposition of the zodiac sign period focusing on the advisability of travel. In London, Wellcome Library, MS 8004 (also known as "The Physician's Handbook"),[14] the perilous days in the month are conflated with; the zodiac period, brontology by the zodiac method, and exposition of dispositions of the zodiac sign with the prognostics from them including specifically medical predictions for when the moon is in the sign. A corresponding part of the text follows, on the times when the Sun is in the sign given using calendar dates (a calendar is provided) and a further prognostic from the dispositions of the sign at those times, also including a medical section.

Warminster, Longleat House, MS 176[15] also refers to the disposition of the zodiac sign period for a prognostic, along with a zodiac nativity and brontology. Manchester, Chetham's Library, MS Mun.A.4.99[16] has two prominent brontologies by the months, combined with; the date of the Sun's entry into the sign, disposition of the sign compared with holy events recorded in the Bible (for January this links Aquarius to the site of Christ's baptism, the River Jordan), nativity, weather forecast from when the sun is in the sign, and medical prediction from when the moon is in the sign. By the end of the fifteenth century, brontology can be found as part of a regimen of health in San Marino, Huntington Library, MS HM 64.[17] This compound text commences with a suitable, humour-balancing drink in January relating to its disposition and the advis-

13 Bodley 591, s. xv^{med}.

14 Wellcome 8004, 1454.

15 Longleat 176, s. xv^{2}.

16 Chetham's A.4.99, s. xv^{2}.

17 Huntington HM 64, s. xv^{ex}.

ability of letting blood, informed by a list of perilous days. These are combined with; a brontology, a mist prognostic,[18] and a general life prognostic for when the moon is in the sign, mentioning travel. Therefore, a number of practices and interests were drawn into these texts with the common elements of planetary influences on the dispositions of the zodiac signs, particularly those of the Sun and Moon.[19] However, these were not collections focused on astronomical or astrological matters but rather practical texts with applications to health and self-care.

Astrological Medical Guides

By the late Middle Ages, medical knowledge was circulating among practitioners outside universities, resulting in an increasingly sophisticated methodology which weighed "contingent and variable factors" in practice, as Arnau de Vilanova put it.[20] This approach is evident from the many and varied prognostic and diagnostic texts, and practical, therapeutic treatments seen in the developed astrological medical manuscripts containing brontologies. In addition to a detailed compound prognostic text which includes brontology, Wellcome 8004 is one of these highly developed examples of grouping of astrological and practical medical texts from the late Middle Ages, which are listed in the Appendix, below. Huntington 64 is another example, shown in the Appendix for comparison. It has fewer individual texts but its sources are from medical textbooks. The attributes of the four humours as explained in Wellcome 8004 and intrinsic to the works of Galen and Hippocrates cited in Huntington 64 are further qualified with visual aids, astronomical charts and tables identifying the positions of the planets. The relative positions of the Sun, Moon, and other planets in both the signs of the zodiac and the houses were thought to augment or reduce the properties of the humours already affected by the nature of each of the planets themselves. This astrological interpretation was then applied to diagnoses and prognoses and reflected in the choice of astrological medical practices, such as bleeding at favourable times and interpreting the state of a patient's health from the appearance of urine.

The wider textual association of items in Wellcome 8004 functions as a diagnostic and prognostic toolkit, dependent upon the humours. University-trained physicians, with skills in astrological computation, could use tables or ephemerides like those in Wellcome 8004, and Chetham's A.4.99, to calculate the exact positions of the planets. In Chetham's A.4.99 these are unusually numerous and cover longer periods like years, several are in the quick-reference form of volvelles, or revolving paper circles loosely attached to the manuscript to allow rotation. Users of these tables could also place the planets in relation to the patient's geographical location through calculating the inter-

18 No reference to another can be found in Voigts, ed., "eTK/eVK2 Project."

19 The Sun and Moon were identified as planets along with the five actual planets known at the time; Mercury, Venus, Mars, Jupiter, and Saturn, see North, "Medieval Concepts," 5–17.

20 Arnau de Vilanova was a scholar from Spain who studied many arts, translated scientific texts from Arabic, and taught at the University of Montpellier. The above phrase is from one of his lectures, "Lecture on the Text 'Life is Short'"; see Wallis, ed., *Medieval Medicine: A Reader*, 211.

section of the zodiac signs with the houses. This built upon concepts introduced in the central medieval period, when physicians encountered the works of Constantine of Africa: *Liber Pantegni* and *Isagoge*.[21] In the former, Constantine explains the variable effects of the Moon on health, in the latter, Galen's theory of critical days for illnesses discussed the movements of the Sun and other planets, in addition to the Moon.[22] This holistic practice was based on careful interpretation of all the available signs, as expounded by Arnau de Vilanova:

> The physician has to modify his tools and practices in accordance with the changes and variations in the illness as well as in the dispositions of the air and other circumstances by which the body is affected.[23]

Here, "dispositions of the air" refers to the state of the weather, and the healthiness of the air, in a given locality. Both of these would make brontology valuable not as a weather forecast but a signifier of long-term changes to the balance of nature caused by thunder events. The study of the wider cosmic effects on future weather, or astrometeorology, was also of great interest in this regard.[24] The most in-depth way of discerning the planetary influences on an individual to judge what medical treatment was appropriate for them, or to investigate their health conditions, was to cast their horoscope. This gave the practitioner a greater insight into the forces active at the time of a person's birth than a simpler birth prognostic. The findings would then be added to enquiries about present planetary influences, those expected in the near future, and the humours affecting them. The skills required to use the necessary tables to carry out this work were taught at university, however, the tables themselves could be reproduced for others, as in the case of Huntington 1336, above. Such computations were attractive to practitioners because they allowed them to produce "more personally tailored and scientifically framed judgements."[25]

Apart from personal horoscopes, calendars also offered practitioners a practical means of applying astronomy to their enquiries with a range of years to work from, allowing forward planning of healthcare and business. These calendars were originally clerical timekeeping tools used to mark saints' feast days and central to the calculation of the date of Easter (based on the variable spring equinox) which had been a major cause of contention between the churches of Britain in the seventh century. Two late-medieval friars, John Somer (in 1380) and Nicholas de Lynn (in 1387) separately produced their own versions of such calendars which included canons for medical application.[26] The canons in general explained how to use the calendar tables and other items relevant to

21 As discussed by Anne Jeavons above (chap. 4 of this volume).

22 Lawrence-Mathers and Escobar-Vargas, *Magic and Medieval Society*, 67–68.

23 Wallis, ed., *Medieval Medicine: A Reader*, 211.

24 For astrometeorology, see Lawrence-Mathers above (chap. 6 of this volume).

25 On the practice of the multi-skilled astrologer and businessman Richard Trewythian, see Page, "Richard Trewythian," 195.

26 *Kalendarium of John Somer*, ed. Mooney; *Nicholas of Lynn*, ed. Eisner.

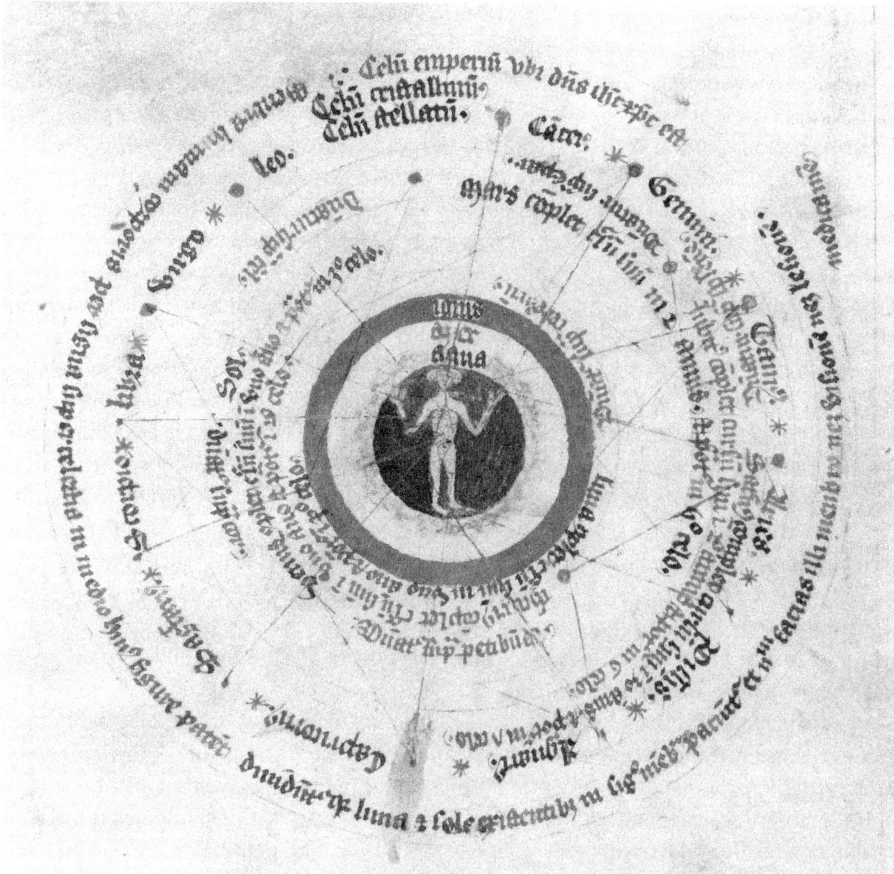

Figure 11.1: "Calendar." London, British Library, MS Sloane 282, fol. 18r. Used with permission © The British Library Board, London.

the calculation of planetary positions through the liturgical year and Lynn, in particular, was interested in medical applications. He treats these in Canons Eleven and Twelve at the end of his calendar and includes a diagram which is considerably more complex than the standard "Zodiac Man" figure. This shows the specific body parts affected by each of the planets and zodiac constellations.[27] Figure 11.1[28] is from the version of Lynn's calendar in Sloane 282, ca. 1400, dedicated to "Lady Joan, Princess of Wales, mother of our lord King Richard the Second after the Conquest."[29] This was probably not just aspirational advertising on the part of Somer, since he was a regular visitor to the court of

27 See *Kalendarium of John Somer*, ed. Mooney, 45.

28 Sloane 282, fol. 18r; calendar, fols. 5r–18r.

29 *Kalendarium of John Somer*, ed. Mooney, 25, 31–32.

Richard II as a representative of the Carmelite convent in Oxford, but a sign of the regard in which his work was held.

Brontology, therefore, sits nicely as an extra dimension of the holistic, astrological medical approach of Arnau de Vilanova. Thunder is certainly dramatic and physically disturbing, whilst in the Bible it is interpreted as an expression of divine will,[30] which provides a safeguard for it against accusations of illicit divination. The potential for prognostics to be regarded as divination had been the subject of debate earlier in the medieval period, especially during the twelfth and thirteenth centuries. There were concerns at the time that prognostics might provide too much foreknowledge of future events thereby compromising the key concept of free will. There was also a lack of clarity about what was judicial astrology, the more problematic branch of the science.[31] However, by the middle of the thirteenth century, scholars like Thomas Aquinas were concluding that astrology which concerns the weather should be accepted and studied for its practical benefit to agriculture, statecraft and public health. Aquinas addressed this in his *Summa theologiae*, judging that weather knowledge was the result of observation and experience.[32] The acceptability of such science was also defined through its technicalities in the near-contemporary *Speculum Astronomiae*,[33] earlier attributed to the scholar Albertus Magnus.[34] The third area of Chapters Four and Five of this work refers to earlier astrological treatises, to give authority to the science of astrometeorology.[35] Also around this time, John Ashenden wrote two brontologies (one using the months, the other the zodiac signs) into his exposition of the effects of thunder and lightning in his work *Summa de accidentibus mundi*.[36]

It seems likely that this holistic humoral thinking, coupled with the possibility that thunder was a form of divine expression, tipped the balance in favour of brontology as an acceptable practice. Over and above this acceptance, the special place of thunder amongst weather prognostics in the original corpus of sixty-six brontologies is evinced by the smaller number of thirteen texts on other types of weather;[37] six sunshine, five wind, one rainbow and one mist. Also, brontology is at the forefront of these groupings

30 God communicates to Moses through thunder and hail, Exodus 9:23; God wills thunder against his adversaries, and sends thunder at Samuel's request, 1 Samuel 2:10, 12:18; God communicates through thunder, Job 37:5, 40:4; God demands attention through the medium of thunder, Ecclesiastes 46:20; thunder heard at Jesus's entrance into Jerusalem is interpreted by some of the crowd as the voice of an angel, John 12:29.

31 For example, the arguments of Bishop Bartholomew of Exeter, see Runciman, "Bishop Bartholomew," 7–8, 265–82.

32 See Lawrence-Mathers, *Medieval Meteorology*, 141.

33 Lawrence-Mathers, *Medieval Meteorology*, 143.

34 See *The* Speculum astronomiae *and Its Enigma*, trans. Zambelli.

35 Lawrence-Mathers, *Medieval Meteorology*, 143.

36 See Johannes Eschuid [John Ashenden], *Summa astrologiae iudicialis*, tract. 2, dist. 7, cap. 2, in 1489 ed., fol. 145r.

37 In the following manuscripts: Sloane 2584, Rawlinson C.814, Egerton 2852, Sloane 282, Ashmole 6, Longleat 174, BL Addit. 27582, Huntington 64, and Digby 88.

of weather texts, although Sloane 282 uses three types of weather for prognosis, thunder, wind and sunshine, framing the others with two brontology texts, the last part of this leaves the reader with the knowledge of what to do in the event of more than one thundering in the year.[38] Brontology is most prominent in the large illuminated heading, incipit and first passage of the compound prognostic text in Chetham's A.4.99,[39] which also contains other weather prognostics further on in the text;

> Hic incipiunt Tonitrua mensium et signo(rum) solis (et) Lune.
>
> Mense Janua(ri), Si tonitruum fit mense Janu(ri) vent(os) valid(os) habund(am) frugu(m) et bellu(m) signif(icat).
>
> (Here begins the thunders of the months and the signs of the sun and the moon.
>
> The Month of January. If it thunders in the month of January, it signifies strong winds, abundant grain and war.)
>
> Whan þond(er) comeþ in Januir(i) þou schalt haue þ(a)t ilke ȝer grete wi(n)ds · Moche fruit and gret werre of folk þ(a)t liuen und(er) sterre.
>
> (When thunder comes in January, you will have great winds that same year, much fruit and a great war for the people who live under the star.)

In professional manuscripts with brontologies, multiples of the same prognostic texts are offered to adapt to individual cases, enabling the selection of suitable preventative and proactive treatments for a range of patients, whereas self-help guides or family reference books usually have only one example. As a result of practitioners creating their own multifunctional texts in this way, the individualized diagnosis and treatment this offered deliberately included brontology. Wellcome 8004 has an example of an alternative brontology. The first brontology is part of a grouping of texts entitled "The Exposicion of the Twelve Signs"[40] and the brontology text appears under the subheading "Aquaryus and hys properties."[41] In this text, Aquarius is described as hot, moist and sanguine, to be understood as a natural influence on the winds, fruit and the likelihood of battle, then if thunder is heard (thunder is a natural force but classed as a medical non-natural)[42] it announces, impacts upon and amplifies these phenomena into great winds, much fruit and certain battle. In this example, thunder is also the harbinger of ill health under two combinations of circumstances:

---

38 Sloane 282, fols. 85v–87r.

39 Chetham's A.4.99, fol. 29r.

40 Wellcome 8004, fols. 33v–41v.

41 Wellcome 8004, fol. 36v.

42 See Jeavons above (chap. 4 of this volume) for naturals and non-naturals and the role of the latter in keeping naturals in balance.

- if heard in June, under the sign of Cancer (described as cold, moist and phlegmatic) many and varied sicknesses are to be expected.[43]
- if heard in August, under Virgo (cold, dry and melancholy), many will fall ill and, unsurprisingly given the pre-fertile nature of Virgo, there will be a number of problems pertaining to women's health and their marriageability.[44]

In the second Wellcome 8004 brontology, the following illnesses are caused by the impact of thunder on the natural world;

- thunder in February signifies much death and from a serious sickness
- thunder in June signifies freak winds causing several ailments, but not of the head.[45]

Similarly, Huntington 64 identifies the culprit of the "great disease and sickness of folk" in February as "the morayne."[46] February is designated as a cold, moist and phlegmatic month and the victims are usually stated as rich men. Several other brontologies in the wider chapter corpus also forewarn of specific diseases,[47] in these cases cough and "scab" (likely to be a form of pox), if thunder is heard in February. These warnings give the medical practitioner specific forewarnings over and above the regular effects of planets on the humours in the month periods in question. Also, it is of note that the variety of presentations of brontology in different textual compilations shows they had not simply been copied into manuscripts along with groupings of texts on weather or health but chosen as a help to astrological medicine. The manuscript contexts they are found in are also varied, as follow;

- within the folios of calendars, or their canons
- portable, folding manuscripts
- university medical textbooks
- handbooks and health regimens for physicians, surgeons, and apothecaries
- household books of useful knowledge

Manuscripts in the first two categories are frequently older than the others and demonstrate early ways of brontology transmission into the late Middle Ages, with calendar manuscripts often shared by an institution or household as a repository of knowledge. The appeal of brontology in subsequent groupings of health texts was the ability to plan

---

43 Wellcome 8004, fol. 38r.

44 Wellcome 8004, fol. 38v.

45 Wellcome 8004, fols. 70r–v.

46 This is a disease of animals in modern terminology, but often refers to plague in humans in the Middle Ages, see *Middle English Dictionary*, s.n. "morein(e", at https://quod.lib.umich.edu/m/middle-english-dictionary/dictionary/MED28633/track?counter=1&search_id=18943118; accessed May 10, 2024.

47 In Cambridge, UL Hh.6.11, cough and scabies in Aquarius; in Digby 95, Trinity R.14.52, and Morgan 775, cough and scab in Aquarius; in Lincoln 91, cough in December; in Ashmole 342, cough in Aquarius.

from knowledge of how health, wellbeing, and business would be affected in the context of the humours over the scope of a year, with the potential to update it should there be another thunder event.

The incipit to the textual grouping with brontology in Huntington 64 explains the holistic approach that the brontology is now part of:

> "Here saythe Galian(us) the goode leche that was, of metis and dryngkis to use in tyme of the yere in every monythe to take and ete and in tyme of bloode Letynge etcetera."[48]
>
> ("Here speaks Galen, the good leech that once was, of seasonal foods and drinks to take each month and at times of bloodletting, etcetera.")

Other Types of Brontology

In addition to the months and zodiac-period brontologies already investigated in this chapter, three other types survive in just six study manuscripts:[49]

- brontology by cardinal directions (needs to be linked to a time marker)
- brontology by liturgical hours
- brontology by the days of Christmas week

All the manuscripts using these multiple texts have the characteristics of reference books and also include a months-brontology. The use of both these markers for brontology seems to have been for thoroughness and comparison, the compiler could use a selection of time periods according to need. The days of Christmas week were the least useful, but potentially considered the most potent due to their association with the time of Christ's birth, because the prognostics from them were fixed for the year ahead, unless the accompanying months-brontologies were to supersede them should there be further thunder. A set of three of these texts, from early fifteenth-century manuscript London, British Library, Sloane MS 989[50] is shown below in a modernized English edition for ease of reference. The third example had an English heading but the rest of the text has been translated from Latin.

> 1) Now it is to know what thunders betoken at diverse times of the year. On Christmas Day thunder betokens the death of the king or some of his children or some other lord close to him by blood. The second day of Christmas, thunder betokens battles and war in that land. The third day betokens there will be no dwelling place. The fourth day, wise men, and mighty men, shall die. The fifth

48 Huntington 64, fol. 79v.

49 Cambridge, UL Gg.1.1, BL Royal 12 C XII, Digby 95, Sloane 989, Longleat 174, BL Addit. 27582.

50 Sloane 989, s. xv^{in}.

> day, many women shall die. The sixth, many fish shall die. The seventh, mayors and dons shall die.
>
> 2) Thunder in January betokens great winds, much corn and great wars in that year. In February, thunder betokens death of many men and namely of mighty men [...].
>
> 3) This betokens thunders throughout the year, set down by the ancients then by ancient teachers. If thunder sounds in the month of January, it signifies there will be strong winds and war that same year.
>
> The month of February, if thunder sounds many men and especially the rich will soon be pronounced dead [...].[51]

For comparison, excerpts from the three brontologies in Warminster, Longleat House MS 174:[52]

> 1) Tokens of thunder as the Jews say and also according to great clerks of astronomy. If it thunders at the time of evensong, four hours after noon, and does not rain, it betokens the birth of a man who will have great lordship and die for God. If it thunders the seventh hour after noon, it betokens mortality of people. If it thunders the first hour after midnight, it betokens war, with great shedding of blood. If it thunders the seventh hour after midnight, it betokens the birth of a king. If it happens at sunrise, it betokens the turning of the seasons and foreigners who destroy the faith. If it happens the seventh hour after, it betokens that year there will be great plenty of many kinds of fruits. If it thunders at the seventh hour, it betokens the growth of corn and oil but sheep, cattle and other four-footed beasts will perish. If it happens at the ninth hour, it betokens great hindrance of the realm or great deeds of arms in the realm. If it thunders at the tenth hour in the east, it betokens the fall of many cities, overthrown by many sinful men. If it thunders in the eleventh hour it betokens a great tempest at sea and war with Saracens in the land.
>
> 2) If it thunders on Christmas Day, it betokens the death of a king or his children. If it thunders the second day of Christmas, it betokens battle in the land. If it thunders on the third day, there shall be no dwelling (places) in the land. If it thunders on the fourth day of Christmas, clever men and poor men shall die. If it thunders on the fifth day of Christmas, many women shall die. If it thunders of the sixth day of Christmas, fish shall die. If it thunders on the seventh day of Christmas, masters who keep the laws shall die that year.

---

51 Sloane 989, fols. 131v–133r.

52 Longleat 174, s. xv^{ex}.

3) If it thunders in January, it betokens great winds and plenty of corn and battles in that year. If it thunders in February, it betokens death of many men and namely rich men [...].[53]

Conclusion

Was a desire to know the physical conditions impinging on health triggered by climatic deteriorations,[54] devastating epidemics and war-borne disease, food insecurity and unrest the reason for a greater interest in weather prognostics in the fifteenth century? If the weather was even more unpredictable than usual in Britain, a greater inclination to prepare for its effects through a range of popular prognostics would be quite understandable. But, despite arising from the weather and references within brontologies themselves to the security of crops, an interpretation of brontology texts as simply popular superstition to help manage the food supply is inadequate, one aspect being these matters were equally of interest to merchants and factors as to estate managers. Brontology could certainly have been used with agriculture in mind, but its numerous appearances with regimens of health and interweaving with astrological prognostics focused on the influences of zodiac signs and planets on earthly humours were at the essence of what was important to managing health and wellbeing in the late Middle Ages. Any medics, merchants or others with the means and interest to commission books were very likely to have been at least functionally Latinate due to a grammar school education (if male) and able to gain access to university derived astrological medical texts to this end, as Robert Taylor did.[55]

The manuscripts discussed above show clear evidence that the predicted effects of visceral, and even deadly, thunder events were noted for their implications to the wider context of health care in professional medical and paramedical contexts. These brontologies were adapted to integrate different needs and interests, for example, the travel information relevant to merchants, travelling scholars and pilgrims in Bodley 591 and Huntington 64, or surgery in Wellcome 8004 and Chetham's A.4.99.[56] The continued consultation of brontology throughout the study period was in the context of comparative prognostics, learned astral charts and concise volvelles.

53 Longleat 174, fols. 81v–82r.

54 Degroot, "Climate Change and Society," 1–20.

55 Degroot, "Climate Change and Society," 17.

56 Degroot, "Climate Change and Society," 11.

APPENDIX

Wellcome 8004 List of Astrological Medicine Texts

- bloodletting, advised against when the moon is full
- perilous days of the month, applicable to bloodletting and other practices which came under a health remit, such as shaving or bathing
- celestial distances and reckoning of times
- what the four elements and four humours consist of[57]
- dispositions (how the humours affect the human experience)
- planetary influences, which planets affect health and wellbeing and in what ways
- Zodiac Man, showing the body parts affected by each constellation
- Vein Man, showing which veins are susceptible to the influence of each constellation
- Regimen of Health, a guide to health and wellbeing based on the theory of the effects of the four humours
- urology, a guide to "reading" urine samples to affect a diagnosis in the context of the four humours
- the "Sphere of Pythagoras" (also known as "The Sphere of Apuleius" or "The Sphere of Life and Death," predicts whether a patient would live or die)[58]
- Declarations of the Abbot of St. Albans (Richard of Wallingford) on the calendar, an explanation of timekeeping for prognostics
- two brontologies, incorporating other prognostics
- physiognomy, how a person's appearance and demeanour is affected by planetary influences from birth and throughout their life
- Huntington 64 list of astrological medical texts:
- a table showing the month, day and hour when the sun enters a sign, which other planets are active, and which parts of the body are affected, at this time
- physical signs of life and death on the body, this text is called an *experimenta*, meaning a practical skill as opposed to a theoretical one
- birth prognostics for children born on each day of the phases of the moon, or days of the month
- "Tokens of Hippocrates," medical diagnosis from symptoms
- *Trotula minor*, on women's health
- Galen's regimen of health, appropriate foods and drinks for the maintenance of health

---

57 See Jeavons above (chap. 4 of this volume), for medieval use of humoral theory.

58 See Edge, "Licit Medicine," 611–32.

- a book of medicines attributed to Galen, Aschofus,[59] and Hippocrates, including correct storage procedures for them
- fifty-five gynaecological recipes, each attributed to an authority, such as Galen, Isaac Judaeus, Dioscorides.

Bibliography

Manuscripts

Chapter Corpus

Cambridge, St. John's College, MS E.9.
Cambridge, St. John's College, MS K.49.
Cambridge, Trinity College, MS R.14.52.
Cambridge, University Library, MS Gg.1.1.
Cambridge, University Library, MS Hh.6.11.
Edinburgh, National Library of Scotland, Advocates Library MS 19.3.1.
Lincoln, Cathedral Library, MS 91.
London, British Library, MS Additional 27582.
London, British Library, MS Royal 12 C XII.
London, British Library, Sloane MS 282.
London, British Library, Sloane MS 989.
London, Wellcome Library, MS 8004.
Manchester, Chetham's Library, MS Mun.A.4.99.
New York, Morgan Library, MS M775.
Oxford, Bodleian Library, MS Ashmole 189.
Oxford, Bodleian Library, MS Ashmole 342.
Oxford, Bodleian Library, MS Bodley 591.
Oxford, Bodleian Library, MS Digby 88.
Oxford, Bodleian Library, MS Digby 95.
Oxford, Bodleian Library, MS Radcliffe Trust e30.
Oxford, Bodleian Library, MS Tanner 407.
San Marino, Huntington Library, MS HM 64.
San Marino, Huntington Library, MS HM 1336.
Warminster, Longleat House, MS 174.
Warminster, Longleat House, MS 176.

Other Manuscripts

London, British Library, MS Egerton 2852.
Oxford, Bodleian Library, MS Ashmole 6.
Oxford, Bodleian Library, MS Rawlinson C.814.
Oxford, Bodleian Library, MS Sloane 2584.

59 Probably Asclepius, ancient Greek god of medicine.

Primary Sources

Ashenden, John [Johannes Eschuid]. *Summa de accientibus mundi.* Venice: Johannes Lucilius Santritter, 1489.

Chaucer, Geoffrey. "The Canterbury Tales." In *The Riverside Chaucer*. Edited by Larry D. Benson, 3–328. 3rd ed. Oxford: Oxford University Press, 1988.

John Somer, *The Kalendarium of John Somer*. Edited by Linne R. Mooney. Athens: University of Georgia, 1998.

Nicholas of Lynn. *Kalendarium*. Edited by Sigmund Eisner. London: Scolar, 1980.

The Speculum astronomiae *and Its Enigma: Astrology, Theology, and Science in Albertus Magnus and His Contemporaries*. Translated by Paola Zambelli. Dordrecht: Kluwer, 1992.

Voigts, Linda Ehrsam, ed. "eTK/eVK2 Project." https://www.nlm.nih.gov/hmd/indexcat/aboutetkevk2.html (accessed May 10, 2024).

Secondary Sources

Barron, Caroline M. "What Did Medieval London Merchants Read?" In *Medieval Merchants and Money: Essays in Honour of James L. Bolton*. Edited by Martin Allen and Matthew Davies, 43–70. London: University of London, School of Advanced Study, Institute of Historical Research, 2016.

Cesario, Marilina. "Weather Prognostics in Anglo-Saxon England." *English Studies* 93, no. 4 (June 2012): 391–426.

Chardonnens, Lázsló Sándor. *Anglo-Saxon Prognostics, 900–1100: Study and Texts*. Leiden: Brill, 2007.

Degroot, Dagomar. "Climate Change and Society in the 15th to 18th Centuries." *WIREs Climate Change* 9, no. 3 (May/June 2018): 1–20.

Edge, Joanne. "Licit Medicine or 'Pythagorean Necromancy?' The 'Sphere of Life and Death' in Late Medieval England." *Historical Research*, 87, no. 238 (November 2014), 611–32.

Heiduk, Matthias, Klaus Herbers, and Hans-Christian Lehner, eds. *Prognostication in the Medieval World: A Handbook*. Berlin: De Gruyter, 2021.

Hicks, Michael A. "The Case of Sir Thomas Cook, 1468." *The English Historical Review* 93, no. 366 (January 1978): 82–96.

Lawrence-Mathers, Anne, and Carolina Escobar-Vargas. *Magic and Medieval Society*. London, Routledge, 2014.

Lawrence-Mathers, Anne. *Medieval Meteorology: Forecasting the Weather from Aristotle to the Almanac*. Cambridge: University Press, 2020.

North, J. D. "Medieval Concepts of Celestial Influence: A Survey." In *Astrology, Science, and Society: Historical Essays*. Edited by Patrick Curry, 5–18. Woodbridge: Boydell, 1987.

Page, Sophie. "Richard Trewythian and the Uses of Astrology in Late Medieval England." *Journal of the Warburg and Courtauld Institutes* 64 (2001): 193–228.

Rawcliffe, Carole. *Medicine and Society in Later Medieval England*. Stroud: Sutton, 1995.

Runciman, David. "Bishop Bartholomew of Exeter (d. 1184) and the Heresy of Astrology." *Journal of Ecclesiastical History* 70, no. 2 (2019): 265–82.

Wallis, Faith. *Medieval Medicine: A Reader*. Toronto: University of Toronto, 2010.

Walls, Janet. "The Relationship of Brontology and the 'Regimen of Health' in the Later Middle Ages." *Reading Medieval Studies* 47 (2021): 153–72.

WONDER AND WONDER WORKING IN MIDDLE ENGLISH ROMANCE

THE *PROSE MERLIN*

VICTORIA FLOOD

THIS CHAPTER EXPLORES the complex role of wonder in distinctions between historical truth and demonic fiction in late-medieval writings on the prophet and wonder worker Merlin, and his incubus father. It takes as its central point of enquiry the first two books of the Middle English *Prose Merlin* (concerning the prophet's birth and childhood), which it approaches as the product of a long Latin and French Arthurian tradition. One of the earliest prose romances in English (at least a decade before Malory), the *Prose Merlin* survives in its fullest form in a single mid-fifteenth-century manuscript, Cambridge, University Library, MS Ff. 3. 11, and is dated roughly contemporary with this.[1] It is for the most part a very close translation of a much earlier French text: the Merlin section of the Old French Vulgate Cycle (also known as the *Lancelot-Grail*), an interconnected body of Arthurian works composed in France in the early thirteenth century, which in turn takes its Merlinian material from the late twelfth-century Arthurian prose work of Robert de Boron. Robert's work is itself an extension of Chrétien de Troyes's unfinished *Perceval*, and a re-imagining of the treatment of Merlin in Geoffrey of Monmouth's *Historia regum Britanniae* (ca. 1138). In some respects, the nature of the demonological interests of the *Prose Merlin* presents a point of disjunction with its fifteenth-century dating. In its engagement with demonic pro-generation, it preserves the interests of its twelfth-century sources, which predate Thomas Aquinas's influential theorisations on the incubus, as well as the early works of witch-theory which positioned sex as a component of the demonic compact.[2] Rather, it stands in the debt of

1 This version of the text is missing three folios from the final quire. There is a second, even less full, copy of the romance: a single leaf bound into the miscellany Oxford, Bodleian Library, MS Rawlinson D. 913. For a codicological discussion of the *Prose Merlin* see Meale, "Manuscripts and Early Audience." Meale suggests that the two manuscripts are related, but neither is directly derived from the other. The Cambridge manuscript contains extensive glosses and annotations and appears to have been enthusiastically read in the sixteenth century by a circle of aristocratic readers, who Meale identifies as belonging to either the Guildford or the Haute family, associated with the Tudor court.

2 Elliott, *Fallen Bodies*, 52–60, 127–56; Cohn, *Europe's Inner Demons*, 34. See further, Bernau, "Bodies and the Supernatural," 99–120. We might note that demonic copulation did not appear to any significant degree in English witch trials until the seventeenth century, see Stephens, *Demon Lovers*, 102.

Victoria Flood is an Associate Professor in Medieval Literature at the University of Birmingham. Her publications include *Prophecy, Politics, and Place in Medieval England* (2016), and *Fantastic Histories: Medieval Fairy Narratives and the Limits of Wonder* (2023).

the demonological theorisations of an earlier time. Its understanding of the incubus, inherited from its earlier source texts, is first and foremost indebted to a line of thought rooted in the deliberations of Augustine of Hippo. Nonetheless, like the works of witch-theorists, the *Prose Merlin* (as was its sources, and indeed Augustine) is engaged with the matter of the incubus in history, beginning with the demon's material trace through his progeny.

While the supernatural interests of the *Prose Merlin* owe more to the twelfth century than the fifteenth, this does not mean that it cannot tell us anything about fifteenth-century understandings of the marvellous and the demonic. I understand the wonder we encounter in this text, on both an aesthetic and affective level, to be aligned with what Caroline Walker Bynum has understood to constitute medieval "literature of entertainment," intended not to shock (the primary characteristic often associated with the early modern marvel) but to intellectually animate, inviting its reader to distinguish knowingly between the credible and the incredible object, person, or event, characterized in predominately secular terms.[3] Yet the *Prose Merlin* also presents an engagement with wonder at the divine workings of history, and its primary intertexts include biblical apocrypha. This chapter asks what the wonder discourse at work in the *Prose Merlin* might reveal about wider cultural conceptualisations of demonic fiction and/or credulity in relation to this loosely historical frame of reference.[4] I follow the cue of earlier scholarship in approaching the Middle English text as "a distinct linguistic version of the [*Merlin*] narrative,"[5] although it is one that must necessarily be located within a multilingual and transhistorical context of cultural production.

The *Prose Merlin* is generally termed a romance, although the classifications romance and history do not always find a neat application to medieval literature, and its source traditions are multi-generic. French Arthurian romances, such as the Vulgate *Merlin*, can be best understood as combining aspects of romance and history, drawing variously on the discursive cues of each. Although English authors were divided as to the historicity of Merlin, in France this part of the Arthurian legend appears to have been received as less complicatedly historical, a broad acceptance carried over to the *Prose Merlin*.[6] Indeed, for the greater part of the Middle Ages, Merlin acted as a signifier not of

---

3 Walker Bynum, *Metamorphosis and Identity*, 40. For other influential discussions on wonder in late medieval literature, see Poirion, *Le merveilleux*; Le Goff, *The Medieval Imagination*, 27–30; Knapp and Knapp, *Medieval Romance*; Lockhart, "'Something Remains'," 45–64; McDonald, "Wonder of Middle English Romance," 13–34; Karnes, "Wonder, Marvels, and Metaphor in the Squire's Tale,"; and Karnes, "Marvels in the Medieval Imagination." This enquiry is extended in Karnes's recent monograph, *Medieval Marvels and Fictions in the Latin and Islamic World* (Chicago: University of Chicago Press, 2022), which was unfortunately not available to me during the period of writing this chapter (completed in late 2022).

4 We might note the absence of any obvious Aristotelian influence in the negotiation of wonder in the *Prose Merlin*, an influence felt deeply from the thirteenth century onwards–a consequence of the early date of its source texts. See further, Daston and Park, *Wonders and the Order of Nature*, 111–20.

5 Stern, "Middle English *Prose Merlin*," 115.

6 For an overview of the mixed Insular reception of the legend of Merlin, as we first find it in the

fiction but of history, for Merlin's magic is first and foremost prophetic revelation.[7] Yet the credibility of medieval prophecy was largely contingent on whether its origins might be said to be divine (truth) or demonic (lies), and Merlin's position was in this respect fraught. We find this from William of Newburgh's rejection of the demonic prophecies of the incubus-sired Merlin in the twelfth century, to the moral panic that saw the denunciation of Merlinian prophecy at the Council of Trent over three hundred years later.[8] Nonetheless, in the Arthurian tradition, even and especially in its historical interests, the credibility of Merlinian prophecy is assured, not in spite of but because of the prophet's demonic parentage. How did this come to be?

The synonymity of the demonic and the false is a consistent and widely diffused medieval position, although in relation to the reading of history it finds one of its most influential medieval articulations in Augustine of Hippo's discussion of wonder in *De Civitate Dei*, Book 21. Augustine draws a distinction between credibly marvellous historical events which might rightly inspire wonder, and demonic delusions or fictions which are sites of false wonder. He discusses the lamps in the shrine of Venus which appear to burn on their own accord, concluding that such a wonder is surely false, the illusion of a demon (a pagan god) if not a manmade experiment with asbestos. In contrast, the ever-burning fires of purgatory (of which Augustine offers an early formulation) present a true source of wonder, affirmed by comparisons to the many worldly marvels of perpetual fire truly attested by the author himself or reliable witnesses, from Mount Etna to the salamander—all testament to the vastness of God's creation.[9] Yet not all apparently demonic occurrences were necessarily illusory. Augustine understood demons to be capable, acting under God, of manipulating natural forces and processes (we might think most famously of his account of the transformation of the rods of Pharoah's magicians in Exodus 7, an acceleration of a natural process of decay),[10] while other demonic phenomena were positioned uncertainly between illusion and material manipulation. In the latter category we find, most notably, the possibility of demonic pro-generation.

Demonic sexuality appears as at once pressing and uncertain in Augustine's writings. While, in a break with patristic commonplace, in *De Civitate Dei* Augustine argues against the angelic identification of the "filii dei" who procreated with the daughters of men in Genesis 6, he suggests that there may be a precedent for the sexual engagements of those angels who fell with Satan, i.e., demons. This is a matter not of biblical evidence but rather popular testimony which functions analogously to it. Augustine writes of the

---

twelfth-century *Historia Regum Britanniae* by Geoffrey of Monmouth see Putter, "Latin Historiography After Geoffrey of Monmouth." For the French reception of Arthurian history see Trachsler, "Question of Time," 23–25.

7 Kieckhefer, *Magic in the Middle Ages*, 111–12. For an important discussion of the relationship of Merlinian romance to the (historical) "unfolding of Christian destiny," facilitated in large part by Merlin's demonic correspondences, see Saunders, *Magic and the Supernatural*, 225–28.

8 Sullivan, "On Recognizing the Limits of Our Understanding," 167–70.

9 Augustine, *City of God*, bk. 21, chap. 6, trans. Green, 7:34–35.

10 For discussion of the false wonders of Pharaoh's magicians, a favourite subject of Augustine across his works, see Wiebe, *Fallen Angels in the Theology of St Augustine*, 136–37.

sexual behaviours of "Silvanos et Panes, quos vulgo incubos vocant" (fauns and pans, commonly called incubi), who have sex with young women; and includes, as an example of the same phenomenon, the Gaulish Dusii, an occurrence so well attested that it cannot be denied. Thus, Augustine concludes, he cannot make any final deliberation regarding the materiality of demonic sexual activity. Indeed, he can only understand its possibility via analogy: he hypothesizes that the spirit's body might act upon the human's like air from a fan.[11] This very brief account is generally considered the "clerical origin statement" of the incubus.[12] Augustine, and the wider medieval tradition which followed from this passage (which was reworked in Isidore of Seville's *Etymologies*),[13] denies the demon's divinity, although demonic sex is theoretically plausible enough.[14] Augustine's uncertainty in this passage created a wider space of discursive indeterminacy with historical implications, regarding demonic conception either as a genealogical event or a demonic trick. Into the later Middle Ages, the genealogical demon appears in historical accounts of the demonic ancestors of the Huns and the Plantagenet kings of England; narratives which were by turns calumnious and invoked as a mark of exceptionality.[15] The ancestral demon became, for some medieval authors writing after Augustine, a historical signifier.

This presents an important context for the treatment of the incubus in the early Arthurian tradition which forms the basis of the *Prose Merlin*. Augustine's deliberations are overtly recalled in the earliest account of the conception of Merlin in Geoffrey of Monmouth's *Historia*. We read of the dilemma of the British king Vortigern, whose building project in Snowdonia is frustrated by unstable foundations revealed—in the full narrative (a component of the episode termed the "Omen of the Dragons" lifted from earlier Welsh prophetic traditions)—to be two dragons, a red and a white, representative of the standards of the Britons and the Saxons, who vie for control of Britain.[16] Vortigern follows the guidance of his *magi*, apparently pagan advisors, who suggest that the foundations might be stabilized with the blood of a boy with no father. Such a child is found in Carmarthen: Merlin, who is understood to be the son of an incubus and a cloistered princess. One *magus*, Maugantius, speculates that Merlin was fathered by one of those sublunary spirits who the second-century author Apuleius terms *daemons*, of whom he has read "in libris philosophorum nostrorum *et in plurimus historiis*" (in the books

11 Augustine, *City of God*, bk. 15, chap. 23, trans. Levine, 4:548–51.

12 Cf. Kiessling, *Incubus in English Literature*.

13 Isidore of Seville, *Etymologies*, trans. Barney et al., 190.

14 Augustine's rejection of the divinity of incubi is found in Augustine, *City of God*, bk. 9, chap. 3, trans. Wiesen, 3:152–55.

15 For discussion of the uses of incubi in medieval historical and pseudo-historical foundation narratives, see Geary, *Women at the Beginning*, 22–27; Elliott, *Fallen Bodies*, 58.

16 For a useful discussion of the *Omen* and Welsh traditions of the prophet Myrddin/Merlin, see Jarman, "Merlin Legend"; Padel, "Geoffrey of Monmouth."

of our philosophers and in very many histories; my italics).[17] Here the incubus enters Arthurian history.

We might ask whether Geoffrey intended us to think of Maugantius as erroneous in his understanding of the prophet's parentage, not least as the *magi* appear to be wrong about much else. The clue to how we might, as a medieval reader, interpret this detail is in the allusion to Apuleius, who finds a particular treatment in Augustine's account of demons in Book 8 of *De Civitate Dei*, Geoffrey's most obvious source for this passage. Augustine writes of the sublunary *daemons* of Apuleius, who the earlier author mistakenly thought might be entreated as a source of human wisdom.[18] A pagan misinterpretation, from the Augustinian perspective Apuleius's work might not be properly called *historia,* as the *magus* terms it. Vortigern's magicians are charged with misrecognition of history, potentially even of a misplaced understanding of the divinity of demons, yet this does not negate the possibility of the prophet's true demonic parentage — for this is a possibility that Augustine does not foreclose in his account of the Gaulish demons. Therefore, we need not assume that the post-Galfridian authors who followed this demonic cue were themselves bad readers of Geoffrey. Rather, like Geoffrey they appear to have been engaged with the historical truth status of marvellous events as a central textual concern, or indeed an intellectual exercise.

* * *

I turn now to the details of the English text itself. The *Prose Merlin* begins (as does its French source) with a council in hell. Following Christ's leading of the righteous pagans out of hell (the events of the apocryphal Gospel of Nicodemus, set in the time between Christ's crucifixion and his resurrection), demons conspire to bring about the birth of Antichrist through the intervention of an incubus. This is understood (as we might expect) as an overt parody of the conception, birth, and life of Christ, and provides a narrative space in which the demons demonstrate—much like the *magi* of Geoffrey's Vortigern—not only improper or false belief, but a failure to comprehend the parameters of history.

The hell-episode not only provides a potted account of apocryphal biblical history; the opening of the chapter is concerned with matters of marvel and belief:

> and whan the fendes sien that, they hadden right grete feer and *gret merveile*; thei assembleden to-gedir, and seiden, "What is he this thus vs supprisith and distroyeth, in so moche that our strengthes ne nought ellis that we haue may nought with-holde hym, nor again hym stonde in no diffence; but that he doth all that hym lyketh, *we ne trowe not* that eny man myght be born of woman, but that he sholde ben oures, and he that thus vs distroyeth, how is he bom in whom we [did] knowe non erthely delyte." (my italics)[19]

---

17 Geoffrey of Monmouth, *History of the Kings of Britain*, bk. 6, chap. 18.

18 Augustine, *City of God*, bk. 8, chap. 14, trans. Wiesen, 3:62–69. The nature of daemons, contra Apuleius, is the subject of Augustine's enquiry across Books 8 and 9 more broadly.

19 *Merlin*, chap. 1, ed. Wheatley, 1:1.

The demons pause on the complex matter of the Incarnation: how might a man be born who is not in the devil's thrall (i.e. without Original Sin)? This would appear to be a variation on the confusion surrounding a virgin birth, which was a familiar topos in representations of pagan credulity and prophetic misperceptions in the later Middle Ages. It is associated with "deceptive prophecy," such as late medieval accounts of Apollo's prophecy to the Romans that the temple of Peace would stand until a virgin gave birth—an event deemed so unlikely that the pagans assumed their temple would last forever and were horrified when it fell at the time of Christ's birth.[20] We might approach this motif as it appears in the *Prose Merlin* in relation to the status of the "merveille" of Middle English romance, as Nicola McDonald has understood it, where the marvel functions as a type of metaphor or riddle, posing "unanswered questions."[21] The demons' disbelief effectively invites considered belief on the part of the reader, an opportunity to pause and marvel at the wonderful nature of the Incarnation as a suspension of the ordinary rules of nature; an event which raises a question which—in terms of its basic mechanics—fundamentally cannot be answered, although it must be believed. We might think here of Steven Justice's formulation of the writing of medieval miracles as a kind of sacred thought experiment, which here we might apply both to the miraculous nature of Christ and the Merlinian marvel presented as its analogue: "shifting, partial, and unregularizable in its cognitive components; reliant on hypothesis and metaphor; sustained by imaginative habits and improvisations, bracing itself against the mind's revanche but also provoking it."[22]

The demons' confusion is in part an act of prophetic misunderstanding. The mystery of the Incarnation has brought to fruition the words of the prophets of the Old Testament, which, we read, the demons had understood to be false. In turn, they devise the conception of Merlin, a man with all the knowledge of demons who can work (false, demonic) marvels. Merlin is intended to "beguile" the men of his own time, just as the devils understand themselves to have been "beguiled" by the Old Testament prophets who forecast apparent impossibilities: "for witeth it wele that soche on myght moche helpe us to be-gile his pepill, like as the prophetes be-giled us, and tolden that we trowe neuer myght haue ben."[23] The terminology used here, "beguile," is a straightforward translation of the French "engignier" (to deceive), and is (similarly) a term often associated with demonic delusion or sleight of hand—we find it, for example, in relation to Satanic temptation in Chaucer's "Man of Law's Tale," and the temptation of Adam in the *York Mystery Plays*.[24] Merlin is not only a double to the

---

20 For a succinct discussion of this prophecy as it appears in the Golden Legend, see Minnis, *Chaucer and Pagan Antiquity*, 49. The term "deceptive prophecy" is Minnis's.

21 McDonald, "Wonder of Middle English Romance," 19. For further discussion on the marvels of Middle English romance, see Karnes, "Wonder, Marvels, and Metaphor in the Squire's Tale," 461.

22 Justice, "Did the Middle Ages Believe in their Miracles?," 13.

23 *Merlin*, chap. 1, ed. Wheatley, 1:2. For a critique of the edition, see Stern, "Middle English *Prose Merlin*," 112–22. It remains, however, the only scholarly edition to date of the text in full.

24 *Vulgate Version of the Arthurian Romances*, ed. Sommer, 2:4. "Beguile," Definition 3a, *Middle*

beguiling prophets of the Old Testament, but Christ (as we would expect of Antichrist, pseudo or otherwise), whose behaviour is characterized as "beguilement" elsewhere in Middle English literature, although his target is the devil. As Lea T. Olsan notes, we read in the *Piers Plowman* C-text that Christ will "bigile the gilour," an application of the principle of the *pharmakon*, "poisonous death poisons itself."[25] This is precisely the kind of ontological, and rhetorical, trick in which the demons of the *Prose Merlin* are ensnared—for Merlin does not direct his wonderful gifts where they expect. The term recurs later in chapter 1, where Merlin's scribe Blaise, fearing that the prophet is indeed Antichrist, agrees to write his book, but only after removing any devilish beguilement, in the name of the trinity:

> "The boke I will gladly make; but I coniure the in the name of the fader, sone, and holy goste that thow have no power me to begyle, ne to make me do soche thynge that god sholde with be displesed." "Alle these thynges," quod Merlyn, "ne mowe the hynder in body, ne in sowle, for never shall I make the do thynge that shalbe ageyn the volente of oure lord Ihesu Cryste."[26]

As in the original French ("engignier"), Blaise echoes, and re-situates, the language employed by the devils of hell—Merlin must not "beguile," and so his narrative, and the wonders contained in the book must be true. Merlin concurs in the name of religious truth, a conscious rejection of the bad belief of the demons, and a defence of the text's wider truth-claim.[27] This serves to legitimate the later events of the narrative, including the Grail legend, and indeed, both Merlin and the Grail have been understood to function as mirrored points of connection between the sacred and the secular.[28]

The historicity or reality of the marvel, in its Augustinian dimensions, is, as we have seen, defined by misrecognitions which might operate on the level of a religious belief that is also historical. The relationship between the demonic or pagan (as we see in Augustine's account of the shrine of Venus, demons were often synonymous with classical gods) and false, or misconstrued, prophecy has a long history.[29] We might note, for example, the concern with the source of prophetic visions, as divine or demonic, that appears in the early writings of the Church Fathers (Augustine included), an interest in spiritual discernment that coloured the broader reception of popular prophets, and the origins of their visions, into the later Middle Ages and beyond.[30] The *Prose Merlin* is closely contemporary with fifteenth-century debates surrounding the visions of Jeanne

---

English Dictionary, s.n. bigīlen at https://quod.lib.umich.edu/m/middle-english-dictionary/dictionary/MED4461/track?counter=1&search_id=17597484; accessed May 10, 2024.

25 Olsan, "Enchantment in Medieval Literature," 183.

26 *Merlin*, chap. 1, ed. Wheatley, 1:22.

27 For discussion of the status of the written word in the *Prose Merlin*, see Cawsey, "Merlin's Magical Writing."

28 Campbell, *Medieval Merlin Tradition*, 30.

29 Kieckhefer, *Magic in the Middle Ages*, 35–36.

30 Kruger, *Dreaming in the Middle Ages*, 50–52.

d'Arc, a paradigmatic example of the vexatious late-medieval question of what was termed the "discernment of spirits."[31] I do not mean to imply a direct correlation here, rather we see the continued topicality of this interest in the time of the *Prose Merlin* as in the earlier period of its sources. While a demonic prophecy may be pure fiction it may also, intended to mislead, prove to be unexpectedly true. This slipperiness is a feature of the presentation of the devils of the *Prose Merlin*. The demons fall afoul not only of Old Testament prophecy but of their *own* prophecy, for Merlin comes to serve God rather than the devil. We read of the demons, "Ffull grete foles were thei whan they wende that oure lorde sholde haue no knowynge of their ordenaunce"; which is to say, as in the Augustinian model, they act with God's permission, facilitating, unknowingly, part of a divine plan.[32] Thus, Merlin's prophetic knowledge, although demonically acquired, acts as divine illumination.

Merlin is consistently authorized by his demonic associations, the malevolent effects of which are forestalled by his baptism. The association of Merlin with Antichrist has a double effect: it explains both Merlin's magic gifts, and his association with prophecy—Antichrist conventionally plays the role of a false prophet and a false wonder worker.[33] Yet Merlin operates beyond the devils' scheme: he is an author of true marvels which refute the demons' best-laid plans for their pseudo-wonder worker. There is a historical rationale to Merlin's refutation of the role of Antichrist: the late-medieval reader knows that the world did not end in the fifth century, and the Last Times are still to come. The demons are therefore engaged in yet another type of historical and prophetic misrecognition: they miscalculate the coming of the End Times. Following Matthew 24:36 "de die autem illa et hora nemo scit neque angeli caelorum nisi Pater solus" (But of that day and hour no one knows: no, not the angels of heaven, but the Father alone), medieval theologians advised against predictions of the arrival of Antichrist. Augustine writes against those who believe that the End Times, contrary to the gospels, have been calculated with some precision, and located in their own historical moment. He alludes to a false prophecy that Christ's disciple Peter, contrived by "maleficia" (sorcery) that Christ's rule would end after three hundred and sixty-five years; a familiar misreading of religious wonder as malevolent magic.[34] This is a heretical misunderstanding, but it is also a misunderstanding of history, which is conceptualized in terms of distinctions between true and false wonder claims.

The *Prose Merlin*'s concern with historical misrecognition must be understood, as Julie Orlemanski has noted in her treatment of medieval fictionality, in relation to "a long tradition in the West of both distinguishing and deriving fictionality from categories of bad belief. As early as the Pre-Socratics, poetic narratives of the gods were the occasion for splitting audiences between the gullible and the sophisticated, which is to say,

---

31 Cf. Elliott, "Seeing Double"; Caciola, *Discerning Spirits*.

32 *Merlin*, chap. 1, ed. Wheatley, 1:3.

33 Cartlidge, "Sons of Devils," 226.

34 Augustine, *City of God*, bk. 18, chap. 53, trans. Greene, 6:80–81.

between those who didn't understand fiction properly and those who did."[35] Orlemanski here refers, among others, to Plato's concerns about the dangers of poets, who fill the gullible with false wonder at artifice and fiction. Augustine's concern surrounding the pseudo-marvels of the shrine of Venus, and indeed, his own suspicions regarding pagan poetry elsewhere in his writings, are born from this tradition—the attentions of audiences to such spectacles are misdirected, and they misunderstand the nature of creation itself. This charge was levelled at groups of "bad" historical readers during the Middle Ages; not least Jews, whose greatest "error" was recognized as a profound misunderstanding, or overly literalized comprehension, of the humanity of Christ (enacted most famously in the "blood libel" charge, and the fabricated Jewish torture of the eucharistic wafer).[36] There may well be a subtextual engagement with the precedent of Jewish misbelief in the *Prose Merlin*, given the demons' interest in the Old Testament prophets, even as they resist the complex reality of the New Testament history there foretold.[37] The sophisticated reader knows fact from fiction, while the unsophisticated reader is incapable of any such distinction—like the Merlinian demons, who are a literalisation of "bad belief".

The treatment of true and false wonder that begins the *Prose Merlin* (as it does Robert de Boron's text) speaks to a particular process of historical reading and misreading. The sophisticated medieval reader can distinguish between fact and fiction, appreciating fundamental truths of Christian history, and its implications for the Christian present and future. The primary historical question here is perhaps, then, not whether a reader is to believe in the reality of Merlin and his father but the sacred history which these events serve to explicate—i.e. a type of reader is anticipated who can separate the history from the romance. Yet Merlin's extra-textual claims are never in question, not least when it comes to the truth of his own prophecies. The text's most direct treatment of Merlinian prophetic material derived from Geoffrey's *Historia* concerns the prophet's interpretation of a singular historical marvel, the "Omen of the Dragons." There is no doubt as to its validity, which, like the account of Merlin's demonic origins, transcends its Arthurian intertext to encompass a wider comprehension of history and apocalypse. The second chapter of the *Prose Merlin* tells of the British king, Vortiger (Geoffrey's Vortigern), who comes to power through the assassination of the previous king, and a pact with Danish invaders. Fearing the anger of the Britons, Vortiger begins building a mountain stronghold in the west of Britain, but—a "merveille"—when his tower reaches a certain height, it falls. The tower's instability cannot be explained by Vortiger's seven wise men, but they tell him that the blood of a boy without a father will strengthen the foundations of the tower, that is: Merlin. Unlike the Galfridian version of the episode, the *magi* (here clerks) make no reference to Apuleuis's *daemons*—presumably because

35 Orlemanski, "Who Has Fiction?," 153.

36 For an important recent publication on medieval Christian perceptions of Jewish misbelief as incomprehension, see Barbezat, "Corporeal Orientation."

37 Antisemitism occupies a familiar place in medieval Antichrist legends: Antichrist was often understood to be born to Jewish parents. Emmerson, *Antichrist in the Middle Ages*, 79–83.

Merlin's history is far less ambiguous in this text than it is in Geoffrey's. Rather, these clerks call for the sacrifice of a fatherless child entirely in order to subvert a prophecy of their own deaths at the hands of such a child as foretold by their "sorte [divination]."[38] Like the demons, the clerks misunderstand or misrecognise prophecy, and here effectively realize the prophecy of their own deaths—although in the final event, Merlin has mercy and the prophecy is proved to be doubly false. A mode of prophecy is here implied that, unlike Merlin's, has no relationship to divine illumination. The Middle English "sort" (lot casting; divination) is a very close translation of the French cognate "sorti' (derived from the Latin *sors, sortis*).[39] It is a term applied to pagan divination and occurs most commonly in Middle English in narratives of the fall of Troy.[40] It rarely bodes well for the diviner in question.

The clerks' imperfect understanding gives way in the text to true prophecy, encoded in terms compatible with biblical revelation. As Jessica J. Lockhart has argued, at the very foundation of the Arthurian tradition (the "Omen" included) are "enigmatic marvels—that is, mysterious and wondrous phenomena that cue in-text and readerly interpretive efforts, much like those required to solve a riddle."[41] While Geoffrey's Merlin interprets the "Omen" as a contestation between the red dragon of the Britons and the white dragon of the Saxons, this Merlin (as in the French) presents a different solution, conflating the "Omen" with a prophecy of the return of Constantine's children which appears separately in *Historia* 8. The red dragon signifies Vortiger, and the white the sons of Constantine who Vortiger has usurped. The white will burn the red ("brenne the with theire power"), and so Vortigern will lose the tower—that is, the kingdom—that was never really his. Beyond its incorporation of content from elsewhere in the *Historia*, this prophecy is a reformulation of the "Omen" in line with the familiar tokens of Apocalypse 12, itself—in the terms of the Latin Vulgate—a "signum," which invites discerning interpretation. Here we encounter the exiled child and the defeat of the satanic red dragon, a series of marvellous signs of a type with Geoffrey's prophecy.[42] This correspondence is by no means a silent or incidental feature of the medieval text. Tellingly, Merlin introduces his account of the marvellous tower: "It was the tokenynge of thinges that were don and also of thinges that were to come." This admonition might be read in the broadest possible sense: of things to come in the Arthurian world of the text, and the tokens which speak to the universal history beyond it. The Merlinian marvel is here history's end.

---

38 *Merlin*, chap. 2, ed. Wheatley, 1:36–41.

39 *Vulgate Version of the Arthurian Romances*, ed. Sommer, 2:31. The French term most immediately refers to lot casting, although in later centuries it also appears to have been applied to sorcery, which is not necessarily prophetic. Veenstra, *Magic and Divination*, 14.

40 "Sort," Definition 2a, *Middle English Dictionary*, s.n. sŏrt at https://quod.lib.umich.edu/m/middle-english-dictionary/dictionary/MED41662/track?counter=10&search_id=17597484; accessed May 10, 2024.

41 Lockhart, "'Something Remains'," 46.

42 For divergent interpretations of this passage in the fifteenth and sixteenth centuries, see Reeves, *Influence of Prophecy*, 491.

Conclusion

The *Prose Merlin* is a case study in the longevity of demonological thought, and its engagements with the true and false marvel, from Augustine to the fifteenth century. It belongs to a textual tradition which drew its inspiration from Augustinian writings on wonder, historical truth, and demonic deception, but was largely unresponsive to late medieval developments concerned with the same—as is often the case in texts which reproduce received narratives rather than theological debate. It is, however, engaged in a topic which was of particular interest into the later Middle Ages: the discernment with which one might approach prophecy as a site of true and false wonders.

The Merlin tradition had a continued topicality. Neil Cartlidge has observed that the figure of Merlin derived from Robert de Boron appears to have informed later representations of Antichrist, presenting a genuinely reflexive relationship between Arthurian imaginings and apocalyptic eschatology.[43] Further, as Laura Chuhan Campbell has noted in her study of the Italian Merlin traditions, versions of the romance of the prophet's early life were found in manuscripts alongside explicitly apocalyptic prophecy depicting the arrival of Antichrist.[44] In many respects, this was facilitated by the always-already historical interests of the Merlin tradition not simply within but beyond its shadow Antichrist narrative, including its Augustinian navigation of the reading of demonic wonders as a fundamentally historical concern. This is an interest which, I suggest, directly informed the discursive positioning of the text in its fifteenth-century English translation, which—like its source traditions—is explicitly concerned with the historicity of wonder.

43 Cartlidge, "Sons of Devils," 227.

44 Campbell, *The Medieval Merlin Tradition*, 10.

Bibliography

Primary Sources

Augustine. *City of God*. Vol. 3. Translated by David S. Wiesen. Loeb Classical Library 413. Cambridge, MA: Harvard University Press, 1968.

——. *City of God*. Vol. 4. Translated by Philip Levine. Loeb Classical Library 414. Cambridge, MA: Harvard University Press, 1966.

——. *City of God*. Vol. 6. Translated by William Chase Greene. Loeb Classical Library 416. Cambridge, MA: Harvard University Press, 1960.

——. *City of God*. Vol. 7. Translated by William M. Green. Loeb Classical Library 417. Cambridge, MA: Harvard University Press, 1972.

Geoffrey of Monmouth. *History of the Kings of Britain: An Edition and Translation of the De gestis Britonum (Historia Regum Britanniae)*. Edited by Michael D. Reeve and translated by Neil Wright. Woodbridge: Boydell, 2005.

Isidore of Seville. *The Etymologies of Isidore of Seville*. Edited and translated by Stephen A. Barney, W. J. Lewis, J. A. Beach, and Oliver Berghof. Cambridge: Cambridge University Press, 2006.

Merlin or the Early History of King Arthur. Edited by Henry Benjamin Wheatley. 4 vols. Early English Text Society, o.s., 10, 21, 36, 102. London: Kegan Paul, Trench, Trübner, 1865, 1866, 1869, 1899.

The Vulgate Version of the Arthurian Romances. Edited by H. Oskar Sommer. 8 vols. Washington, DC: Carnegie Institute, 1908–16.

William of Newburgh. *The History of English Affairs: Book 1*. Edited and translated by P. G. Walsh and M. J. Kennedy. Oxford: Aries and Philips, 1988.

Secondary Sources

Barbezat, Michael D. "The Corporeal Orientation: Understanding Deviance Through the Object(s) of Love." In *The Routledge History of Emotions in Europe, 1100–1700*. Edited by Andrew Lynch and Susan Broomhall, 119–32. London: Routledge, 2020.

Bartlett, Robert. *The Natural and the Supernatural in the Middle Ages*. Oxford: Oxford University Press, 2008.

Bernau, Anke. "Bodies and the Supernatural: Humans, Demons, and Angels." In *A Cultural History of the Human Body in the Medieval Age*. Edited by Linda Kalof, 99–120. Oxford: Berg, 2010.

Caciola, Nancy. *Discerning Spirits: Divine and Demonic Possession in the Middle Ages*. Ithaca: Cornell University Press, 2006.

Campbell, Laura Chuhan. *The Medieval Merlin Tradition in France and Italy: Prophecy, Paradox, and "Translatio"*. Cambridge: Brewer, 2017.

Cartlidge, Neil. "Sons of Devils." In *Heroes and Anti-Heroes in Medieval Romance*. Edited by Neil Cartlidge, 219–36. Cambridge: Brewer, 2012.

Cawsey, Kathy. "Merlin's Magical Writing: Writing and the Written Word in *Le Morte Darthur* and the English Prose *Merlin*." *Arthuriana* 11, no. 3 (2001): 89–101.

Cohn, Norman. *Europe's Inner Demons: The Demonization of Christians in Medieval Christendom*. London: Pimlico, 1970. Reprint, 2005.

Daston, Lorraine and Katherine Park. *Wonders and the Order of Nature 1150–1750*. New York: Zone, 1998.

Elliott, Dyan. *Fallen Bodies: Pollution, Sexuality and Demonology in the Middle Ages.* Philadelphia: University of Pennsylvania Press, 1999.

——. "Seeing Double: John Gerson, the Discernment of Spirits, and Joan of Arc." *American Historical Review* 107, no. 1 (2002): 26–54.

Emmerson, Richard K. *Antichrist in the Middle Ages: A Study of Medieval Apocalypticism, Art, and Literature.* Seattle: University of Washington Press, 1981.

Geary, Patrick J. *Women at the Beginning: Origin Myths from the Amazons to the Virgin Mary.* Princeton: Princeton University Press, 2006.

Le Goff, Jacques. *The Medieval Imagination.* Translated by Arthur Goldhammer. Chicago: University of Chicago Press, 1992.

Jarman, A. O. H. "The Merlin Legend and the Welsh Tradition of Prophecy." In *The Arthur of the Welsh: The Arthurian Legend in Medieval Welsh Literature.* Edited by Rachel Bromwich, A. O. H. Jarman, and Brynley F. Roberts, 117–45. Cardiff: University of Wales Press, 1991.

Justice, Steven. "Did the Middle Ages Believe in their Miracles?" *Representations* 10, no. 1 (2008): 1–29.

Karnes, Michelle. "Marvels in the Medieval Imagination." *Speculum* 92, no. 2 (2015): 327–65.

——. "Wonder, Marvels, and Metaphor in the Squire's Tale." *English Literary History* 82, no. 2 (2015): 461–90.

Kieckhefer, Richard. *Magic in the Middle Ages.* Cambridge: Cambridge University Press, 2014.

Kiessling, Nicholas. *The Incubus in English Literature: Provenance and Progeny.* Pullman: Washington State University Press, 1977.

Knapp, James F., and Peggy A. Knapp. *Medieval Romance: The Aesthetics of Possibility.* Toronto: University of Toronto Press, 2017.

Kruger, Steven F. *Dreaming in the Middle Ages.* Cambridge: Cambridge University Press, 1992.

Lockhart, Jessica J. "'Something Remains Which Is Not Open to My Understanding:' Enigmatic Marvels in Welsh Otherworld Narratives and Latin Arthurian Romance." In *Cultural Translations in Medieval Romance.* Edited by Victoria Flood and Megan G. Leitch, 45–64. Cambridge: Brewer, 2022.

McDonald, Nicola. "The Wonder of Middle English Romance." In *Thinking Medieval Romance.* Edited by Katherine C. Little and Nicola McDonald, 13–34. Oxford: Oxford University Press, 2018.

Meale, Carol M. "The Manuscripts and Early Audience of the Middle English *Prose Merlin*." In *The Changing Face of Arthurian Romance: Essays on Arthurian Prose Romances in Memory of Cedric E. Pickford.* Edited by Alison Adams, Armel H. Diverres, Karen Stern, and Kenneth Varty, 92–11. Woodbridge: Boydell, 1986.

Minnis, Alastair J. *Chaucer and Pagan Antiquity.* Cambridge: Brewer, 1982.

Olsan, Lea. "Enchantment in Medieval Literature." In *The Unorthodox Imagination in Late Medieval Britain.* Edited by Sophie Page, 166–92. Manchester: Manchester University Press, 2010.

Orlemanski, Julie. "Who Has Fiction? Modernity, Fictionality, and the Middle Ages." *New Literary History* 50, no. 2 (2019): 145–70.

Padel, O. J. "Geoffrey of Monmouth and the Development of the Merlin Legend." *Cambrian Medieval Celtic Studies* 51 (2006): 37–65.

Poirion, Daniel. *Le merveilleux dans la littérature française du Moyen Age.* Paris: Presses Universitaires de France, 1982.

Putter, Ad. "Latin Historiography After Geoffrey of Monmouth." In *The Arthur of Medieval Latin Literature: The Development and Dissemination of the Arthurian Legend in Medieval Latin.* Edited by Siân Echard, 85–108. Cardiff: University of Wales Press, 2011.

Reeves, Marjorie. *The Influence of Prophecy in the Later Middle Ages*. Notre Dame: University of Notre Dame Press, 1993.

Saunders, Corinne. *Magic and the Supernatural in Medieval English Romance*. Cambridge: Brewer, 2010.

Stern, Karen. "The Middle English *Prose Merlin*." In *The Changing Face of Arthurian Romance: Essays on Arthurian Prose Romances in Memory of Cedric E. Pickford*. Edited by Alison Adams, Armel H. Diverres, Karen Stern, and Kenneth Varty, 112–22. Woodbridge: Boydell, 1986.

Stephens, Walter. *Demon Lovers: Witchcraft, Sex, and the Crisis of Belief*. Chicago: University of Chicago Press, 2003.

Sullivan, Karen. "On Recognizing the Limits of Our Understanding: Medieval Debates About Merlin and Marvels." In *Uncertain Knowledge: Scepticism, Relativism, and Doubt in the Middle Ages*. Edited by Dallas George Denery, Kantik Ghosh, and Nicolette Zeeman, 161–84. Turnhout: Brepols, 2014.

Trachsler, Richard. "A Question of Time: Romance and History." In *A Companion to the Lancelot-Grail Cycle*. Edited by Carol Dover, 23–32. Cambridge: Brewer, 2003.

Veysseyre, Géraldine. "Metre en roman: *Les prophéties de Merlin*: Voies et détours de l'interprétation dan trois traductions de l'*Historia Regum Britannie*." In *Moult obscures paroles: Études sur la prophétie médiévale*. Edited by Richard Trachsler, Julien Abed, and David Expert, 107–66. Paris: Presses de l'Universite de Paris–Sorbonne, 2007.

——, ed. *L'estoire de Brutus: La plus ancienne traduction en prose française de l'"Historia regum Britannie" de Geoffroy de Monmouth*. Paris: Garnier, 2015.

Veenstra, Jan R. *Magic and Divination at the Courts of Burgundy and France: Text and Context of Laurens Pignon's "Contre les devineurs" (1411)*. Leiden: Brill, 1997.

Walker Bynum, Caroline. *Metamorphosis and Identity*. New York: Zone, 2001.

——. "Wonder." *American Historical Review* 102, no. 1 (1997): 1–26.

Wiebe, Gregory D. *Fallen Angels in the Theology of St Augustine*. Oxford: Oxford University Press, 2021.

ALCHEMICAL POETRY, ALCHEMICAL PRACTICE

ZACHARY MATUS

> "Ah, nay, Let be, the Philosopher's Stone
> Called elixir, we seek it earnestly, each one of us;
> For if we had it, then we would be very well off.
> But unto God of heaven I make avow
> Despite all of our craft, when we have all done,
> And for all our skill, he will not come us to."[1]
>
> Chaucer, *The Canon's Yeoman's Tale*

THIS CHAPTER EXAMINES medieval alchemical thought through the lens of alchemical poetry. Medieval alchemical poems number far fewer than those of early modernity (the same could be said of prose treatises) and the aims of medieval poets differed from their early modern successors.[2] Medieval alchemical poems, however, tell us a great deal about how the West's first alchemical authors approached their art even if little about their content is surprising. They hew fairly closely to standard medieval alchemical ideas. Poetry's gift to the historian, however, is that these verses say rather a great deal about how their authors conceptualized their craft. Poetry answers the question of *how* alchemists thought alchemy more than *what* they thought alchemy was. Poetry, I argue, was superior to prose as a means of communicating the experiences of alchemists who practised an art that empirically could not achieve its loftiest aims.

Not all poems highlighted in this chapter were written by alchemists, but both the *The Romance of the Rose* and Chaucer's *The Canon's Yeoman's Tale* are highly informed

1 For references to Chaucer, I have elected to use Harvard's excellent Chaucer site, which is open access and based on the work of Larry Benson. The site includes original text and translation, though I will hew to translations only. Geoffrey Chaucer, *Canon's Yeoman's Tale* (*Canterbury Tales*, Fragment 8), lines 862–66, https://chaucer.fas.harvard.edu/pages/canons-yeomans-prologue-and-tale.

2 Kahn, "Alchemical Poetry...Part II–Synthesis," 63–69, 71.

Zachary Matus is an Associate Professor at Morrissey College of Arts and Sciences, Boston College, MA. His research interests include the intellectual and cultural history of Europe during the Middle Ages, with a focus on intersections between religious, magical, and scientific activities. His book, *Franciscans and the Elixir of Life: Religion and Science in the Later Middle Ages* (Philadelphia: University of Pennsylvania Press, 2017) examines how various members of the Franciscan Order justified alchemical practice as a quintessentially Christian endeavour, in spite of increasing ecclesiastical suspicion that alchemy was either fraudulent or demonically inspired.

about alchemical theory and practice as well as highly influential. Other poems come from working alchemists. Those of the English tradition—George Ripley, Thomas Norton, and John Lydgate—are fairly well known. Less famous in the Anglophone world is the German alchemist (whose verses are in Latin), Johannes Ticinensis. The medieval practice of alchemy was nestled in a complicated and often quite messy tangle of historiographical issues. It remains loosely analogous to modern chemistry and physics as a *scientia* of the physical composition of the world. At the same time, it diverged from many mainstream philosophical pursuits since many initiates viewed alchemical knowledge as secret. Secrecy was a function of alchemists themselves who wished to guard valuable knowledge by hiding processes and ingredients with code names. It was also a function of the art itself, which many, but not all, practitioners claimed was transmitted by God or other spiritual powers. And, while one would find geometry, optics or other physical sciences taught at a university, alchemy was not part of the curriculum. To its adherents, alchemy offered the power to turn other metals into gold or silver and even make remarkable medicines to prolong human life. To its detractors, it was mere chicanery and the refuge of forgers and confidence men. Though alchemists did manage to whiten metals, distill alcohol and develop complex apparatus for processing metals, salts, acids, and other caustics, we also know that they frequently failed to meet the grandest objectives of their art. Sometimes this was due to the empirical impossibility of transmutation, and sometimes it was the result of unstable substances, lack of skill, and imperfections in their equipment.

Any contemporary study of alchemical poetry owes a debt to Didier Kahn, whose two pioneering articles synthesizing alchemical poetry ("Alchemical Poetry in Medieval and Early Modern Europe: A Preliminary Survey and Synthesis, Parts I and II") remain required reading.[3] Kahn provides a broad outline of the major works, specific traditions within major linguistic groups (Latin and vernaculars), and development from medieval to the early modern. This chapter departs from Kahn, though, in some important ways. I explore new ideas about the "function" of medieval alchemical poetry, which Kahn identifies as "primarily to condense doctrinal points and thereby render them memorable [...]. The mnemonic function, widely represented in all languages (most of all in German), is often stated in the texts themselves [...]."[4] Kahn's argument about the stability of poetry is well taken and he provides a nuanced discussion of other probable motives including aesthetic preference and patronage. Aude Mairey, in a study of English poets Thomas Norton and George Ripley, has argued along similar lines, though she has also importantly highlighted that alchemists may have been attracted to poetry because both rely on metaphor.[5] I argue in what follows, however, that poetry was superior to prose

3 Kahn, "Alchemical Poetry...Part I–Preliminary Survey," 249–74; Kahn, "Alchemical Poetry...Part II–Synthesis," 62–77. It is worth noting here Anke Timmermann's fine study of a body of medieval English alchemical poetry, Timmermann, *Verse and Transmutation*, which largely agrees with Kahn on the didactic nature of alchemical poetry and the utility of poetry as mnemonic device.

4 Kahn, "Alchemical Poetry...Part II–Synthesis," 64.

5 Mairey, "Entre littérature, science et politique," 251.

as a means of communicating the kind of empirical difficulties and occasional triumphs faced by practicing alchemists. Poetry was a means of crafting rhetorical and intellectual strategies to cope with empirical failure and preserve scientific truth as they understood it. Further, poetry offered the possibility of performing alchemical knowledge on the page. Performing with an alembic was, after all, far more fraught with the possibility of failure.

I make no claim that what follows is in any way encyclopedic. This is not a review of *all* alchemical poetry. Nor is this a synthesis of alchemical poetry. The poets I have selected have different aims, and some of them are critical, or even outright hostile, towards the practice of alchemy. I am suggesting, however, there are particular ideas or consequences that can be communicated via poetry that fail to obtain if reduced to cold, unyielding prose. Poetry offered a way to communicate alchemical truths that may have been less easily conveyed through the kind of philosophical prose embraced by natural philosophers, not to mention the dialectic of the schools. Poetry, at least in its best renditions, allows the poet and the reader to imagine multiple meanings. It is the language of ambiguity and paradox. Ambiguity and paradox were, for most practitioners of the alchemical arts, inherent features of their craft, and while I chart some similarities and trends, I make no claim that every poem or every poet shared the same aims or ideas.

Two Kinds of Knowledge

Literary studies of alchemy have focused alchemical imagery and symbolism and the work they perform in texts, courts, and culture. And, while it is something of a truism, it bears repeating that genre affects the ideas presented.

> For instance, I could write thusly
> About alchemical science justly
> As a science, art and alleged hope
> Of friar, freeman, and even a pope.

I am tempted to continue writing this chapter in doggerel, convention aside, but my priorities as an author would have to change significantly in order to achieve this. Rather than trying to present complex ideas as clearly as possible, I would, at the very least, have to attend to rhythm, rhyme, and meter. Moreover, many stylistic sins best avoided by poets appear forgivable in academic writing. But medieval philosophers clearly understood that poetry and prose served different purposes.

Early in his *Commentary on the Sentences*, Thomas Aquinas takes up the question of poetry and its ability to convey truth. "Poetry is the science of those things which, because of their deficiency of truth, cannot be grasped by reason; whence it is necessary that reason be seduced, as it were, by certain metaphors [...]."[6] Paul Murray has argued

---

6 "poetica scientia est de his quae propter defectum Veritatis non possunt a ratione capi; unde oportet quod quasi quibusdam similitudinibus ratio seducatur." From Aquinas, *Scriptum super*

that what Aquinas means in this instance is that poetry "resists abstraction."[7] Poetry speaks in a way that evades the kind of dialectic or philosophical discourse favoured by medieval philosophers. Poetry is still entirely capable of producing truth, but cannot do so in the way that prose does. It must use allusion and metaphor rather than direct speech. Aquinas, of course, considers poetry a lesser mode of expression than the kind of logic of the schools where abstraction, deduction, and speculation reign.

All of that said, Aquinas cannot escape the fact that poetry also yields knowledge of the highest order, i.e., theological knowledge, where metaphors are also crucial—not least because so many spiritual truths are paradoxical that metaphor is one's only recourse.[8] Thus, even if it is largely inferior to logic, poetic thinking and expression are often the only way to discuss certain qualities that cannot be contained in prose. A later Dominican, Meister Eckhart states this more positively: "All the ancient theologians and poets generally used to teach about God, nature and ethics by means of parables. The poets did not speak in an empty and fabulous way, but they intentionally and very attractively and properly taught about the natures of things divine, natural and ethical by metaphors and allegories. This is quite clear to anyone who takes a good look at the poets' stories."[9]

While alchemy is not theology (well, not usually anyway), it does force its adherents to cope with paradox. Every scholar of alchemy is well acquainted with the existence of paradoxical statements that abound in the alchemical corpus, but let me focus briefly on a few of those made by the alchemical poet Johannes Ticinensis who makes many of the standard kinds of statements about the existence of the Philosopher's Stone. It is at once an indivisible (*inscindibilem*) substance, yet from it three substances can be exhumed (*fodiuntur*). It cannot be dissolved (*nulla pars dimittetur*), but can be moistened, rubbed smooth and otherwise manipulated.[10] Ticinensis revels in oppositions, tensions, and ambiguities. The existence of paradoxes also obtunds the use of the kind of deductive logic championed by Aquinas and other logicians. If multiple, conflicting premises are true and not true at the same time, then it is impossible to use reason to ferret out truths. Hence, Ticinensis tells his readers that "You who wish to seek and chase/ The precious art's founding base/ With intuition (*sensui*) you detect it."[11]

While Ticinensis's poem is, in fact, fairly descriptive, or at least would be for an initiate, it is clear that he does not believe he is just transmitting instructions in meter and verse, even if some of his later readers read him in just this way.[12] Ticinensis argues

---

Sententiis, lib. 1, q. 1, art. 5, ad. 3, https://aquinas.cc/la/en/~ST.I.Q1.A5.

7 Murray, "Aquinas on Poetry and Theology," 65.

8 Murray, "Aquinas on Poetry and Theology," 67–68.

9 Meister Eckhart, *Essential Sermons*, trans. Colledge and McGinn, 93. Quoted from Murray, "Aquinas on Poetry and Theology," 67.

10 Ticinensis, "Processus de lapide philosophorum," ed. Roth-Schultz, 610–12.

11 "Tu qui velis indagare/ Fundamentum artis carae/ Sensui edissere." From Ticinensis, "Processus de lapide philosophorum," ed. Roth-Schultz, 610.

12 For example, the sixteenth-century alchemist Lorenzo Ventura does not dwell on the distinction

that alchemy is a truth one apprehends by feel or by intuition. Hence poetry is a more suitable vehicle. What is more, Ticinensis likens the revelation of alchemical truth to religious truth. Alchemy is an extension of spiritual knowledge, and he thinks of his own poem as a kind of hymn. "I attempt to all make plain/ The hidden method to explain/ By means of scripture's melody."[13] This verse in particular points at Ticinensis's desire to deploy a multitude of meanings. The over reading is Ticinensis's claim that what follows is meant to echo a hymn. But there is more to it than that. This verse recalls earlier ones where he calls upon God and angels to aid him. In this line, he is calling not upon God, but upon a different kind of Christian power: Scripture. Scripture, i.e., God's word, is the ultimate expression of Truth. By singling out Scripture, he is likely also alluding to the Book of the World. This Book of the World was an idea common to theologians, natural philosophers and alchemists who believed that nature could be read as a kind of scripture, albeit not as clearly as the Word of God itself. The fact that he is dealing with Scripture's *melody*, however—asserts at the same time that there is something important about poetry and song itself. There is something beyond prose to which the alchemist must attend.

One must be careful not to take this too far, however. Alchemists more often wrote in prose than they did in verse, with the possible exception of late medieval English alchemists. (Poetry was the mode of all sorts of scientific writing in English.) And, for his part, Ticininesis did write prose works on alchemy.[14] It is important to keep in mind Aquinas's notion of poetry as revealing a kind of truth that cannot be abstracted, while philosophical prose allows for speculation and logical inference. Ticinensis does not claim that alchemy can *only* be understood through poetry—one can communicate ideas and instructions in prose as well. And, indeed, when he works in prose, he does so quite clearly. That said, the sum of Ticinensis's work suggests a tension between what can be expressed in prose and what can be expressed in poetry.

A further example of this tension between alchemical prose and poetry comes from a fourteenth-century manuscript, Oxford, Bodleian Library, MS Ashmole 1384, which binds together a number of alchemical treatises, but one of the most curious comes at the end of an alchemical text attributed to a certain "Sarne"—possibly William of Tunis. In any case, Sarne's *Lily* is a prose treatise on the Philosopher's Stone, but just after its explicit, one finds a set of sixteen verses (in the same hand) also on the Philosopher's Stone. While Sarne's treatise dwells on the relations of planets to metals and other scientific or philosophical aspects of alchemy, the verses that follow are highly evocative, calling the stone "a dragon of the deeps" and warning that it easily escapes the grasp of the alchemist "At its first opportunity it shall fly off, unless every crack in its den is

---

of poetry and prose. In arguing about the temperature of a flame, he quotes a dozen or more passages from prior alchemists, all of which are in prose save for a few verses from Ticinensis. Ventura, "Liber Lapidis Philosophici," 302.

13 "Totum conor propalare,/ Artis callem enodare/ Scripturae modulamine." From Ticinensis, "Processus de lapide philosophorum," ed. Roth-Schultz, 610.

14 Telle, "Johannes von Teschen," 774–76.

sealed off."[15] The metaphor in this case is quite clear—make sure your alembic and other alchemical vessels are sealed and without flaw, but the juxtaposition of this verse with the more staid treatise ahead of it is suggests a playfulness and an ambiguity inherent in alchemical practice. The poem reinforces the potentiality of failure while at the same time affirming the possibility of the alchemical science, but does so in a way that is evocative rather than proscriptive. By using poetry to talk around the subject of the foregoing treatise, the poem destabilizes the clarity of the earlier work. The poem is not simply cloaking a straightforward chemical reaction in mysterious or hyperbolic language. Rather, it is subtly insisting that alchemy is an art that relies on logic and empiricism, but also at times transcends or frustrates them.

The Poetry of Failure

Medieval alchemy's great critic, Chaucer, was well acquainted with the idea of alchemical failure. He is certainly familiar enough with alchemy to have sought out training in the art itself, though he seems ultimately, like the teller of *The Canon's Yeoman's Tale*, to have abandoned its practice.[16] The first part of *The Canon's Yeoman's Tale* is a comical screed against alchemy from a former practitioner who has lost wealth and status as a result of his misguided attempts to transmute base metals into gold. The array of alchemical terminology Chaucer employs is staggering, but so is the litany of failures. Alchemical vessels explode, investments are lost, and practitioners tumble into a state of obsession: "Yet of that art they can not be satisfied,/ For unto them it is a bitter sweet—/ So it seems—for had they nothing but a sheet/ Which they might wrap themselves in at night,/ And a rough cloak to walk in by daylight,/ They would sell them and spend it on this craft./ They can not stop until nothing is left."[17] Catastrophe or even disappointment are not consequences of a lack of expertise or knowledge, but rather the natural product of taking up an art which is doomed to failure. Failure also compounds itself since the art of alchemy itself is never to blame. It is the product of a cracked alembic, an impure ingredient, or a wayward alchemical text. It is not so much the strength of Chaucer's critique that interests me, but rather the fact that Chaucer seems to have set off a trend of poetic descriptions of alchemical failure among practicing alchemists.

In one sense, failure was part of the alchemical lexicon before Chaucer. Alchemists were known for denigrating the work of their fellows. And, by the fifteenth century, practicing alchemists had begun to critique and criticize what might be deemed the classic works of alchemy.[18] In his preface to his English translation of pseudo-Aristotle's *Secret of Secrets*, the monk and alchemist John Lydgate takes up this trope and adds his own twist, namely that failure is inevitable for those of a certain class: "There

15 "Evolat in primis, nisi clausis undique rimis [...]." MS Ashmole 1384, fol. 74v.

16 Gabrovsky, *Chaucer the Alchemist*, 22.

17 Chaucer, *Canon's Yeoman's Tale*, lines 877–83.

18 Bernard of Treves, *De Chymico*, 6.

is of ryght a greete difference,/ Tween a Princes royall Dignite,/ And twen Commons rude Intelligence [...]."[19] Lydgate goes on to explain that not only is failure inevitable for middling and lower social classes, but that said failure is just. The pursuit is to be limited to nobles as well as those "Clerkys whiche have Experience." Yet Lydgate also engages in the very complaint levelled against alchemy by Chaucer and other English alchemists. Far from making money, alchemy is the source of financial woe and ruin. It empties coffers and ravages the mind with equal fervor.[20] And yet, Lydgate writes regardless.

Lydgate's description of (pseudo-)Aristotle and *The Secret of Secrets* is a study in contrasts. He constantly sets up oppositions: smart and stupid, rich and poor, noble and common, truth and lie. Aristotle himself does not escape this treatment as he is described as feeble and impotent, yet also courageous and "trew in his entent."[21] The antitheses do not just echo the alchemical contradictions discussed in the previous section. They amplify and extend them. Failure and success are themselves a contradiction, entangled in this array of seemingly antithetical qualities. No aspect of alchemical work can escape this ambiguity. One cannot have the truth without the lie, the success without the failure. This is, to be sure, a rhetorical flourish. It is not only rhetoric, however. It expresses a fundamental problem. Alchemy is a true science, but it cannot be readily performed. Writing on Lydgate, Carolyn Collette argues, "The lost knowledge of the science is actually lost truth. The conceptual umbrage in which alchemists work signifies an impoverished world."[22] Lydgate is coping with the intangibility of an art that relies on the senses to both perform and confirm.

Similar themes emerge in the fourteenth-century *Confessio Amantis* of John Gower. Gower's short section on the Philosopher's Stone has a threefold structure. The first and longest part details the practice of alchemy, defining key terms and providing some rather vague instructions, which would be, quite typically for an alchemical text, no help at all to someone uninitiated to the art. Second follows a section that echoes Chaucer in that Gower complains that alchemy, rather than making one wealthy or hale, will in fact leave one penniless. Finally, however, in the third section we get something rather different. Gower says the following about alchemical treatises from the past: "There be many now today/That little know of what they mean/It is not one to know or think/ in the form of words they have inked/ But yet they fail to obtain."[23] Gower goes on then to suggest that the failure of alchemy is not due to a failure of the science, but rather in an imperfect understanding of it. Gower's perfect medicine is "grounded in nature," but mastery for latter day practitioners may be doomed to fail. Like Carolyn Collette, Clare

19 Lydgate, "Introduction to *Secreta Secretorum*," ed. Ashmole, 397.

20 Lydgate, "Introduction to *Secreta Secretorum*," ed. Ashmole, 401.

21 Lydgate, "Introduction to *Secreta Secretorum*," ed. Ashmole, 401

22 Collette, *Species, Phantasms, and Images*, 139.

23 "There ben full manie now a day,/That knowen litle that tei mene,/It is not one to wite and wene,/ In form of words thei it trete;/ But yet thei failen of beyet." Gower, "Concerning the Philosopher's Stone," 372–73.

Fletcher has argued, rightly, I think, that this owes to a general sense of *senectus mundi*.[24] Practices and truths once accessible are now closed.

For Gower, the poetics of alchemy again point to its fundamental ambiguity. His poetry is more than a mere mnemonic and indeed something more than an aesthetically pleasing means of conveying information about science. Gower lists a number of ancient authorities whom he regards as having unlocked alchemy's secrets—Hermes the Thrice Great, Geber or al-Jabir, Morienus, Avicenna, etc. With the exception of the emerald tablet ascribed to Hermes, all of these texts existed in Latin translation as standard prose treatises (the tablet circulated in many different translations and is so brief that it is in many ways analogous to poetry). Yet, Gower claims that it is impossible to understand the formal prose treatises of alchemy via "the forme of words they [...] trete." The certitude reflected in their prose does not hold up. Fletcher also focuses on Gower's view that the loss of alchemical knowledge is a problem with language itself. "Gower's contemporaries actively converse about the 'Philosopher's Stone' but none possess knowledge of the true nature or essence of the thing itself. The 'signifier,' therefore, and the 'signified' have become estranged and the relationship has thus been contaminated. They know the name but true cognizance of the object has perished with the decline of language and the world."[25] Whether the failure of contemporary language pushes Gower to a poetic rather than a prose response is difficult to say, since his critique centers on "words" in general, but his concern about the ability of language to convey alchemical thought suggests his choice of verse was intentional.

Not all poetic descriptions of failure suggest that alchemy is impossible. In fifteen stanzas, found at the end of his poem, the *Compound of Alchemy*, George Ripley elaborates at length on the trope of alchemical failure: a narration of the various missteps he has met in the course of his attempts to make the Philosopher's Stone. Yet, at the end of the poem Ripley reminds that he has, in one single case, succeeded. He has made the Philosopher's Stone. "I never saw true worke truly but onse/of which in this treatise the truth I have told."[26] If you are not failing, again and again and again, you must be doing something wrong. Failure is to be expected and success is ephemeral. Ripley too points to a problem with language. In spite of having "rosted and boylyd as one of *Gebers* Cooks" Ripley finds that recipes have not availed him. "For I was dyscevyd wyth many falce Books."[27] What is most intriguing about the insufficiency of language here is that it turns on its head the standard view of poetry as the "deficient" (*defectum*) form of expression and reasoning when compared to prose.[28] Like Gower, Ripley does not claim

24 Fletcher, "Alchemy in John Gower's *Confessio Amantis*," 121.

25 Fletcher, "Alchemy in John Gower's *Confessio Amantis*," 126.

26 Ripley, "Admonition," ed. Ashmole, 192.

27 Ripley, "Admonition," ed. Ashmole, 191.

28 Aquinas, *Scriptum super Sententiis*, lib. 1 q. 1 art. 2, ad 3 (https://aquinas.cc/la/en/~ST.I.Q1.A2).

that poetry is superior, but the insufficiency of language itself suggests that alchemical truth will not be found through traditional philosophy.

Failure was a part of alchemical practice. And alchemical practice, being an art that relied on empirical observation, constantly confronted its adherents with uncomfortable observations. Medieval alchemists could hardly ignore the evidence before them, nor were they necessarily gullible rubes. And while their alchemical failures could push them toward skepticism, this was a far cry from embracing modern scientific principles. Instead, they crafted rhetorical and intellectual strategies to cope with empirical failure and preserve scientific truth as they understood it.

Performing Alchemical Knowledge

Given the frequency of failure in alchemical practice, writing about alchemy offered a more certain means of demonstrating's one knowledge. Writing was a means of performing mastery that did not require success with an alembic, but it presented its own particular challenge: another alchemist could check your work. Thus, performing alchemy was something of a balancing act. George Ripley's student, Thomas Norton, the author of the 1477 *Ordinall of Alchemy*, attempts to strike this balance by being both prolix and strikingly vague.[29] In a verse poem that stretches to seven chapters in more than one hundred printed pages, the *Ordinall* is an elegy not only to alchemy, but also to the generosity of Norton himself for deigning to present alchemical knowledge to laypersons of lesser means as well as to the elite.

The proem and first chapter are, as noted above, a kind of ode to alchemy, peppered—like any alchemical treatise worth its salt—with insults against other alchemists and their lack of clarity.[30] Alchemical instruction ranges from the simplistic (i.e. metals are underground) to the confused, i.e., recapping other alchemical works without really betraying much in the way of understanding them conceptually. An example of the latter is Norton's retelling of a pseudo-Lullian work itself written as an allegory. Here is Norton:

> But holy Alkimy of right is to be loved,
> Which treateth of a precious Medicine,
> Such as trewly maketh Gold and Silver fine:
> Whereof example for Testimonie,
> Is in a Citty of Catilony.
> Which Raymond Lully, Knight; men suppose,
> Made in seaven Images the trewth to disclose;
> Three were good Silver, in shape like Ladies bright,
> Everie each of Foure were Gold and did a Knight:
> In borders of their Clothing Letters like appeare,

29 Mairey, "Entre littérature, science et politique," 249.

30 Norton, *Ordinall of Alchemy*, 2–17.

Signifying in Sentences as it sheweth here.

1. Of old Horshoes (said one) I was yre,
   Now I am good *Silver* as good as ye desire.
2. I was (said another) Iron fet from the Mine,
   But now I am *Gould* pure perfect and fine.
3. Whilome was I *Copper* of an old red pann,
   Now I am good *Silver*, said the third woman.
4. The fourth saide, I was *Copper* growne in the filthy place,
   Now am I perfect *Gould* made by God's grace.
5. The fift said, I was *Silver* perfect through fine,
   Now am I perfect *Goulde*, excellent, better than prime.
6. I was a Pipe of *Leade* well nigh two hundred yeare,
   And now to all men good *Silver* I appeare.
7. The seventh said, I *Leade* am *Gould* made for a Maistrie,
   But trewlie my fellowes are nerer thereto then I.[31]

The description goes on for several more verses, but there is no incisive commentary nor explanation. Those laypersons for whom Norton claims to write would only get the sense that Norton had in fact himself read a book about alchemy that was no more elucidating than what they were presently reading. Norton here is performing, albeit rather poorly, his own mastery of alchemical knowledge. While it is entirely possible that other initiates who had read the same book as Norton would be able to decipher the language, Norton never transforms the language into concrete steps that could be followed. The fact that he unceasingly laments this sin in others is apparently forgotten for the moment.

Norton is, above all, performing his erudition. The principal object of his performance is the royal court, but also lay readers of various classes.[32] But alchemical poems perform more than just the knowledge of their authors. They also perform as a source of entertainment, enjoyment, and wonder. Poetry as a source of pleasure runs through the commentary of both Avicenna and Averroës and, via the Latin translation of Hermannus Alemannus, to Aquinas and other western scholastics.[33] The idea of alchemical poetry as existing, first and foremost, as fun should not surprise us. Indeed, the earliest identified original alchemical verse in a western vernacular comes from Jean de Meun's *Roman de la Rose*. Didier Kahn argues that the alchemical section of the poem (about a hundred verses) operates as a didactic poem.[34] This is certainly true. One could learn quite a bit

31 Norton, *Ordinall of Alchemy*, 20–21.

32 Mairey, "Entre littérature, science et politique," 250, 253–54.

33 Malette, "Beyond Mimesis," 585–86.

34 Kahn, "Alchemical Poetry...Part I–Preliminary Survey," 252.

about the theory of alchemy from this section.[35] At the same time, the *Roman de la Rose* did not become the most widely read French poem for than two centuries because it was didactic. It gained popularity because it was witty, it brimmed with irony, and, above all, because it was enjoyable to hear and read.

The alchemical section comes just before Nature's "confession" to her priest (who is not a priest, but the character Genius, who sheds his priestly raiment just as soon as the section concludes). The confession itself, argues Charles Dahlberg, is ironic. "It also serves at the outset to establish the nature of the parody by assuring the reader of Genius's false credentials."[36] Even before we get to Nature's confession to Genius, we are treated to a discussion of Nature and her poor cousin, Art, who "imitates her like a monkey (*Et la contrefait comme singes*)."[37] The critique of art compared to nature is itself nothing new, but the tone is mocking, even self-mocking. "Bien la vous vousisse descrire/ Mais mi sens n'I porroit souffrire./ Mi sens? K'ai je dist? C'est du mains!/ Non-feroit voir nus sens humains."[38] How much more amazing and beautiful is nature when compared to art? Well, the poet cannot really say since art cannot equal nature. It's a good joke.

So, however didactic the alchemical portion may be—and indeed, it was copied out from the *Roman* to serve just this purpose—the context of the piece is about entertainment. More specifically, the contradiction at the heart of alchemical practice also seems to be a source of humor. The discussion of alchemy begins in the context of Art's many failures, going on to say that she could know as much as there is to know about alchemy and be able to manipulate and colour metals, but she would die before she ever managed to actually transmute something.[39] Then, however, the poet says something unexpected, namely that alchemy is nevertheless an *"art veritable"* capable of transmutation since all things are made from prime matter and can be reshaped after being returned to this primordial state: *"Car tuit par diverses manieres/ Dedenz leur terrestres minieres/ De souffre et de vif argent nessent* (for all are born, in various ways beneath their earthly appearances, from sulfur and from quicksilver)."[40] This is standard alchemical doctrine, and it is easy to see why such a piece might be excerpted by other alchemical writers, especially since it is followed by a passage that decrees the many amazing feats that can be performed by the truly learned. They can make gold, either from silver or dross; they can make silver too. All of this, however, is really just the lead up to another joke.

35 For a full exegesis of the alchemical ideas present in the *Roman*, see Newman, *Promethean Ambitions*, 77–82.

36 Dahlberg, "Introduction," 10. All English translations come from Dahlberg's edition. French translations come from Strubel's edition.

37 Lorris and de Meun, *Rose*, line 16035.

38 Lorris and de Meun, *Rose*, lines 16169–72. "I would willingly describe her to you, but my sense is not equal to it. My sense! What have I said? That's the least one could say. No human sense would show her, either vocally or in writing."

39 Lorris and de Meun, *Rose*, lines 16069–72.

40 Lorris and de Meun, *Rose*, lines 16125–27.

After raving about the potency of alchemists, the final stanza drips with irony. "*Mais ce ne feroient cil mie/ Qui oevrent de sophisterie:/ Travaillent tant com il vivront, Ja nature n'aconsivront.* (But those who work with sophistry would never do this. They work just as they will live; they will never catch up with nature.)"[41]

Having begun the passage with a discussion of Art's resolute failure to fully emulate Nature, and having ended the discussion of alchemy with a nod to sophists and perhaps even fraudsters, the poet is, I think, insinuating that sophists and fraudsters are exactly the kind of people who are practicing alchemy. Here, it seems as though the poet is poking fun not just at confidence men, but also at the high-minded *philosophes* whose efforts yielded results that hardly compared to the grandiose claims they made. No doubt there were a few of these at court. Whatever the poet's position on the philosophical basis of alchemy that makes up the central passage, the goal is entertainment. Alchemy may have been a true science, but it was important not to take it too seriously. Verse once again destabilized alchemical philosophy by pointing at the inherent contradiction of a science that cannot realize its aims.

Conclusion

Alchemy was easily theorized, but as the poets above attest, practice seldom lived up to theory. While failure could be easily enough conveyed by prose, such a strategy left little room for explanation beyond either the shortcomings of the alchemist or, even more troubling, the invalidity of alchemy itself. Poetry better communicated the intellectual problems that arose in the context of empirical experience. While we would be remiss to forego other aspects of poetic function—didacticism, appeals to patrons, aesthetic preference—it would also be problematic to overlook the fact that poetry is a useful vehicle for communicating paradox and contradiction. For practicing alchemists as well as their audiences these paradoxes may have been theoretical, but they could also be practical. The poetry of failure is invested with the emotion of real alchemical results—explosions, wasted time and money, and obsession. No wonder poets like Gower felt that language could not properly convey truths that could not be replicated. If empirical failure destabilized alchemy as a science, poetry destabilized prose treatises as vehicles of truth. Wordplay and metaphor claimed value on par with clarity and philosophical cohesiveness. Whether as a critique or as a performance of alchemical and poetical skill, these poems display a playful intent, a desire to negotiate the ambiguous spaces between discursive truth, empirical failure, and cosmological wonder.

41 Lorris and de Meun, *Rose*, lines 16149–52.

Bibliography

Manuscripts

Oxford, Bodleian Library, MS Ashmole 1384.

Primary Sources

Bernard of Treves. *De Chymico Miraculo.* Basel: Dionys Zecharius, 1563.

Chaucer, Geoffrey. *The Canterbury Tales.* Harvard's Geoffrey Chaucer Website. https://chaucer.fas.harvard.edu/.

Guillaume de Lorris, and Jean de Meun. *The Romance of the Rose.* 3rd ed. Translated by Charles Dahlberg. Princeton: Princeton University Press, 1995.

——. *Le Roman de la Rose.* Edited by Armand Strubel. Paris: Librairie générale française, 1992.

Johannes Ticinensis. "Processus de lapide philosophorum." In *Deutches Theatrum Chemicum.* Vol. 3. Edited by Friedrich Roth-Schultz. Nürnberg: Felßecker, 1732.

Lydgate, John. "Introduction to *Secreta Secretorum.*" In *Theatrum Chemicum Britannicum.* Edited by Elias Ashmole. London: Brooke, 1652.

Meister Eckhart. *Essential Sermons.* Translated by E. Colledge and B. McGinn. London: Paulist, 1981.

Norton, Thomas. *The Ordinall of Alchemy.* London: Edward Arnold, 1928.

Ripley, George. "Admonition." In *Theatrum Chemicum Britannicum.* Edited by Elias Ashmole. London: Brooke, 1652.

Thomas Aquinas. *Scriptum Super Sententiis.* Edited by The Aquinas Institute. https://aquinas.cc/la/en/~Sent.I.

Ventura, Lorenzo. "De ratione conficiendi lapidis philosophici liber." In *Theatrum Chemicum.* Vol. 2. Strassbourg: Zetzner, 1602.

Secondary Sources

Collette, Carolyn P. *Species, Phantasms, and Images: Vision and Medieval Psychology in The Canterbury Tales.* Ann Arbor: University of Michigan Press, 2001.

Dahlberg, Charles. "Introduction." In Guillaume de Lorris and Jean de Meun. *The Romance of the Rose.* 3rd ed. Translated by Charles Dahlberg, 1–27. Princeton: Princeton University Press, 1995.

Fletcher, Clare. "'The Science of Himself Is True': Alchemy in John Gower's *Confessio Amantis.*" *South Atlantic Review* 79 (2014): 118–31.

Gabrovsky, Alexander. *Chaucer the Alchemist: Physics, Mutability, and the Medieval Imagination.* New York: Palgrave Macmillan, 2015.

Kahn, Didier. "Alchemical Poetry in Medieval and Early Modern Europe: A Preliminary Survey and Synthesis: Part I–Preliminary Survey," *Ambix* 57 (2010): 249–74.

——. "Alchemical Poetry in Medieval and Early Modern Europe: A Preliminary Survey and Synthesis: Part II–Synthesis," *Ambix* 58 (2011): 62–77.

Mairey, Aude. "Entre littérature, science et politique: Les œuvres alchimiques de Thomas Norton et George Ripley." *Revue Historique* 313 (2011): 243–63.

Malette, Karla. "Beyond Mimesis: Aristotle's *Poetics* in the Medieval Mediterranean." *PMLA* 124, no. 2 (March 2009): 583–91.

Murray, Paul. "Aquinas on Poetry and Theology." *Logos: A Journal of Catholic Thought and Culture* 16 (2013): 63–72.

Newman, William R. *Promethean Ambitions: Alchemy and the Quest to Perfect Nature*. Chicago: University of Chicago Press, 2004.

Telle, Joachim. "Johannes von Teschen." In *Die deutsche Literatur des Mittelalters. Verfasserlexikon*. Edited by Wolfgang Stammler and Karl Langosch, 4:774–76. Berlin: de Gruyter, 1978–2008.

Timmermann, Anke. *Verse and Transmutation: A Corpus of Middle English Alchemical Poetry*. Leiden: Brill, 2013.

ENCOUNTERING THE WONDER IN NATURE

THE SCIENCE OF THE SACRED IN THE EARLY-MODERN CONSTRUCTION OF THE NATURAL WORLD

HELEN PARISH

> The vast Ocean presents a wonderful spectacle [*admirabile spectaculum*] to every nation in its swirling waters [...]. In this broad expanse of fluid Ocean, receiving the seeds of life with fertile growth, as sublime nature ceaselessly gives birth, an abundance of monsters is found.[1]

WONDERS AND MARVELS dominated Olaus Magnus' *Description of the Northern Peoples* (1555). Here, Olaus Magnus added a layer of explanatory detail to his earlier *Carta marina et descriptio septemtrionalem terrarum ac mirabilium*, a detailed and richly illustrated map of the northern lands and waters. The sea monsters depicted in both works were consciously labelled as wonders, physical objects that were capable of eliciting a mental response that ranged from curiosity to fear to ambition. The early modern lexicon of the wondrous incorporated miracles, portents and prodigies, and marvels in nature, a challenging and shifting category in which "sensibilities overlapped and recurred like waves." The history of wonders has been conceptualized as the history of "objects of natural inquiry," a history of the orders of nature embedded in and emerging from the individuals and communities that exchanged knowledge of natural philosophy.[2] The pages of early modern natural histories expose both the fluidity of this natural philosophy, and the complexity of the interactions between the human and nature in this period. Descriptions of the wonders of the oceans, such as those contained in Olaus Magnus' work, were constructed by a dialectical relationship between culture, observation, and memory. This was a polyvalent approach to the objects and wonders of nature that was positioned on a permeable boundary between the material, observational, and

1 Olaus Magnus, *Historia de gentibus septentrionalibus* (1555 ed.), 729.

2 Daston and Park, *Wonders*, 11, 14.

Helen Parish is a Visiting Professor in History at the University of Reading, and a Fellow of Worcester College, Oxford. Major publications include book-length studies of clerical marriage during the English Reformation, the history of clerical celibacy and clerical marriage in the Latin West between 1100 and 1700 (both published with Ashgate) and a study of representations of the medieval church during the Reformation. More recently she has written on medieval and early modern debates over superstition, magic and priestcraft, the history of witchcraft, and the intersections of religion, natural history, and the supernatural in the late medieval and early modern period.

philological.[3] As a result, it was entirely possible for physical encounter, mental encounter, and spiritual encounter to coinhere on the same page of natural histories as different strands within the same process of description.[4]

Olaus Magnus was a Roman Catholic priest, later bishop of Uppsala, who travelled widely across Sweden and Norway propagating the faith and acquiring first-hand knowledge of the land and water. Christian missionaries who compiled natural histories were a pivotal part of the (global) circulation of knowledge in this period, transmitting information, interpreting the seen and the unseen, and overlaying observational detail with a language of enquiry and belief that made clear the meanings that underpinned the natural and the wondrous. Natural philosophy and Christian evangelism were far from mutually exclusive interpretative lenses; the observation and interpretation of the natural world in this period retained much of its religious language and motive.[5] But that language was also shaped by mercantilism, and by the accompanying expansion of the known world. Navigators, cartographers, and sailors contributed to the formation of a vocabulary that could be used to reconcile the old and the new, to shape the social and cultural networks within which knowledge exchange took place, and to give voice to the emerging connections between natural knowledge, collecting, and commerce.[6]

The variegated nature of the knowledge economy encouraged an approach to natural philosophy in which multiple meanings could reside within the same object, text, or image. That capacity for multiple meanings invites a closer reading of wonders in nature, and the *admirabile spectaculum* that Olaus Magnus described. The seeing and the interpretation of wonders in this period sheds light upon the emergences of new textual forms in natural histories, the complexity of the material, emotional and intellectual interactions that were created by—and created—wonders in nature, and the cultural context in which knowledge of the natural world was acquired and shared. The breadth and depth of that knowledge is explored here in two case studies which illustrate the content and form of the conceptualized and contextualized wonder. The first, the cartographic work of Olaus Magnus, alongside his detailed textual commentary, offer insights into the connections between image and text, mission and mercantilism, fact, and fiction. The second, Edward Topsell's *History of Four-footed Beasts and Serpents*, exemplifies the process by which knowledge could be collected and collated, interrogated and inspected, in an encyclopaedic approach to nature and its wonders. In both cases, we can chart the evolution of ideas and attitudes, and the emergence of a syncretic approach which multiple interpretations could co-exist on a single page.

That evolution in the meaning and function of facts and evidence, including wonders and miracles, across the medieval and early modern period has been well studied.[7] Lor-

3 Müller-Wille and Charmantier, "Natural History and Information Overload"; Mulsow, "Antiquarianism and Idolatry"; Pinon, "Conrad Gessner."

4 Parish, "None of Them Could Say."

5 Field and James, eds. *Renaissance and Revolution*.

6 Findlen, "Inventing Nature."

7 Daston, "Marvelous Facts."

raine Daston invited us to see miracles as a form of evidence that was both evident to the senses but dependent upon intention. Wonders and prodigies, and their interpretation, were deeply rooted in *scientia* and natural knowledge. But neither perception nor classification were static categories, and the compartmentalization of the natural, preternatural, and supernatural was intellectually rigid but materially permeable. The "preternatural" category in particular was open to reinterpretation, with prodigies and portents occupying a contested space as both "signs" and conceptually neutral facts. In the hands of evangelical theologians and polemicists, the heterogeneity of the Christian miraculous opened up the possibility that miracles might be feigned or constructed, and eroded the assumption that as a pure form of evidence they required no interpretation.

Neither of these thought processes excluded the possibility that the supernatural might intrude into the early modern natural world. As Alexandra Walsham has demonstrated, the Christian God was "an assiduous, energetic deity who constantly intervened in human affairs". Providentialism presented a means by which meaning might be found in natural disaster, and an explanation offered for the otherwise inexplicable. Signs and wonders in nature—monstrous fish, strange weather, fire, flood, and disease—provided a means by which mankind might come to encounter and know God. A theocentric view of the universe framed wonders and prodigies in terms of human sin; for the scientific movement such phenomena invited a re-framing of the boundary between the natural and the supernatural.[8] There was no conflict here between a knowledge of nature and a knowledge of God; it was entirely possible for science, nature, religion, and legend to continue to occupy space in the narrative accounts of God's intervention in the world, and in natural histories, throughout the early modern period. The wonders and portents that punctuated the mental and material world were embedded in written and visual sources, but also in the conceptual understanding of natural philosophers, cartographers, sailors, and believers. Neither the aberrations of nature nor its inexplicable wonders were accidental. Enticing or fascinating, perhaps, and certainly capable of inducing emotional and intellectual wonder that acted as a spur to inquiry and curiosity. The "history of marvels" lay at the heart of Francis Bacon's understanding of a new natural philosophy, and wonders—and the wonder that they induced—occupied a space at the physical edge of the known and the unknown, and at the mental frontiers of philosophy, theology, and observation.[9] The continued presence of wonder within English Protestantism demonstrated its capacity for contextual adaptation, and the acceptance of a syncretic approach to the supernatural that allowed seemingly "superstitious" events to act as a vehicle for the transmission of moral and theological meaning.[10] Providence neither shattered belief in the capacity of supernatural forces to shape events, nor negated the obligation to interpret the meaning that inhered in such occurrences.

---

8 Walsham, *Providence*, 2.

9 Daston and Park, *Wonders*, 13.

10 Walsham, "The Fatall Vesper"; Walsham "*Vox Piscis*"; Walsham, "History, Memory and the English Reformation"; Lake and Questier, *The Antichrist's Lewd Hat*; Hall, *Worlds of Wonder*.

Such belief in God's providential interventions in human affairs and in the natural world is deeply rooted within Judaeo-Christian tradition, and within the history of the interactions between the created world and the divine. Nature was both visible and readable, capable of conveying material and metaphorical messages and meaning. In the book of Job, instruction is given to "ask the animals, and they will teach you, or the birds of the air, and they will tell you; or speak to the earth, and it will teach you, or let the fish of the sea inform you" (Job 12:7–10). Creation imparted the will of God, and a knowledge of creation had the potential to bring knowledge of the divine. The world, on the sixth day of its creation, was the perfect work of God; animals lived peacefully together, they ate grass, leaves, and herbs (Genesis 1:30), and man, in God's image, held "dominion over the fish of the sea, and over the fowl of the air, and over the cattle, and over all the earth, and over every creeping thing" (Gen. 1:26). But as sin entered into God's creation, the nature of the relationship between God, man and animals changed. Fear became real, on both sides. God used animals—the plagues of Egypt, the quails that fed Israel in the desert—to punish sinful man but also to succour him. The natural world was "God's great book in folio" in which miracles, wonders and providences shaped the conceptualization of human relationships with creation and with the divine.[11] Religious language permeated natural histories, and human accounts of the wonders and providences of nature found their way into pastoral and polemical literature.

This co-constructed book of nature provided mankind with a means of understanding and interpreting the world around it. Conrad Gesner, in the *Historia Animalium* (1551–1558) reflected upon the process by which knowledge was created, and upon the ways in which man might come to understand the world in which he lived. "Reason and experience are the two pillars of scientific work" he argued, "reason comes to us from God, experience depends upon the will of man. Science is born of the collaboration of the two." Knowledge of nature and a knowledge of God fashioned a rich tapestry of religious belief, myth, legend, natural history, and *scientia*. Observation and encounter, described in a shared vocabulary distilled from ancient sources, and perpetuated by each additional retelling, created a complex picture of the natural world. With the advent of popular print, contemporary wonders and providences communicated through nature could be overlaid on an older palimpsest of portents and their interpretation.

A common verbal and visual lexicon shaped the description of flora and fauna in early modern natural histories. Assumptions about the connections between animals and religion asserted a firm anchor in authoritative texts, and became a self-referential and self-perpetuating means of constructing a confessional and cultural identity and moralising through cheap print, rousing sermon, and striking imagery.[12] Theology and religious belief provided a mortar for an imbrication of natural histories that cemented the connections between *scientia* and the sacred, classification and catechesis.[13] Religion

11 Fudge, *Perceiving Animals*; Walsham, *Providence*; Thomas, *Man and the Natural World*.

12 Walsham, *Providence*.

13 Mackenzie, "Guillaume Rondelet's Sea-Monsters"; Ogilvie, "Natural History"; Glardon, "L'Histoire naturelle du XVIe siècle."

turned nature into a potent and profitable commodity, whether in satisfying curiosity, or providing comfort.[14] In this arena, natural histories could collide with religious texts, particularly on the occasions when the communication of God's will was purported to take place not through natural irregularities, but through man-made signs and symbols, hybrid creatures that bore the mark of human rather than divine intervention. The marvellous, the wondrous, and the curious not only invited a theological interpretation, but also encouraged a more pragmatic form of human creativity, in which nature was bought and sold, fashioned and fabricated. In his *Historia Animalium* (1558) Conrad Gesner described "apothecaries and others who usually dry rays and shape their skeletons into varied and wonderful forms for the ignorant." The natural world was the creation of God, but still vulnerable to reinvention by man, twisting the relationship between knowledge, faith and wonder.

Human efforts to imbue animals with soteriological or eschatological meaning are certainly visible in early modern natural histories. A confident articulation of providential meaning is not always apparent in the writings of Gesner, Rondelet, Belon, and Topsell, but neither is a total rejection of the possibility that animals, with or without human intervention, might communicate a religious message. The symbolism of the sacred existed alongside the interrogation and classification of nature in such texts, in a careful balancing of the "vanity" of men's opinion against the veracity of God's word and value of canonical texts.[15] Accounts of nature and natural irregularities could swiftly become part of the accepted corpus, finding their way into the pages of the natural histories of Conrad Gesner and Edward Topsell, whose account of the whale (like most other beasts) was informed not by personal encounter and observation, but by the writing of Pliny, the framework of medieval bestiaries, and early modern investigations of nature. Gesner's encyclopaedic discussions of nature were likewise derived from ancient texts and personal observation, and punctuated by references to contemporary discussions, debates, catalogues and cartographies.[16]

The continued presence of sea monsters and divinely ordained aberrations in nature in early modern print culture exposes the extent to which such eclecticism was accepted and embedded in many narratives. Representation was visual as well as verbal. The *Carta Marina*, Olaus Magnus' wood-block map printed in Venice in 1539, is perhaps the most famous example of the genre. But his *Historia de Gentibus Septentrionalibus* demonstrated the scope and the desire to provide a detailed verbal description and explanation. Both works included images of animals that are recognisably real, and others that are more difficult to identify. Their purpose was more than decorative; fearsome creatures amply demonstrated the dangers of the sea, especially those parts that sat on the margins of cartography and navigation. A combination of narrative and imagination fashioned sea creatures that emerged from a fertile natural world in which forms of life on land were mirrored by forms of life in the sea. Aquatic monsters in uncharted waters

14 Findlen, "Inventing Nature," 301ff.

15 Rondelet, *Libri de Piscibus Marinis*.

16 Ogilvie, *The Science of Describing*, 74ff; Hendrikx, 'Monstrosities from the Sea," 126.

were no less real than the familiar animals that walked the land. The ziphius, for example, with the head of an owl was capable of "mischief," slicing into ships with a dorsal fin that was as sharp as a sword, and feeding on sea-life, including sailors.[17] The Norwegian Sea was densely populated with such monstrous creatures, each of which had a story to tell. But their presence also carried an economic purpose, and the terrifying creatures of the deep could be harnessed to deter sailors and merchants from entering these waters. Olaus Magnus was charting the unknown, populating unfamiliar waters with creatures whose existence could be neither proved nor disproved. The mapping of the fullness of God's creation also mapped the limits of human understanding, combined to create a curiosity, a sense of the marvellous, and a reminder of the invisible depths of the undomesticated oceans.

In the maps of the seas, monsters and strange fish filled the waters, perhaps as decoration, but also as a means of explaining how God used such monsters to communicate with man. Magnus labelled each monster on the map with a letter, accompanied by a more detailed description in the key in the lower left corner. Several, he explained, were to be read as omens of trouble and upheaval, or warnings from God of the potential consequences of human sin. After describing the "monstrous Fish" that had been sighted off the coast of England in 1532, Magnus noted that a "monstrous Hog [...], was found afterwards, Anno 1537, in the same German Ocean, and it was a Monster in every part of it. For it had a Hog's head, and a quarter of a Circle, like the Moon, in the hinder part of its head, four feet like a Dragon's, two eyes on both sides of his Loyns, and a third in his belly inkling toward his Navel; behind he had a Forked-Tail, like to other Fish commonly." Descriptions of "sea-pigs" predate Olaus Magnus' work; his commentary in the *Historia* overlaid familiar imagery with contemporary allegory. The source was almost certainly a 1537 pamphlet, *Monstrum in oceano Germanico* in which the sea pig was interpreted as a sign of God's displeasure. Olaus Magnus imbued the detailed description in the pamphlet with a polemical meaning, using the appearance of the sea pig to make a pointed attack on Protestantism. The sea pig "can properly be displayed as a symbol to the unclean men of this wretched age, urging them to recoil from monstrous habits and to embrace goodness." Drawing upon the 1537 pamphlet, Olaus Magnus suggested that the individual parts of the beast "show how heretics generally pursue a swinish existence."[18] In God's great book in folio, the description of the Hog, with its forked tail, was a sign and story of God's judgement on Lutheran heretics who were no better than swine.

Other sea monsters on the map were distilled from narratives of creatures in the deep provided by sailors, or perplexed spectators who saw them washed up on land, overlaid with suitably providential vocabulary. Most famous among them was the Sea-serpent, or Sea Orm, which in the *Carta Marina* sits in its three-hundred-foot long splendour just below a terrifying maelstrom. The map key describes the Orm "wrapping itself

17 Van Duzer, *Sea Monsters*; Conrad Gessner, *Nomenclator aquatilium animantium*; Olaus Magnus, *Historia de gentibus septentrionalibus*.

18 Olaus Magnus, *Carta Marina* (1572 ed.).

around a big ship and destroying it" citing evidence presented by "they who in Works of Navigation, on the Coasts of Norway, employ themselves in fishing or Merchandise." In oral and cartographic tradition, the Orm was "wont to live in Rocks and Caves toward the Sea-coast about Berge: which will go alone from his holes in a clear night, in Summer, and devour Calves, Lambs, and Hogs, or else he goes into the Sea to feed on Polypus [octopus], Locusts [lobsters], and all sorts of Sea-Crabs." Hair hung from its neck, its scales were sharp, and its eyes flaming. "He hath commonly hair hanging from his neck a Cubit long, and sharp Scales, and is black, and he hath flaming shining eyes." The accompanying note that the Orm's appearance "disquiets the shippers" may be putting it rather mildly, particularly given that the serpent's appearance was understood to signify some wonderful change in the terrestrial kingdoms, or tumultuous war. But such creatures remained a key part of the way in which early modern Europeans imagined themselves within the natural world, and the intentions of its creator.[19] The observational experience of the senses continued to be refracted through the prism of assumptions about the hand of God in creation, and ongoing divine interventions in the world. Assertions and rejections of the reality and nature of creatures described in the pages of earlier natural histories did not fundamentally undermine the assumption that the hand of God was still at work in the world.

Images borrowed from *Carta Marina* were reproduced in later maps, including Gerard Mercator's 1541 *Globe*, and richly illustrated cartographies prepared by Sebastian Münster and Abraham Ortelius, who filled the Pacific Ocean with mermaids and sirens and hungry whales who preyed upon passing ships. From the *Carta Marina*, the Great Orm image found its way into Munster's *Monstra Marina et Terrestria*, and (reversed) into Gesner's *Natural History*, and from there into Edward Topsell's *History of the Serpents*. Gesner was clear in his attribution of the visual depiction and verbal description of the Orm to Olaus Magnus, refusing to be drawn into debate over the accuracy of either word or image. Erich Pontoppidan, Bishop of Bergen, was eventually convinced of the reality of the Orm's existence by multiple reports received from "creditable and experienced" fishermen and sailors.[20] Removed from the original map, but still recognisable, the Orm appeared in John Johnston's *Historia Naturalis* (1657).

Edward Topsell's *The History of Four-Footed Beasts and Serpents* was published in 1658. Topsell was a clergyman, and made no claim to be a naturalist. His information came not from his own travels, but from a list of sources that incorporated "divine scriptures, fathers, philosophers, physicians and poets" as well as Conrad Gesner's *Historia Animalium*. His purpose was to collect visual and textual narratives of the physical and cultural characteristics of animals "to profit and delight the reader, whereinto he may look on the holiest deities." Topsell provided his reader with detailed descriptions of mammals, reptiles, amphibians, insects, and marine life, accompanied by detailed images, proverbs, myths, and Christian writing in which they featured. Alongside these "natural" visible creatures sat a variety of mythical beasts and animals. The Hydra appears with

19 Daston and Park, *Wonders*.

20 Pontoppidan, *Natural History of Norway*.

two claws, a curled serpent's tail, and seven small mammalian heads; the Lamia with a cat-like body, hooves on the hind feet, claws on the front, and a human woman's face and hair; the Mantichora with a lion's body and mane, a man's face and head of hair, and a grotesquely smiling mouth. We learn that dragons might come in various forms, and that their preferred food is lettuce, but only wild lettuce which does not induce a stomach-ache. Topsell, repeating ancient legends, assigned exotic attributes to animals. Weasels, for example, give birth through their ears, lemmings graze in the clouds, Elephants worship the sun and the moon and become pregnant by chewing on mandrake, and Apes are terrified of snails. This approach to the natural world was simultaneously practical, pragmatic, and pastorally driven, informed by a respect for authoritative texts and a sense that the unusual physical characteristics of such creatures were the handiwork of God. The beasts and serpents that inhabited the pages of Topsell's work were a conduit for God's communication with mankind in moral terms; their behaviour could be described and explained with reference to authoritative ancient texts, but also served as a physical reminder of the bigger questions of sin and redemption. Mutations and the monstrous, Topsell argued, "signifie the mutation or change of worldly affairs" in an already degenerate Christian world.[21] The description of living creatures, was shaped by a language which communicated a view of nature that was moralized rather than mechanical, and firmly focused upon the relationship between man and God.

But the presence of mythical and imagined creatures in *The History of Four-footed Beasts* should not be assumed to imply that Topsell was entirely uncritical in his reading of the recorded natural world. In his discussion of the Hydra, for example, Topsell incorporated not only an image taken from Gesner's *Historia*, but also some of the scepticism that accompanied the description. The "water-serpent with seven heads" in Gesner's account was reported to have been brought to Venice from Turkey in 1530. The creature had been put on public display, a detail that was perhaps intended to provide proof that the Hydra had been seen with the eye, and not simply reported in text and speech. But Gesner also noted that those who were "knowledgeable about nature" were convinced that the Hydra was not a natural creature, but "ein erdichter körpel" a fictional or invented body.[22] Topsell followed Gesner's lead here, suggesting that it was no less "unpossible" for the Hydra to be real than for "armed men to be created from dragon's teeth."[23] Such narratives emerged at the convergence of teratology, portents and providences, a potent mix of ideas that was not confined to the printed page. When a leviathan was stranded at the mouth of the Humber River in 1595, the crowd that gathered knew not "what to saye or judge therof, but onely resolveth themselves that it was sent of God for some great purpose."[24] When a "marvellous straunge fishe" was brought

21 Topsell, *The History of Four-Footed Beasts and Serpents*, 2:736. See title page of *Septiceps Lutherus* (Leipzig: Johannes Cochlaeus, 1529), in which a Luther / Hydra embodies the seven deadly sins—Wiedermann, "Cochlaeus as a Polemicist," 196.

22 Parish, "Every Living Beast."

23 Topsell, *The History of Four-Footed Beasts and Serpents*, 2:735.

24 *The Diary of Ralph Josselin*, ed. Macfarlane, 60; Anon., *A most certaine report of a monster borne*

to Billingsgate in 1569, an indeterminate "many" came to wonder at its shape and size. A printed pamphlet *A most strange and true report of a monsterous fish* (1604) described the sighting of a creature that was half fish, half woman, in 1604 off the coast at Pendine, Carmarthenshire. The detailed account of the "mermaid" was accompanied by a list of witnesses who would all vouch for the authenticity of the written account. Natural history was intermingled with visibility of God's wrath in the natural world, intermingled with personal testimony, local memory, and an evolving religious culture.

Encountering the wonder in nature was a central and consistent part of the way in which early modern Europeans envisioned themselves and the natural world.[25] And as Alexandra Walsham rightly warns, there is a danger in exaggerating the extent to which natural prodigies and providences were demythologized in the early modern period. Even divorced from their association with sin, unnatural fish and distorted animals could still present evidence of the power of nature and the God that created it.[26] Wonder inhabited a conceptual space that was elastic enough to accommodate such beliefs in multiple forms, and to syncretize rather than suppress competing interpretations. The natural histories of the Renaissance did not force open a deep fracture between past and present.

The broad chronology of this collection of the essays provides us with a narrative and interpretative structure in which the natural and the supernatural are permeable; human and animal, sacred and secular, time and space. Interactions between the natural and the supernatural described above are polytemporal, simultaneously elusive and ever-present in the medieval and early modern cultural and theological world view. The topography of the natural and the supernatural is punctuated by a conscious interaction between the medieval and early modern, shared points of reference in which wonder and marvel take a material form. Within this context, continuity and change do not take a linear form, or a single direction of travel. The lens through which we view the wondrous may change—for example with the advent of religious pluralism, or the interactions between magic, medicine and natural knowledge—but there is no single irretrievable point of seismic separation with the past. Any assertion of the existence of an epistemically consistent community is hard to accommodate within a multiform model of culture and belief; the notion that the magical and mysterious were banished from the mental and physical world by the birth of modern science is too simplistic in its construction.[27] The supernatural and the wondrous continued to inhabit natural histories, narratives of wonders and the mental cosmos beyond the age of reformations, undermining the assumptions that this period marked a watershed in the relationship

at Oteringham in Holdernesse [...] Also of a most strange and huge fish, which was driven on the sand at Outhorn (1595), sig. B1^v.

25 Daston and Park, *Wonders*.

26 Walsham, "*Vox Piscis*: Or The Book-Fish".

27 Scribner, "The Reformation, Popular Magic and the 'Disenchantment' of the World"; Walsham, "The Reformation and the Disenchantment of the World Reassessed"; Schroeder, *Max Weber and the Sociology of Culture*; Spierenburg, *The Broken Spell*; Weber, *The Protestant Ethic and the Spirit of Capitalism*.

between the natural and the supernatural, or a neat and linear progression into a modern scientific world view. The interpretation and representation of the natural world occurred in layers rather than lines; knowledge was projected onto the culture of belief, but in a moralized universe that projection was never unidirectional. Wonders remained confessionally, intellectually, economically and emotionally charged, open to a multiplicity of meanings and conflicting interpretations in which science and the supernatural could coinhere without collapsing into one other.

Bibliography

Primary Sources

Anon. *A most certaine report of a monster borne at Oteringham in Holdernesse [...] Also of a most strange and huge fish, which was driven on the sand at Outhorn.* London [?]: P.S., 1595.

Gessner, Conrad. *Nomenclator aquatilium animantium.* Zürich: Froschauer, 1560.

Josselin, Ralph. *The Diary of Ralph Josselin, 1616–1683.* Edited by Alan Macfarlane. London: British Academy, 1976.

Olaus Magnus. *Carta marina et descriptio septemtrionalem terrarum ac mirabilium.* Rome: Antoine Lafréry, 1572.

——. *Historia de gentibus septentrionalibus, earumque diversis statibus, conditionibus, moribus, ritibus, superstitionibus, disciplinis, exercitiis, regimine, victu, bellis, structuris, instrumentis, ac mineris metallicis, & rebus mirabilibus, necnonuniversis pene animalibus in Septentrione degentibus, eorumque natura.* Rome: Giovanni M. Viotto, 1555.

Pontoppidan, Erik. *Natural History of Norway.* London: Linde, 1755.

Rondelet, Guillaume. *Libri de Piscibus Marinis.* Lyon: Matthias Bonhomme, 1554.

Topsell, Edward. *The History of Four-Footed Beasts and Serpents: Describing at Large Their True and Lively Figure, Their Several Names, Conditions, Kinds, Virtues (Both Natural and Medicinal) Countries of Their Breed, Their Love and Hatred to Mankind, and the Wonderful Work of God in Their Creation, Preservation, and Destruction.* London: for G. Sawbridge, 1658.

Secondary Sources

Daston, Lorraine. "Marvelous Facts and Miraculous Evidence in Early Modern Europe." *Critical Inquiry* 18, no. 1 (1991): 93–124.

Daston, Lorraine, and Katharine Park, *Wonders and the Order of Nature, 1150–1750.* New York: Zone, 1998.

Field, J. V. and Frank James, eds. *Renaissance and Revolution: Humanists, Scholars, Craftsmen, and Natural Philosophers in Early Modern Europe.* Cambridge: Cambridge University Press, 1997.

Findlen, Paula. "Inventing Nature: Commerce, Art and Science in Early Modern Cabinets of Curiosities." In *Merchants and Marvels: Commerce, Science and Art in Early Modern Europe.* Edited by Paula Findlen and Pamela Smith, 297–323. New York: Routledge, 2002.

Fudge, Erica. *Perceiving Animals: Humans and Beasts in Early Modern English Culture.* Chicago: University of Illinois Press, 2002.

Glardon, Philippe. "L'Histoire naturelle du XVIe siècle: Historiographie, methodologie, et perspectives." *Gesnerus* 63 (2006): 280–98.

Hall, David D. *Worlds of Wonder, Days of Judgement. Religious Popular Belief in Early New England*. Cambridge, MA: Harvard University Press, 1990.

Hendrikx, Sophia. "Monstrosities from the Sea. Taxonomy and Tradition in Conrad Gessner's (1516–1565) Discussion of Cetaceans and Sea-Monsters." *Anthropozoologica* 53 (2018): 125–37.

Lake, Peter, and Michael Questier. *The Antichrist's Lewd Hat: Protestants, Papists and Players in Post Reformation England*. New Haven: Yale University Press, 2002.

Mackenzie, Louisa. "Guillaume Rondelet's Sea-Monsters and Bruno Latour's Modern Constitution." In *Animals and Early Modern Identity*. Edited by Pia F. Cuneo, 29–49. Burlington: Ashgate, 2014.

Müller-Wille, Staffan, and Isabelle Charmantier, "Natural History and Information Overload: The case of Linnaeus. Studies in History and Philosophy of Science." *Studies in History and Philosophy of Biological and Biomedical Sciences*, Part C 43, no. 1 (2012): 4–15.

Mulsow, Martin. "Antiquarianism and Idolatry. The *Historia* of Religions in the Seventeenth Century." In *Historia: Empiricism and Erudition in Early Modern Europe*. Edited by Gianna Pomata and Nancy G. Siraisi, 181–210. Cambridge, MA: MIT Press, 2005.

Ogilvie, Brian. "Natural History, Ethics, and Physico-Theology." In *Historia: Empiricism and Erudition in Early Modern Europe*. Edited by Gianna Pomata and Nancy G. Siraisi, 75–1048. Cambridge, MA: MIT Press, 2005.

——. *The Science of Describing: Natural History in Renaissance Europe* (Chicago: University of Chicago Press, 2006).

Parish, Helen. "'Every Living Beast Being a Word, Every Kind Being a Sentence': Animals and Religion in Reformation Europe." *Religions* 10, no. 7 (July 2019): item 421 (20 pp.).

——. "'None of Them Could Say They Ever Had Seen Them, but Only Had It from Others': Encounters with Animals in Eighteenth-Century Natural Histories of Greenland." *Animals* 10, no. 11 (2020):2024. https://doi.org/10.3390/ani10112024.

Pinon, Laurent. "Conrad Gessner and the Historical Depth of Renaissance Natural History." In *Historia: Empiricism and Erudition in Early Modern Europe*. Edited by Gianna Pomata and Nancy G. Siraisi, 241–68. Cambridge, MA: MIT Press, 2005.

Scribner, Robert W. "The Reformation, Popular Magic and the 'Disenchantment' of the World." *Journal of Interdisciplinary History* 23, no. 3 (1993): 475–94.

Schroeder, Ralph. *Max Weber and the Sociology of Culture*. London: Sage, 1992.

Spierenburg, Pieter. *The Broken Spell: A Cultural and Anthropological History of Preindustrial Europe*. London: Macmillan, 1991.

Stern, Karen. "The Middle English *Prose Merlin*." In *The Changing Face of Arthurian Romance: Essays on Arthurian Prose Romances in Memory of Cedric E. Pickford*. Edited by Alison Adams, Armel H. Diverres, Karen Stern, and Kenneth Varty, 112–22. Woodbridge: Boydell, 1986

Thomas, Keith. *Man and the Natural World*. London: Allen Lane, 1983.

Van Duzer, Chet. *Sea Monsters on Medieval and Renaissance Maps*. London: British Library, 2013.

Walsham, Alexandra. "'The Fatall Vesper': Providentialism and Anti-Popery in Late Jacobean London." *Past and Present* 144 (1994): 36–87.

——. "History, Memory and the English Reformation." *Historical Journal* 55 (2012): 899–938.

——. "The Reformation and the Disenchantment of the World Reassessed." *Historical Journal* 51, no. 2 (2008): 497–528.

——. *Providence in Early Modern England*. Oxford: Oxford University Press, 1999.

——. "*Vox Piscis*: Or, The Book Fish: Providence and the Uses of the Reformation Past in Caroline Cambridge." *English Historical Review* 114 (1999): 574–606.

Weber, Max. *The Protestant Ethic and the Spirit of Capitalism*, 2nd ed.(London: George Allen & Unwin, 1976.

Wiedermann, Gotthelf. "Cochlaeus as a Polemicist." In *The Seven-Headed Luther: Essays in Commemoration of a Quincentenary*. Edited by Peter Newman Brooks, 195–205. Oxford, Oxford University Press, 1983.

INDEX

Printed and bound by CPI Group (UK) Ltd, Croydon, CR0 4YY

13/09/2026

14961067-0001